KNOWING GOD BY EXPERIENCE

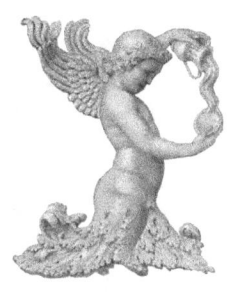

KNOWING GOD BY EXPERIENCE

The Spiritual Senses in the Theology of William of Auxerre

BOYD TAYLOR COOLMAN

The Catholic University of America Press
Washington, D.C.

Copyright © 2004
The Catholic University of America Press
All rights reserved
Printed in the United States of America

The paper used in this publication meets the minimum requirements of American National Standards for Information Science—Permanence of Paper for Printed Library materials, ANSI Z39.48-1984.
∞

LIBRARY OF CONGRESS CATALOGING-IN-PUBLICATION DATA
Coolman, Boyd Taylor, 1966–
Knowing God by experience : the spiritual senses in the theology of William of Auxerre / Boyd Taylor Coolman.— 1st ed.
p. cm.
 Includes bibliographical references and index.
 ISBN 0-8132-1368-1 (alk. paper)
 ISBN 978-0-8132-2916-4 (pbk : alk. paper)
 1. Guillermus, Altissiodorensis, d. 1231. Summa aurea. 2. God—Knowableness—History of doctrines—Middle Ages, 600–1500. 3. Experience (Religion)—History of doctrines—Middle Ages, 600–1500. 4. Senses and sensation—Religious aspects—Christianity—History of doctrines—Middle Ages, 600–1500. I. Title.
 BT98.C66 2004
 230´.2´092—dc21
 2003012007

For Anna, *who arrived to see this project begun.*

In memory of Velma and Florence, *who departed too soon to see it completed.*

For Nancy, *who first taught me to taste and see that the Lord is good.*

CONTENTS

Acknowledgments ix
Abbreviations xi

1 Introduction 1

PART I BEATIFIC FRUITION AS SPIRITUAL APPREHENSION

2 A Synaesthetic Beatific Vision 21

PART II THE OBJECTS OF SPIRITUAL APPREHENSION

3 The Manifold Effects of the Metaphysical Good 53
4 The Trinity as Manifold Delectable 72
5 Creation: The Manifestation of the *Delectabilia Divina* 91

PART III THE VIRTUES OF SPIRITUAL APPREHENSION

6 Faith: Knowledge of God in a Visual Mode 111
7 Charity: Love of God in a Tactile Mode 139

PART IV THE FORMS OF SPIRITUAL APPREHENSION

8 Symbolic Theology: Exterior Perception of God's Effects 161
9 Mystical Theology: Interior Perception of God's Effects 184
10 Taste and See: The Spiritual Senses and the Eucharist 218

Conclusion. Spiritual Apprehension: The Spiritual Senses and the Knowledge of God 235

Bibliography 241
Index 249

ACKNOWLEDGMENTS

THIS BOOK ORIGINATED as my 2001 doctoral dissertation at the University of Notre Dame. It is a pleasure to acknowledge the assistance, support, and encouragement without which it would not have been possible. I would like to thank the faculty of the Department of Theology for their high standards, collegiality, and, in many cases, their friendship. In particular, I would like to thank Brian Daley and Larry Cunningham for their careful reading; Rabbi Michael Signer for his good will and affection; Father Thomas O'Meara for his wisdom and guidance; and especially my dissertation advisor, Joseph Wawrykow, for his patient direction, keen sensibilities, and constant support. I am also grateful to Steven P. Marrone, of Tufts University, for his thoughtful review of the manuscript, and to Ellen Coughlin, copy editor for the Catholic University of America Press, for her careful editorial eye and for her patience. Finally, I wish to convey my appreciation to Holly Taylor Coolman, who read the manuscript too many times, but always with care. Whatever defects remain are my own doing.

ABBREVIATIONS

CCCM	*Corpus christianorum continuatio medievalis.*
CCL	*Corpus christianorum, Series latina,* Turnhout.
CSEL	*Corpus scriptorum ecclesiasticorum latinorum,* Vindobonae.
DH	H. Denzinger et Cl. Bannwart, *Enchiridion symbolorum, definitionem et declarationum de rebus et morum,* Friburgum Brisgoviae et Roma.
Lyranus	*Biblia sacra cum Glossa interlineari, ordinaria et Nicolai Lyrani Postilla,* Venetiis, 1588.
PG	*Patrologie Cursus completus, Series graeca,* ed. J.-P. Migne.
PL	*Patrologie Cursus completus, Series latina,* ed. J.-P. Migne.
SA	*Summa Aurea.*

KNOWING GOD BY EXPERIENCE

CHAPTER 1

INTRODUCTION

A REMARKABLE FEATURE of medieval scholasticism is the use by its practitioners of metaphors drawn from sense perception to characterize both theological expression and Christian experience. Scholastic authors often take up the language of the senses to differentiate theological endeavor from other modes of discourse and forms of experience. In his *Summa theologica*,[1] for example, "Alexander" of Hales distinguishes philosophy from theology by comparing the former to sight and the latter to taste. A half-century later and in a similar vein, Giles of Rome argues in his *Expositio in Canticum canticorum* that philosophical contemplation delights spiritual sight and hearing, while the "spiritual contemplation of the theologians gives delight to taste, smell, and touch."[2] An especially prominent use of metaphors drawn from physical sensation emerges in the varied scholastic employment of the doctrine of the spiritual senses of the soul,[3] an ancient Christian tradi-

---

1. "Alexander" of Hales, *Summa Theologica*, Intro., q. 1, c. 4, art. 2, cited in A. J. Minnis and A. B. Scott, eds., *Medieval Literary Theory and Criticism c. 1100–c. 1375: The Commentary-Tradition*, rev. ed. (Oxford: Oxford University Press, 1991), p. 216.

2. Giles of Rome, *Exposition on the Song of Songs*, cited in Denis Turner, *Eros and Allegory* (Kalamazoo, Mich.: Cistercian Publications, 1995), p. 364.

3. This doctrine considers the interplay among the human person's sensate, volitional, and intellectual faculties in the knowledge of God. In particular, it posits the existence of certain capacities or operations within the spiritual dimension of the person for the perception (in the widest sense of the term) of divine realities, a perception which is in some way analogous to that of the physical senses. The relation between these forms of sensation has been variously conceived: as radical opposition, as separate parallelism, in some cases as a transformative evolution from physical to spiritual sense perception. Whatever the case, behind the notion of the spiritual senses is the tension between the affirmation, on the one hand, that finite human beings are deeply, if not inescapably, bound to sensa-

tion reaching back at least to the third century. Among the scholastics, Bonaventure's teaching on the matter is the most celebrated,[4] but a merely partial list of other scholastics who took up this doctrine includes William of Auvergne, Albert the Great, Roger Bacon, Thomas Aquinas,[5] and Rudolph of Biberach.[6]

The focus of this book is the doctrine of the spiritual senses of the soul in the theology of William of Auxerre, scholastic master at the University of Paris in the early thirteenth century. The following chapters consider William's conception of human knowledge of God in relation to his fundamental claim that human persons can know God in a manner analogous to physical sensation. William's utilization of this doctrine is in fact the first in the period of classical scholastic theology, and one must go back perhaps as far as Origen of Alexandria to find a similarly extensive treatment of this theme. After William, the doctrine can be found in the writings of theologians and spiritual writers stretching into the sixteenth century and beyond.[7]

---

tion and imagination and, on the other hand, that the transcendent God is in some way knowable by human persons. Mariette Canévet, "Sens Spirituel," *Dictionnaire de spiritualité ascétique et mystique doctrine et histoire*, ed. Marcel Viller, assisted by F. Cavallera, J. de Guibert, et al. (Paris: Beauchesne, 1937), vol. 15, pp. 598–617.

4. See Fabio M. Tedoldi, *La dottrina dei cinque sensi spirituali in San Bonaventura* (Rome: Pontificum Athenaeum Antonianum, 1999); Karl Rahner, "The Doctrine of the 'Spiritual Senses' in the Middle Ages," in *Theological Investigations* 16 (New York: Seabury, 1979), pp. 104–34; Hans Urs von Balthasar, *Studies in Theological Style: Clerical Styles*, vol. 2 of *The Glory of the Lord, A Theological Aesthetics* (San Francisco: Ignatius, 1984), pp. 260–362, esp. 309–26.

5. Cited in Rahner, "The Doctrine of the 'Spiritual Senses,'" p. 109.

6. Rahner, "The Doctrine of the 'Spiritual Senses,'" pp. 104–34.

7. Ibid. Although the most sustained treatments of the doctrine of the spiritual senses occurred in the patristic and medieval periods, it is significant that in the twentieth century Karl Rahner and Hans Urs von Balthasar were particularly interested in the doctrine. Each undertook a sustained analysis of this doctrine in the thought of St. Bonaventure, though they drew rather different conclusions. Thirty years separate their respective studies: Rahner's work dates to the early 1930s, when he published two articles in *Revue d'ascétique et de mystique*, both of which were subsequently revised and republished in *Theological Investigations* as "The 'Spiritual Senses' According to Origen," and "The Doctrine of the 'Spiritual Senses' in the Middle Ages"; Balthasar's work dates to the early 1960s; see citation in note 4. For an analysis of the differences between the two authors, see Stephen Fields, S.J., "Balthasar and Rahner on the Spiritual Senses," *Theological Studies* 57 (1996), pp. 225–41. Both of these thinkers argued that the doctrine of the spiritual senses reflected an important, often neglected aspect of Christian theology as well as of human knowing: the irreducible role of matter and sensation, and the images drawn from them. In his brief

While William's doctrine of the spiritual senses has been noted, it has not been studied, nor has its full significance for his theology been considered. In part, this is because the doctrine can be described as capillary—pervasive, yet easily overlooked due to its subtle dispersion throughout. In its most basic form, the argument of this study is that the doctrine of the spiritual senses is central to William's conception of human knowledge of God, especially so in the next life, but in the present life too. So crucial is this doctrine for William that it consummates his account of Christian theology and the knowledge of God.

Spiritual Apprehension

As a symphony's first notes introduce the tonality of the score, so the key to William's *Summa Aurea*—its signature concerns and overriding themes—is found in its Prologue. At the same time, the final tractate of the *Summa Aurea* is not merely the last topic treated; it is also the denouement of the whole work, summing up all that precedes. A proper introduction to William's thought, therefore, begins with these two tractates.

In the final treatise of his *Summa Aurea,* William describes the goal of human existence: an experiential apprehension of God in the next life *(in patria).* To capture the fullness of this encounter, he employs the ancient doctrine of the spiritual senses of the soul. His description of beatitude, accordingly, includes references to a spiritual *sensorium:* the *visio Dei* entails not only the seeing of divine *pulchritudo,* but also hearing,

---

study of the history of the spiritual senses, Rahner noted perceptively that "if religious, and especially mystical, experience seeks to express the inexpressible despite all the obstacles that lie in the way, then inevitably it must go back to images which come from the realm of sense knowledge." Balthasar, for his part, spoke more pointedly about the implication of the Incarnation for the role of matter and sensation in the knowledge of God: namely, that in Christ, matter and form are known together. Thus, he notes how "in an extravagant way (since other words are lacking) sensory experiences can be adduced to shed light on the ineffable." For both authors, tracing the doctrine of the spiritual senses as it emerged in Christian history yielded insights into the encounter between human beings and God, as well as revealing the assumptions of various epochs or schools concerning the natures of the participants. This suggests that the study of the doctrine of the spiritual senses—both in individuals and across historical epochs—has value both as a source for theological reflection and as a means of investigating the form, style, and content of a given theology.

smelling, tasting, and touching the divine *simphonia, odor, dulcedo, suavitas,* respectively. For the careful reader of the *Summa Aurea,* these descriptions of fruition are no surprise. For William construes not only beatitude in this way; throughout the *Summa Aurea* he depicts knowledge of God in the present life similarly. Faith too is a vision *(visus)* of divine beauty; charity is a touching *(tactus)* of divine suavity. Progress in the knowledge of God increasingly entails the taste of divine sweetness and, in the reception of the Eucharist, the believer delights in the presence of Christ through all the spiritual senses. The spiritual yet sensuous beatific vision is the culmination, then, of a process begun in this life and of an experience foretasted here.

In the Prologue, William programmatically outlines the steps in this process as he describes the fundamental structure and process of Christian theology. It moves from basic knowledge *(scientia),* to understanding *(intellectus),* to wisdom *(sapientia).* This triad contains the fundamental elements in William's concept of the knowledge of God. Theology is a science and an understanding which comes to fruition in wisdom. More precisely, beginning with a divine illumination of the creedal articles, faith moves progressively to an increasingly experiential perception *(sensus)* of God and divine things. The process thus leads to that spiritual sense-perception which constitutes beatitude.

The term adopted here to refer generally to William's conception of the knowledge of God is "spiritual apprehension."[8] The choice of words must be explained. Throughout the *Summa Aurea,* as intimated above, William depicts knowledge of God in two ways: it is, on the one hand, a form of spiritual, even mystical, *aesthesis,* a perception *(percipere)* or sensation *(sentire)* of the manifestations of the divine nature. As such, a cer-

---

8. Medieval thinkers employed a variety of terms (including *scientia, cognitio, intellectus,* and *ratio*), each possessing different shades of meaning and connotation, to describe what in a vague and general way might be termed "knowledge" in English. Perhaps the most frequently used Latin term for knowledge is *scientia,* which translates the Greek *episteme.* This can refer to an organized body of knowledge. It can also refer to knowledge derived through a certain methodology, as in the Aristotelian sense of *scientia.* The German *Wissenschaft* is perhaps a closer equivalent. Medieval thinkers were also familiar with the Augustinian distinction between *scientia* and *sapientia,* the former pertaining to knowledge of created realities, the latter to knowledge of God. Timothy Potts, *Conscience in Medieval Philosophy* (Cambridge: Cambridge University Press, 1980), p. 75.

tain aesthetic pleasure characterizes the knowledge of God. As the physical senses experience a unique delectation in the perception of their proper objects, so spiritual sensation of the *delectabilia divina*—the diverse modes in which the Trinity reveals itself—entails diverse forms of spiritual pleasure. Here then, paradoxically, knowledge of God may be described as "spiritually sensuous." Yet, for William, knowledge of God is also fundamentally noetic and conceptual. Flush with increasingly ascendent Aristotelian thought and its strong claims for certain knowledge *(scientia, episteme)*, he is unabashed about the intellectual nature of Christian theology. To know God is to cognize *(cognoscere)* the divine nature through theological concepts—in particular the doctrines contained in the creedal articles of faith. This dimension entails knowledge *(scientia)* and understanding *(intellectus)*. In short, then, for William knowledge of God consists of both theological concept and spiritual percept.

Significantly, William not only posits a theological noetic and a spiritual aesthetic, but integrates them. Consistently, his descriptions of the knowledge of God combine the act of *cognoscere*[9] with those of *percipere* and *sentire*.[10] So much is this the case that this triad comprises a unified form of knowing. Its members are less discrete, rigidly demarcated categories and more points along a continuum of apprehending. Here, it must be noted that these components correspond generally to the basic structure of theology outlined in the Prologue of the *Summa Aurea*, described above: as *cognoscere*, theology entails *scientia* and *intellectus*;[11] as *percipere* and *sentire*, it corresponds to *sapientia*. For William, theology

---

9. Potts argues that there is no ready English equivalent for this Latin term and this is emphatically so in the case of William of Auxerre. Also pertinent here is Potts's observation that: "[*cognitio*] is much wider than '*scientia*' and even includes perception." Ibid., p. 76.

10. These verbs and their cognates will be translated by the English terms "perceive" and "sense" along with their derivatives.

11. According to Potts, "thought" is probably the nearest English equivalent to this term, which translates the Greek *nous*. He notes, though, that this English term does not normally mean the ability to think, what he considers to be the basic idea expressed by the Latin term. Potts also judges the term "understanding" too narrow. While William often uses this term to refer to a particular power or capacity in the soul, he also uses it to mean the act of that power and its result. In the former case, it will simply be transliterated in this study as "intellect"; in the later case, the verb "understand" will be employed to describe the act of the intellect and the noun "understanding" to refer to the result. Potts, *Conscience*, p. 76.

entails a progression from *scientia,* to *intellectus,* to *sapientia;* from *cognoscere,* to *percipere,* to *sentire.* Knowledge of God proceeds from an affirmation of creedal doctrines, through a deeper understanding of their meaning and coherence, to a direct and experiential perception of divine realities. In light of this wedding of theological cognition and spiritual perception, "spiritual apprehension" is both apt and felicitous.[12]

Of great import is that in the process of spiritual apprehension a specific relationship arises between doctrine and experience. Spiritual experience does not abandon doctrinal formulation; prior forms of knowing are not left behind by, or radically dissociated from, later forms. Rather, knowledge is subsumed into the subsequent sensation of God. Spiritual percept is mediated by theological concept. The speculative penetration of doctrine, the progressively deeper *intellectus fidei,* is inseparable from the spiritual experience that such theological labor makes possible: understanding informs and transforms experience. The spiritual hearing of Christ speaking within Scripture, for example, progresses from catching the fragrance of the meaning of the Incarnation and tasting its salvific significance, to in some way touching the divine nature itself. Thus, the spiritual perception of divine realities is mediated by theological reflection on central Christian doctrines, by *scientia* and *intellectus.* S*cientia-cognoscere* structures and informs *sapientia-sentire,* while *sapientia-sentire* subsumes and consummates *scientia-cognoscere.* As noted, William sums up this knowledge of God under the title "wisdom" *(sapientia),* whose linguistic root, *"sapio,"* connotes both savoring and understanding, thus evoking the "tasted knowledge" which with William integrates scholastic speculation and mystical perception.

Thus, rather than overlaying spiritual experience with theological doctrine, or privileging experience over second-order speculation, William's method moves in the opposite direction. The starting point is not spiritual experience, but the creedal summary of revelation found in Scripture. Experience presumes the preparatory, informing, and enabling function of theological science, and theology is integral and vital

---

12. This English term seems appropriate, given its literal meaning of "to grasp" or "to seize" and its extended meanings, which include "to grasp the meaning of; understand, esp. intuitively; perceive." *Webster's Encyclopedic Unabridged Dictionary of the English Language,* 1989 ed., s.v. "apprehend."

to the lived experience of the encounter with God. Furthermore, though spiritual experience is personal, it is far from privatized or individualistic, precisely because it is mediated generally by the communally affirmed Creed and in the particular sense that it arises out of the communal enterprise of scholastic discourse, which draws its life from that broader theological tradition. Experience is indeed interiorized, but not at the expense of the corporate. William, thus, unites theology and spirituality in a uniquely scholastic fashion.

Here, finally, it must be noted that in a general way William seems to have transposed a monastic model of reading Scripture into a scholastic key. Where earlier exegetes moved from the *sensus litteralis*, the surface meaning of the text, to a *sensus allegoricus*, the deeper theological meaning of the text, and finally to a *sensus spiritualis*, where the very presence of the Word is known experientially, tasted and touched, William's theology, *mutatis mutandis*, envisions a movement from the *articulos fidei* to an *intellectus fidei*, and from there finally to a *sensus spiritualis* where the *delectabilia divina* are perceived and sensed. The initial level pertains to the historical events of salvation history, the Incarnation and Passion especially. The *intellectus fidei* pursues the deeper meaning and significance of these events. The *sensus spiritualis*, finally, offers an experiential sense-perception of the divine nature. Similarly, William has taken up certain categories and concerns, for example, moral formation (exterior, active life) in the service of spiritual experience (interior, contemplative life), but incorporated them within a different intellectual milieu. Rather than juxtaposing knowledge *(scientia* and *cognitio)* and experience *(experimentum)*, as some previous authors had done,[13] he integrates them. Through the spiritual senses—by uniting *cognoscere* and *sentire*—*experimentum* emerges out of *cognoscere*. This is perhaps best exemplified in William's description of the Eucharist, where faith penetrates from the material forms of bread and wine, to a theological understanding of Christ's Incarnation and Passion and their salvific significance, and finally to a spiritual delectation in the very presence of Christ through the spiritual senses.

13. See Brian Stock, "Experience, Praxis, Work, and Planning in Bernard of Clairvaux: Observations on the *Sermones in Cantica*," in *The Cultural Context of Medieval Learning*, ed. John E. Murdoch and Edith D. Sylla (Dordrecht, Holland: D. Reidel, 1975), pp. 219–68.

In ways, therefore, that have not yet been appreciated the doctrine of the spiritual senses is central to William of Auxerre's view of the knowledge of God. The doctrine is a leitmotif in his theology. It shapes his presentation of other, major doctrines, guiding the presentation of his theological system, forming his theological sensibilities, and giving his entire theological endeavor a unique savor. His thought cannot be appreciated adequately without taking it into consideration.

William of Auxerre in Historical Perspective: A Brief Sketch

Secular master of theology at the University of Paris in the early thirteenth century, William of Auxerre is the best known of several medieval "Williams" from Auxerre. Surprisingly little, though, is known concerning his life. According to quite conjectural evidence, he was born between 1140 and 1150, most likely in Auxerre. There is some evidence that he was already well known as a teacher as early as 1189, but it is not certain whether he was working in grammar, arts, or theology. Sometime before 1228, he had become a master in theology at Paris. It is also known that at some point he became Archdeacon of Beauvais. Throughout his academic life, William was involved in administrative or diplomatic tasks on the part either of the University of Paris, King Louis IX, or Pope Gregory IX. These tasks involved at least one journey to Rome and perhaps a stay there of more than a year, which would have taken place during the years 1230–31. In 1231, William was appointed by Pope Gregory IX to a commission charged with correcting the works of Aristotle in order to make them more amenable for use by Christian thinkers. This project came to naught, perhaps due to William's death sometime late in 1231.[14]

Though at the middle of the twentieth century it could be claimed that "William of Auxerre is no unknown quantity in the history of scholastic theology,"[15] at the turn of the twenty-first century this better expresses a hope than a reality. The current state of research on William

---

14. Walter Principe, *William of Auxerre's Theology of the Hypostatic Union*, vol. 1 of *The Theology of the Hypostatic Union in the Early Thirteenth Century*, Studies and Texts no. 7 (Toronto: Pontifical Institute of Medieval Studies, 1963), pp. 14–16.

15. Johannes Beumer, "Die Theologie als *intellectus fidei*: Dargestellt an Hand der Lehre des Wilhelm von Auxerre und Petrus von Tarantasia," *Scholastik* 17 (1942): p. 34.

of Auxerre provides a rather telescoped and truncated picture of his thought. In standard histories of scholastic theology and philosophy, William typically merits a short remark, usually concerning his above-noted appointment by Pope Gregory IX to expunge questionable material from the newly discovered *"libri naturalium"* of Aristotle.[16] The prevalent scholarly estimation of William can be stated briefly: he is a pioneer who falteringly, hesitantly, initiates and anticipates the flowering of the scholastic genius among his successors. In one respect, this is an accurate assessment and, indeed, it is hoped that this study will further clarify the ways in which William's work—bridging as it does a transitional period in the evolution of scholastic theology—receives and shapes earlier developments and influences later trends. At the same time, another objective of this book is to offer a fuller picture of William's theology in its own right, rather than simply as an important but tentative step in the evolution of scholastic theology or as a contribution to the development of a particular doctrine. It will also be suggested that, at least in some respects—perhaps especially in his doctrine of the knowledge of God—William represents something of a scholastic "road not taken."

William of Auxerre in Context

With his *Summa Aurea*, William stands at a significant juncture in the evolution of medieval theology: at a moment of intellectual, ecclesial, and spiritual ferment. Venerable patristic traditions are present in his thought, yet he is one of the first medieval thinkers to grapple with the fuller presentation of Aristotle's philosophy rapidly emerging in his day. At the same time, vibrant currents of popular devotion and significant shifts in medieval religion shape his sensibilities. It will be helpful, if only superficially, to locate him within these contexts.

Although the meaning and usefulness of the designation has been intensely debated, the term "Augustinian" remains a generally appropriate label for William's theology.[17] In terms of epistemology, for example,

---

16. Stephen Brown, "The Intellectual Context of Later Medieval Philosophy: Universities, Aristotle, Arts, Theology," in *Routledge History of Philosophy*, 3, *Medieval Philosophy*, ed. John Marenbon (London: Routledge, 1986), p. 191.

17. T. Heitz, *Essai historique sur les rapports entre la philosophie et la foi: de Bérenger de*

William espouses a form of illuminationism. He is familiar, moreover, with the African bishop's distinction between *scientia* and *sapientia* (though he does not adopt it). With respect to faith-psychology, his concern with an affective dimension in Christian theology (especially his interest in *delectatio*) is reminiscent of Augustine, as is his (intriguingly muted) use of psychological triads (memory, understanding, and will) in his theological anthropology and trinitarian theology. Much of this "Augustinianism," though, is filtered through the lens of William's twelfth-century predecessors, especially the great Cistercian writers, Bernard of Clairvaux, William of St. Thierry, and the anonymous author of the *De spiritu et anima*. The *Summa Aurea* is then largely Augustinian in its ideas, arguments, and method.[18]

Another patristic influence on William, also mediated by twelfth-century thinkers, is the pseudo-Dionysian corpus. William shares with twelfth-century authors such as Abelard, the Chartrians, Gilbert of Poitiers, and Alan of Lille a Dionysian-inspired sensitivity to divine transcendence of human language and concepts. Moreover, he appears to derive his metaphysics of the good and his insistence that knowledge of God is mediated by God's created effects from the Dionysian corpus. But he has little interest in negative theology as such, and is far more cataphatic in his theological method than many of his contemporaries.[19] In this regard, William must be distinguished from a particular medieval Dionysian tributary which thrived in his time, namely, an "affectivized" Dionysian theology. The twelfth century witnessed various attempts to

---

Tours à S. Thomas d' Aquin (Paris: Libraire Victor Lecoffre, 1909), pp. 92–98. The term "Augustinian tradition" is used here advisedly, without any attempt to enter into the debate over the precise meaning of the term. For a discussion and bibliography regarding this debate, see Steven P. Marrone, *William of Auvergne and Robert Grosseteste: New Ideas of Truth in the Early Thirteenth Century* (Princeton, N.J.: Princeton University Press, 1983), pp. 3–23.

18. Johannes Beumer, *Theologie als Glaubensverständnis* (Würzburg: Echter, 1953), pp. 71–72.

19. For a helpful discussion of the influence of Dionysian traditions in the medieval period generally, see Paul Rorem, *Pseudo-Dionysius: A Commentary on the Texts and an Introduction to Their Influence* (Oxford: Oxford University Press, 1993), pp. 216–19. For a more focused treatment of that influence in the twelfth and thirteenth centuries, see Tugwell's discussion in Simon Tugwell, O.P., *Albert and Thomas: Selected Writings* (New York: Paulist Press, 1988), pp. 39–95.

supplement the strongly apophatic and intellectualist character of the Dionysian mystical theology with an affective dimension, inspired in large measure by a mystical reading of the Song of Songs.[20] The pinnacle of the mystical ascent in Dionysius' *Mystical Theology* was the entry into the dazzling darkness of complete and utter "un-knowing." For Dionysius' medieval readers, however, love is higher than knowledge, and (in the words of Hugh of St. Victor) "one loves more than one understands, and love enters and approaches where knowledge stays outside."[21] An interesting exponent of this view is the thirteenth-century Victorine, Thomas Gallus (d. 1246), a near contemporary of William. Gallus was persuaded of the harmony between the Dionysian unknowing and the affective approach based on the Song of Songs. For him, there is an affective or loving knowledge of the affection that is above the knowledge of the intellect. Though William shares with this tradition a concern with the affect, his is a very different conception, both of the relation between the love and the knowledge of God, and of how the highest knowledge of God is to be characterized. In sum, then, while William is familiar with the Dionysian corpus, and takes up certain Dionysian themes, he does not incorporate Dionysius' theological method in any significant sense.

It is widely acknowledged that William occupies an important place in the development of early scholastic theology. As Jules St. Pierre notes, "it is becoming clear that William occupies a key, pivotal position between the earlier scholastic theology of the twelfth century and the full flowering of the scholastic genius in the thirteenth."[22] Martin Grabmann speaks of William, along with Philip the Chancellor, Godfrey of Poitiers, and William of Auvergne, as "impressive forms in the antechamber of high scholasticism."[23] William's significance is largely due to the influence of his major work, the *Summa Aurea*, written between 1215

---

20. Rorem, *Pseudo-Dionysius*, pp. 216–19.

21. Hugh of St. Victor, *In hierarchiam caelestem S. Dionysii*, 1.10.3, PL 175.1038D, cited in Rorem, *Pseudo-Dionysius*, p. 229, n. 21.

22. Jules St. Pierre, "The Theological Thought of William of Auxerre: An Introductory Bibliography," *Recherches de théologie ancienne et médiévale* 33 (1966): p. 147.

23. Martin Grabmann, *Die Geschicte der katholischen Theologie seit dem Ausgang der Väterzeit* (Freiburg, 1933), pp. 57–59.

and 1225,²⁴ a work which represents a new stage in the evolution of scholastic theology. Though it generally follows the organization of the Lombard's *Sentences*, it is neither a gloss nor a commentary on the Lombard's text, but an independent work with its own organization and method.²⁵ Accordingly, it inaugurates a new genre of theological literature, systematically bringing together the speculative substance of Christian theology in a true *summa theologica*. Johannes Beumer speaks of the "the ripe and good-quality fruit of the preparatory work of the early-scholastic authors," which in the *Summa Aurea* receives a uniform shape.²⁶ With the *Summa* of Praepositinus of Cremona, William's *Summa* is frequently quoted among later scholastics. Dom Odo Lottin has noted some twenty-six medieval theologians who are known to have used the *Summa Aurea*.²⁷ Its influence on subsequent thirteenth-century scholastics such as Alexander of Hales, Hugh of St. Cher, and Thomas Aquinas has also been noted.²⁸ Megivern, for example, suggests that William is an important link between the Lombard and Aquinas; William is cited several times by Thomas.²⁹ With regard to William's influence on subsequent developments in theology, Principe mentions, among other things, issues of theological method, problems in psychol-

---

24. William also wrote a *Summa de officiis ecclesiasticis*, a treatise dealing with the sacraments and the liturgy in general but also including many historical details about the Parisian liturgy of the period. See Principe, *Hypostatic Union*, p. 15.

25. Martin Grabmann, *Die Geschichte der scholastischen Methode* (Graz, 1957): "Wilhelm von Auxerre hat in seiner Summa Aurea sich wieder an das Einteilungsschema des Lombarden ohne diese Ausmerzung von Dispositionsmängeln, indessen mit zeimlicher Selbständigkeit, gehalten"; pp. 369–70. "Protois bezeichnet als die erste uns bekannte Sentenzenerklärung die Summa Aurea des Wilhelm von Auxerre. Doch dies ist nicht richtig. Denn wie im dritten Bande sich zeigen wird, ist die Summa Aurea kein Sentenzenkommentar, sondern eine selbstäntige, wenn auch in ihrer Struktur und Doktrin vom Lombarden vielfach abhänige theologische Summa. Fernerhin hat er schon vor den Zeiten Wilhelm von Auxerre Kommentatoren der Sentenzen gegeben"; p. 393.

26. Beumer, *Theologie als Glaubensverständnis*, p. 58.

27. O. Lottin, *Psychologie et morale au XII et XIII siècles*, 6 vols. (Louvain and Gembloux, 1942–60), vol. 4, pp. 846–47.

28. Grabmann, *Die Geschichte der katholischen Theologie*, p. 57. "The *Summa Aurea*, which was fundamental in particular in the moral and sacramental doctrines and also fertilized theological terminology, was greatly influential (as the uncommonly large dispersion of manuscripts shows) and extremely much read and analyzed by Albert the Great and Thomas Aquinas."

29. James J. Megivern, *Concomitance and Communion: A Study in Eucharistic Doctrine and Practice* (Freiburg: University Press, 1963), p. 174.

ogy and moral doctrines, and various points regarding the sacraments, in which William "either opened new paths or markedly advanced the old."[30]

William must also be seen within the context of the early-thirteenth-century struggle to assimilate a fuller understanding of Aristotelian philosophy within theology. The early thirteenth century witnessed a major transformation not only in its sources, with the introduction of new Aristotelian texts, but also in its forms, methods, and criteria of thought. William is one of the first medieval theologians to wrestle with the implications of Aristotle's thought for theology.[31] In this, moreover, he initiates a new period of theological activity. The *Summa Aurea* is greatly affected by Aristotelian dialectic and the new method of theological disputation minted under its influence. This is especially evident in relation to theological discourse and language, as William applies in an intensified manner the conceptual framework and language of Aristotelian philosophy to the doctrines of the faith and the terminology employed therein.[32]

For our purposes, the most important intersection of Aristotelian philosophy and Christian theology involves the question of knowledge or science *(scientia)*. Of momentous significance was the embracing of the Aristotelian model of science *(scientia)* in the context of the newly emerging universities in the early thirteenth century. It became the paradigm of cognitive certitude, the undisputed ideal of all disciplines, and the unquestioned yardstick according to which the disciplines were to be evaluated. Increasingly what counted for knowledge was only that which could be known with absolute certainty, namely that which had been arrived at by means of strictly logical demonstration from indubitable and self-evident first principles, as described in the *Posterior Analytics*. The-

---

30. Principe, *Hypostatic Union*, p. 16.

31. Grabmann, *Die Geschichte der katholischen Theologie*, p. 59: "In the *Summa Aurea* the first quotations and effects of the new Aristotle appear." Though explicit citations of Aristotle in the *Summa Aurea* are relatively rare, there are more of them than in the work of William of Auvergne; cf. Heitz, *Essai historique*, pp. 92–98.

32. Chenu notes that William is familiar with the Aristotelian notion of a *habitus*, though perhaps he has not penetrated its meaning deeply, and the Augustinian psychology compromises the Aristotelian notions. M.-D. Chenu, "Pro fidei supernaturalitate illustranda," in *Xenia Thomistica*, ed. Sdoc Szabó, (Rome, 1925), vol. 3, pp. 300–301.

ology, accordingly, was forced to ask itself whether it was a true science. How? In what sense? And, if so, what were its first principles and how was further knowledge to be derived from them? William is one of the first to tackle this question, arguing strongly for the scientific nature of theology and thus charting a course for subsequent scholastic thinkers. In this respect, he has been called "the thirteenth-century apostle of deductive theology."[33]

William must also be briefly located within the various currents of medieval spirituality and devotion present in his day. The great religious upheavals of the twelfth century, spawned at least in part by the Gregorian reforms initiated in the eleventh, represent a surge in popular interest in more authentic and meaningful expressions of Christian life. The quest for the true *vita apostolica*, exemplified in the proliferation of new religious orders, especially the Cistercians, Carthusians, and Augustinians, along with various women's movements *(Frauenbewegungen)*, is ample evidence of the widespread interest in authentic forms of the Christian life. But the impulse was not limited to religious orders. Increasingly, the laity sought greater participation, as is evident in such groups as the Cathars, Albigensians, and Waldensians in France and the Humiliati of north Italy. These initiatives continued with vigor into the thirteenth century with the rise of the mendicant orders associated with Francis and Dominic. These various impulses provided the impetus for the invocation of the Fourth Lateran Council, which can be seen as an institutional response to popular religious movements, attempting to provide ecclesiastical direction and clarification to new quests for authentic Christianity.[34]

---

33. Brown, "The Intellectual Context of Later Medieval Philosophy," p. 198. Stephen Brown, "Declarative and Deductive Theology in the Early Fourteenth Century," in *Was ist Philosophie im Mittelalter*, ed. Jan A. Aertsen and Andreas Speer (Berlin: Walter de Gruyter, 1998), 649–50: "The procedure of deducing new truths or conclusions from premises that are articles of the faith antecedes Thomas Aquinas. William of Auxerre, for example, started with the articles of the faith that were most immediate to our senses and went on to further conclusions that were based on them." See also E. Krebs, *Theologie und Wissenschaft nach der Lehre der Hochscholastik*, Beiträge zur Geschichte der Philosophie und Theologie des Mittelalters (Münster: Aschendorff, 1912), vol. 11, pp. 3–4.

34. R. N. Swanson, *Religion and Devotion in Europe, c. 1215–1515* (Cambridge: Cambridge University Press, 1995), pp. 10–135.

Written in the period just after Lateran IV, William's *Summa Aurea* and its theology reflect many of these currents of spirituality and devotion. Two are especially important. The first is the still vibrant and powerful current of monastic spirituality and thought, especially that emanating from Cistercian circles, with its strong emphasis on the "interior man," affectivity, a direct encounter between God and soul, bridal mysticism, and an orientation toward the humanity of Christ. The second is the emerging devotion to the Eucharist as a primary locus for an experiential encounter with Christ, as well as for theological reflection.

The Doctrine of the Spiritual Senses

William's place within scholastic reflections on the doctrine of the spiritual senses was noted above. Something further, though, should be said about the doctrine's development before and after William. The Christian doctrine of spiritual senses, the inspiration for which lies in the language of Scripture,[35] finds its roots in the patristic period with Origen, Gregory of Nyssa, and others in the East, and with Augustine and Gregory the Great in the West. Its proponents span the medieval period from Gregory the Great to Ignatius of Loyola, Teresa of Avila and John of the Cross, reaching a zenith with Bonaventure—though, as noted above, Bonaventure's achievement must be viewed in the light of William's contribution.

Traditionally, the notion of "senses" (Greek: *aisthesis,* Latin: *sensus*) connoted not only a form of perception, but also a form of comprehension or knowledge, often an immediate, nondiscursive operation of the intellect, with an emphasis on the experiential dimension of knowledge. Hence, the spiritual senses were associated with the discernment of spiritual realities and with the experience of fruition. Typically, the spiritual senses were considered the possession of the mature or the perfect, and a "hierarchy of senses" could be established in order to chart the soul's progress toward maturity. Faith and moral purity were understood to be necessary conditions for their operation. Furthermore, the objects of the spiritual senses were conceived in various ways, often depending on the

---

35. Several biblical passages are perennial favorites in relation to the spiritual senses: Ps 18:9, Ps 33:9, Prv 2:5, Mt 5:8, Jn 6:23, 2 Cor 2:15–17, 2 Cor 12:2, Heb 5:14, 1 Jn 1:1.

particular "spiritual sense" involved. Frequently, a Christological orientation emerged, as the Incarnate Christ in both human and divine natures was viewed as susceptible to human perception, both physical and spiritual. Alongside this Christological emphasis, however, was an emphasis on the important role played by the Holy Spirit in relation to the spiritual senses.[36]

After the patristic period, the doctrine of the spiritual senses emerged again with vigor in the twelfth century (here Bernard of Clairvaux,[37] William of St. Thierry,[38] and Alcher of Clairvaux are noteworthy). This is due in part to the influence of several important patristic texts. First, a comment of Origen's pertaining to the spiritual senses from his Third *Homily on Leviticus* is quoted in the *Glossa ordinaria* in relation to the text of Leviticus 3:7.[39] In the third book of his *Sentences*, Peter Lombard, apparently contradicting the saying of Origen, states that in Christ, the head of the mystical body, all the senses are to be found, while the saints only possess the sense of touch. This apparent contradiction stimulated discussion of the topic among later scholastic commentators.[40] Second, Augustine's comparison, in *Letter 187*, of the five prudent virgins from the gospel parable with the five spiritual senses was important for scholastic speculation on this topic. Third, Gregory the Great's references in his *Moralia* to the *sensus mentis, sensus animi, sensus interni,* and

---

36. See Canévet, "Sens Spirituel," *Dictionnaire spiritualité*, vol. 20, pp. 598–617.

37. Bernard developed this theme extensively in his writings on the spiritual life, especially in his well-known sermons on the Song of Songs. For him, the object of the spiritual senses appears to be Christ, the Bridegroom, who is encountered by the soul as it moves progressively through deeper levels of understanding of the biblical text. The spiritual senses are frequently engaged when Bernard is treating the moral sense of scripture. In one sermon, for example, he refers to the "smell" of the Bridegroom's spices, the "feel" of his ointments, and "taste" of his wine; Sermon 23:6–8. See Bernard McGinn, *The Growth of Mysticism*, vol. 2 of *The Presence of God: A History of Western Christian Mysticism* (New York: Crossroad, 1994), pp. 185–90.

38. William of St. Thierry made use of the notion of the soul's spiritual senses in his understanding of the *sensus amoris*, that is, love's own ability to understand or perceive God. See McGinn, *The Growth of Mysticism*, pp. 255–58.

39. *Glossa ordinaria*, ed. Léandre de Saint-Marten, t. 1, anvers, 1634, col. 956, cited in Aimé Solignac, "Oculus," in *Dictionnaire de spiritualité ascétique et mystique doctrine et histoire*, ed. Marcel Viller, assisted by F. Cavallera, J. De Guibert, et al., vol. 18 (Paris: Beauchesne, 1937), p. 593.

40. Cited in Rahner, "The Doctrine of the 'Spiritual Senses,'" p. 106, n. 11.

his reference in his *Homilies on Ezekiel* to the *occuli cordis* were also influential.⁴¹

Rationale and Method

In the interest of presenting William's teaching on the spiritual senses fully and faithfully, two approaches present themselves: on the one hand, a synthetic composition in which the major elements of various doctrines are pulled together from their disparate places in the text and organized into a coherent whole; on the other hand, a predominately analytic exposition more attentive to the details in themselves and to their origin than in their place within the whole. Both approaches have their advantages and risks. The clarity and brevity of the first might come at the cost of a certain infidelity—it would be tempting to reconstruct William's thought to some extent. The second might come at the cost of a certain loss of comprehension of the whole. Perhaps unavoidably the two approaches have been combined here, not with the vain hope of retaining all benefits and eliminating all drawbacks, but because this strategy was unavoidable.⁴² Throughout, it has been necessary to give a close analytic reading of various tractates of the *Summa Aurea* in order to render their contents adequately. At the same time, some synthesis of elements (those which his teaching on the spiritual senses either presumes or engenders) found scattered throughout the *Summa Aurea* has been required in order to present William's thought with clarity and precision. Furthermore, it was found necessary to establish the theological and philosophical assumptions which underlie the doctrine, to analyze the necessary conditions for the operation of the spiritual senses along with their proper objects, to chart their development and progress, and to locate them within the overall trajectory of William's theology. The organization of this work thus involves the imposition from without of a certain form and structure, though without compro-

---

41. For Augustine, see note 39 above; for Gregory the Great, see *Moralia* VI c. 33 (PL 75.973) and *Homilies on Ezekiel* II, homily 1, n. 18 (PL 76.948B), cited in Rahner, "The 'Spiritual Senses' According to Origen," p. 103, n. 164.

42. This approach is inspired by that of J.-P. Torrell's *Théorie de la prophétie et philosophie de la connaissance aux environs de 1230: La contribution d'Huges de Saint-Cher* (Spicilegium Sacrum Lovaniense, fasc. 40) (Louvain, 1997), pp. 149–50.

mising, it is of course hoped, the essential nature of William's theology.

An appreciation of William's *Summa Aurea* as a literary work, and of the theological vision expressed therein, is enhanced when viewed from the end, that is, from the vantage point of his account of ultimate beatitude. The same is true with his doctrine of the spiritual senses. Like Christian thinkers before and since, William affirms that the chief end and vocation of human persons is the beatific *visio Dei* in the next life. Therefore, although beatitude is of course the climax of the knowledge of God, and although William accordingly treats it at the conclusion of the *Summa Aurea*, it will be analyzed here first. This proves helpful for several reasons. First, William's most sustained treatment of the doctrine of the spiritual senses occurs in his discussion of beatitude. The states of life *in via* and *in patria*, moreover, are linked. The activity of the spiritual senses *in patria* is the culmination of a progressively greater knowledge of God which builds upon other forms of that knowledge begun *in via*. Hence, the beatific activity of the spiritual senses is not unrelated to their possible activity in this life. More importantly, with this discussion in the foreground, William's often terse references to the doctrine or its components in other contexts will be more intelligible and their significance more apparent.

The following chapters are organized into four parts. Part I considers William's doctrine of the spiritual senses in the context of beatitude. The remaining parts consider his teaching in relationship to the present life: Part II treats the objects of spiritual apprehension; Part III, the virtues of spiritual apprehension; and Part IV, the forms of spiritual apprehension.

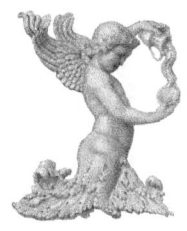
PART I
BEATIFIC FRUITION AS
SPIRITUAL APPREHENSION

CHAPTER 2

A SYNAESTHETIC BEATIFIC VISION

WILLIAM OF AUXERRE'S DOCTRINE of the spiritual senses receives its fullest elaboration in his descriptions of the beatitude experienced by the blessed in the next life *(in patria)*. For William, beatitude is realized precisely through the activity of the spiritual senses; the doctrine, in fact, stands at the heart of his understanding of the *visio Dei*. Furthermore, his conception of beatitude through the spiritual senses contains the fundamental structure and constitutive components of William's general conception of human knowledge of God and is thus paradigmatic of all such knowledge.

William's treatment of beatitude occurs in the fourth and final book of the *Summa Aurea*, in the eighteenth and final tractate: "On the Effects of the Sacraments or On the Resurrection." This dual designation is not accidental, for it reflects the tractate's function within Book IV. The first seventeen tractates contain his analysis of the sacraments; as Tractate 18's title suggests, William understands the resurrected life *in patria* to be closely connected to the effects of the sacraments in this life *(in via)*. The significance of the last tractate, however, transcends its connection to the sacraments. Tractate 18 also functions as the summation of the entire *Summa Aurea*. Beatific knowledge of God is not merely the last topic in the *Summa Aurea*; it is the climax. Throughout, William's theology is oriented toward the final encounter with God, and he posits important continuities between this life and the next. An appreciation of his doctrine of the spiritual senses and its significance for all human knowledge of God, accordingly, must begin here.

In order to appreciate fully the role of the spiritual senses in the beatific knowledge of God, a detailed exposition and analysis of Tractate 18 is necessary. Such an approach will not merely facilitate an introduction to the topic; it will also highlight the other aspects of William's theology which the doctrine of the spiritual senses presumes and entails. This, in turn, will provide a rationale for the organization of the subsequent examination of the doctrine of the spiritual senses throughout William's theology.

A Foundation for Beatitude: The Beatific Endowments of the Soul

William's understanding of beatitude through the spiritual senses is founded upon his conception of the constitution of resurrected persons, which he describes in terms of the notion of endowments *(dos, dotes)*. He divides the endowments of resurrected persons into two kinds: four of the body—beauty or clarity *(claritas)*, impassibility *(impassibilitas)*, subtlety *(subtilitas)*, agility *(agilitas)*; and three of the soul—cognition *(cognitio)*, love *(dilectio)*, fruition *(fruitio)*. While he treats both kinds, he allots the bulk of his analysis to the latter.

As found in William's thought, the doctrine of the *dotes* represents an intriguing chapter in the development of medieval theology.[1] In its origin, the term *"dotes"* was associated with marriage rights in Roman law, and eventually made its way into medieval canon law.[2] The literal sense of the term *"dotes"* referred in its social setting to wedding gifts exchanged between bridegroom and bride. This meaning, in turn, facilitated the term's figurative use among theologians, who conceived of the church as the *sponsa Christi* and emphasized Christ's role as eternal Bridegroom and the church as bride. Here, the Incarnation establishes a

---

1. Nicholas Wicki, *Die Lehre von der himmlischen Seligkeit in der mittelalterlichen Scholastik von Petrus Lombardus bis Thomas von Aquin*, (Freiburg: University Press, 1954), p. 202. William himself does not invent the notion of the endowments. Yet its use prior to him is not clearly delineated. Such a conception is not found in Scripture, though some early church authors seem to have used the term in a similar way. Tertullian, for example, speaks of the resurrected body as the *dos* of the soul; *De resurrectione carnis*, c. 63, PL 2.933, cited in Wicki, *Seligkeit*, p. 209, nn. 35–37.

2. Ibid., pp. 209–10, especially n. 34.

marital relation between Christ and the church, which serves as the basis for the reception of *dotes*.[3] The Incarnate Christ is not merely the Object of beatitude, but in a crucial way also its Donor, equipping his bride with her *dotes*. This doctrine thus entails a unique perspective on beatitude,[4] grounding it in ecclesiology and Christology.[5]

This spousal conception of the beatific endowments undergirds William's justification of the soul's three endowments of *cognitio, dilectio*, and *fruitio*.[6] "An endowment is that gift which the bridegroom gives to the bride, in order that by it she may live. . . . And since by these three [endowments] the soul lives immediately—for by these three the soul is moved immediately into God—only these three warrant the status of an endowment."[7] The endowments, then, are a special kind of virtue, namely, those given to the soul-bride in order to facilitate her beatific marriage. These virtues are distinguished from other kinds of virtues by

---

3. Ibid., pp. 209–12.

4. Ibid., pp. 41–43. According to Wicki, the doctrine of the *dotes* enjoyed considerable success among later thirteenth-century scholastic theologians, in no small measure due to William's influence. In his *Magisterium divinale*, William's colleague at the University of Paris, William of Auvergne, is influenced by him in this regard. The first Dominican master at the University of Paris, Roland of Cremona, transfers William's doctrine of the *dotes* unchanged into his *summa*. The *Sentence Commentary* of Hugh of St. Cher also betrays William's influence.

5. Wicki, *Seligkeit*, pp. 217–19. An important implication of the ecclesiological orientation of the doctrine of the *dotes* is its communal aspect. Many early thirteenth-century treatments of this doctrine reflect this: beatitude *in patria* is presented as the church's possession. The church is the bride of Christ and thus the recipient of *dotes*. The individual elect possess the right to beatitude not in themselves as individuals, but from the strength of their affiliation to the church. Wicki cites a *Quaestio de dotibus*, originating from the circle of Guiard of Laon, in this regard. Wicki also speculates that perhaps under the influence of progressive theological systematization, the doctrine of the *dotes* became less connected to Christology and ecclesiology. In his treatises *De resurrectione* and *Quaestio de dotibus sanctorum in patria*, Albert treats them together, but neither Bonaventure nor Thomas Aquinas do so, though both treat the *dotes* in detail.

6. The appropriate translation of the first two members in this triad is problematic, and so for now they will be left untranslated. *Fruitio* is the least ambiguous and will be rendered below as either "fruition" or "delight." The other two, however, contain various nuances, whose meanings depend upon context. With respect to *dilectio*, William has in mind a whole complex of terms and concepts associated with the concupiscible power, including *desiderium, amor, affectio,* and *caritas*. At present, the English word "love" will be used. An even greater complexity revolves around *cognitio*. William's meaning here will also emerge below. For now, the English "knowledge" will render it.

7. SA IV 18.3.3.1: 497,6ff.

the fact that they facilitate an immediate and direct encounter between the soul and Christ.

As he proceeds, William integrates his doctrine of the endowments with other aspects of his teaching on beatitude. First, he loosely correlates them with the rational, concupiscible, and irascible powers of the soul. Not surprisingly, he aligns *cognitio* with the rational power and *dilectio* with the concupiscible power,[8] while the irascible power is relegated to performing exclusively this-worldly functions.[9] He asserts, moreover, that the endowments of *cognitio* and *dilectio* are the beatific perfections of the theological virtues of faith and charity, respectively.[10] Third, he argues that properly speaking fruition, the third endowment, is the product of the simultaneous acts of *cognitio* and *dilectio*. "Perfect beatitude consists in the rational power through *cognitio* and in the concupiscible power through *affectio* or perfect *dilectio*, and in these two simultaneously through *fruitio*."[11] As the synthesis of the endowments of rational and concupiscible powers, fruition is the consummation of both. For, in fruition, both *cognitio* and *dilectio* delight in the beauty of the Bridegroom. "For God is beauty, as it is said in the Canticle: *Your beauty and your comeliness, delight me* (Cant 1:15): beauty pertaining to divinity, comeliness to humanity." And so William concludes, "therefore,

---

8. SA IV 18.3.3.1: 498,49.

9. SA IV 18.3.3.1: 499–500,105ff. The issue of how to distribute the individual *dotes* to the different powers of the soul provoked considerable discussion in the late twelfth and early thirteenth centuries. In taking this position on the question, William deviates significantly from his immediate predecessors. The division of the soul into the rational, concupiscible, and irascible powers finds its nearest source in the influential *De anima et spiritu* of pseudo-Alcher of Clairvaux, which was then attributed to Augustine. While there was a general consensus in assigning *cognitio* to the rational power and *dilectio* to the concupiscible power, a question arose over the third endowment, whether or not it should be assigned to the irascible power. As it turns out, William's account is the most detailed presentation of the thesis that the irascible power is not a recipient of an endowment. His view will be adopted by William of Auvergne, the *Filia Magistri,* Roland of Cremona, and John of Treviso. The anonymous *Basler Summa* also substantially reproduces William's views; see Wicki, *Seligkeit,* pp. 43–44. Other authors, such as Stephen Langton, Hugh of St. Cher, Alexander of Hales, Guerric of St. Quentin, Albert the Great, and Bonaventure, did however assign an endowment to the irascible power. See Wicki, *Seligkeit,* pp. 232–37.

10. SA IV 18.3.3.1: 498,55f.

11. SA IV 18.3.3.1: 499,98. *Unde perfecta beatitudo consistit in vi rationabili per cognitionem, et concupiscibili per affectionem vel per dilectionem, et in duabus simul per fruitionem.*

the delight by which we delight in God will not only be in love, but also in vision."[12] Using a common scholastic distinction, William argues that *cognitio* and *dilectio* constitute the material aspect of beatitude, while fruition constitutes its formal aspect.[13]

But William does not maintain fruition's symmetrical relation to *cognitio* and *dilectio*. Fruition must be more proper to one or the other, and in the end he sides with *cognitio*, which he associates with spiritual vision.[14] "Properly speaking, there will be fruition in vision alone.... For if fruition were properly in love, then there would be equal reward in love and in vision and the Lord could have as equally said: this is eternal life, that they may love, as *this is eternal life that they may know you* (Jn 17:3)."[15] William thus grants to *cognitio* a clear priority over *dilectio*, on the basis of Jesus' words in John 17. Having taken this stand, however, he immediately attempts to give as great a place to love as possible. "Delight pertains both to vision and to love: ... to vision as that in which *(in qua)* there is delight, to love as that by which *(a qua)* delight is grasped and augmented. For love tends toward this, namely, that through vision it

---

12. SA IV 18.3.3.1: 501,146ff. *Delectabimur in visione pulcritudinis Dei. Est enim pulcritudo, sicut dicitur in Canticis: <<Tu>> pulcher, dilecte mi, et decorus. Pulcher secundum divinitatem, decorus secudum humanitatem. Ergo delectatio qua delectabitur in Deo, non erit tantum in dilectione, sed etiam in visione.*

13. SA IV 18.3.3.1: 501,137ff. William knows of other configurations: if there are only two powers that relate directly to God, there should be only two endowments, namely, cognition and love. Again, it seems that fruition is simply the delight found in both cognition and love, rather than something separate from them. If so, then there ought to be a different fruition for each one. Or, if there is only one fruition, it ought to be associated with love on account of Augustine's well-known definition: "to have fruition is to adhere to something in love for its own sake" (*De doctrina christ.* I, c.4 [PL 34.20]). It should be noted that the editors of the critical edition of the *Summa Aurea* have tried to identify the actual sources of William's references to his predecessors. I cite these identifications in my notes. The reader should be aware that in many cases these are only probable sources, since the text quoted by William often does not correspond well with the text as it is found in modern critical editions.

14. Wicki notes that the exact constitution of beatitude was actively debated at this time. Initially, scriptural and patristic texts determined the prevailing views. Augustine's comment in relation to Psalm 90—"the vision of God will be the whole reward" (*Enarratio in psalmum* 90, n.13 [PL 37.1170])—articulated the regnant view in the early scholastic period, in which vision was dominant among the various acts of beatitude. Gradually, however, this hegemony was weakened and an equality emerges between the acts. See Wicki, *Seligkeit*, pp. 175–82.

15. SA IV 18.3.3.1: 501–2,157ff.

may delight in loving."[16] A particular structure in the relationship between knowledge and love thus begins to emerge. *Cognitio* is primary; it is that *in which (in qua)* there is fruition or delight, properly speaking. *Dilectio*, in some sense, follows from it, as that *by which (a qua)* delight is augmented; yet *dilectio* can also be seen as a cause of delight in as much as it provides the impetus, as it seeks, hungers, and desires the fruition that comes from *cognitio*. As William puts it: "those who eat through vision, will hunger through charity. For they will have hunger, that is, the desire of charity, so that they may eat delectably; and so it is clear that love augments the delight, which will be in vision." Knowledge is not independent of love; rather it brings about the fulfillment of love's desire. The delight found in the eating, to which knowledge is compared, is itself the result of love's unsatiated hunger: *the one who eats me will yet hunger* (Eccl 24:29). This somewhat circular relationship between knowledge and love is fundamental for William and governs the nature of the soul's relationship to God.

The foregoing forms the foundation for beatitude. As a member of the church, united to Christ by a common nature through the Incarnation, the soul receives beatifying endowments *(dotes)* from her divine Spouse. These are the components of beatitude. Materially, it consists in the acts of *cognitio* (the virtue and perfection of the rational power) and *dilectio* (the virtue and perfection of the concupiscible power); formally in their simultaneous *fruitio*. *Cognitio* is oriented toward the vision of divine beauty, and delight or fruition properly pertains to it. Yet, *dilectio* is also integral to fruition. As a kind of hunger, it desires to obtain and to increase delight. As that in which *(in qua)* there is fruition or delight, cognition has a certain priority; yet, as that from or by which *(a qua)* fruition emerges, love's hunger brings it about. These, then, act in concert with one another in the experience of fruition: the one desiring and hungering, the other perceiving and delighting, but only in proportion to the desire. Precisely in this loving knowledge, fruition emerges.[17]

16. SA IV 18.3.3.1: 502,164ff.
17. SA IV 18.3.3.1: 499,100f. William offers a memorable allegory for this union of love and knowledge. Recalling the relationship between the prophets Elijah and Elisha, he remarks: "This is the twofold spirit, namely *intellectus* and *affectus*, which Elisha, that is, the Church, sought from Elijah, that is, from Christ, as he was ascending into heaven. His

The Spiritual Senses

How precisely do the soul's endowments experience beatific fruition? At this juncture, William introduces his doctrine of the spiritual senses. As will be seen, these in fact are essentially the means by which *cognitio* and *dilectio* arrive at fruition. The doctrine, therefore, lies at the heart of his teaching on beatitude.

William begins his treatment of the spiritual senses with a common scholastic question regarding beatitude: whether the blessed will see God with bodily eyes. By his time the question is largely settled against bodily vision (though there is some ambiguity) and William does not deviate from this opinion.[18] The spiritual senses are exclusively associated with the immaterial, spiritual dimension of the human person. While not lingering on this issue, he introduces an anthropological consideration that will be foundational for his doctrine of the spiritual senses. Arguing against a bodily vision of spiritual realities *in patria*, he employs the Pauline distinction between the "outer man" and the "inner man" to clarify the point: "the Apostle said: *but though the outer man is corrupted, yet the inner man is renewed day by day* (2 Cor 4:16), that is, reason advances day by day in the knowledge *(agnitio)* of God." Accordingly: "the exterior man does not advance in the knowledge of God; for corporal eyes do not now see God. But spiritual sight will only be perfected by that in which it now advances."[19] Here, William distinguishes between the spiritual senses and the physical senses,[20] according to the Pauline

---

response to him [was]: *if you see me when I am taken from you, you will have what you have asked* (2 Kgs 2:10). For the one who sees Christ at the right hand of the Father, at which he sat down after his ascension into heaven, has the twofold spirit, namely, perfect *intellectum* and perfect *affectum*."

18. William refutes an argument which speaks of an exchange of the physical and spiritual abilities regarding their objects: with spiritual eyes, not only spiritual but also physical things are seen, therefore glorified bodily eyes will see not only physical but also spiritual objects. Against this, he invokes the Boethian principle that a superior power can do whatever an inferior power can do, but not vice versa. See Wicki, *Seligkeit*, pp. 107–8.

19. SA IV 18.3.3.2.1: 503,20. *Exterior autem homo non proficit in agnitione Dei; oculis enim corporalibus modo non videt Deum. Set visus spiritualis non perficietur nisi in eis in quibus modo proficit.* William continues: "For just as the grace of God is the perfection of nature, so the glory [of God] will be the perfection of grace.... that is, begin to see God through faith in order that afterwards you may see God by sight."

20. Although for William the *visio Dei* will be enjoyed by the "inner man," he yet

28 · Beatific Fruition as Spiritual Apprehension

distinction between the "outer" and "inner" man;[21] identifies the "inner man" with the soul; and suggests that its progressive renewal entails an advancement in knowledge of God through spiritual sight. In this way, he introduces the crucial link between spiritual perception and knowledge of God generally.

The distinction between the "outer" and "inner" man in place, William begins his *ex professo* treatment of the spiritual senses. He introduces the topic with a quotation from Origen's third *Homily on Leviticus*, wherein the Alexandrian describes the spiritual senses:[22]

In that authority five spiritual senses are distinguished through which we have fruition of God. With spiritual vision we will be delighted by the fullness of God; and with spiritual hearing we will be delighted by the symphony of God.

---

stresses that corporal eyes will see the humanity of Christ: "For [corporal sight] will see the glorified body of Christ, which will be like the sun in its infinite brightness, and we will see other glorified bodies, and in this will consist the perfection of corporal sight" (SA IV 18.3.3.2.1): 504, 34. Some of his contemporaries (e.g., Alexander of Hales) are content with the statement that God cannot be seen with physical eyes, while others also stress that the glorified bodily eyes have their own proper object *in patria*. Hugh of St. Cher suggests that the vision of God with bodily eyes can be spoken of by way of accidents. Albert the Great argues similarly. In general, there seems to be a consensus on this question. Stephen Langton, John of Treviso, Hugh of St. Cher, and Albert the Great all provide essentially the same answer as William: the eyes of the resurrected body will see the glorified humanity of Christ, the eye of the soul will see his divinity. See Wicki, *Seligkeit*, pp. 107–13.

21. The relation between the spiritual senses and the "interior man" is present in William's first explicit mention of the spiritual senses in this tractate. Responding to an objection concerning the superfluity of physical hair *in patria*, William argues that physical hair will be an ornamentation "of the exterior man in the same way that the hair of the soul, that is good thoughts *(bone cogitationes)*, decorate the soul. For the interior man, namely the soul, has its sight *(visum)*, its hearing *(auditum)* and so forth" (SA IV 18.1.3:475,173).

22. According to Rahner, William knows Origen's text through the *Glossa ordinaria* (in Lev 6:3, Lyranus I, 223r). In Book III of his *Sentences* (dist. 13), the Lombard, apparently contradicting the saying of Origen, stated that in Christ, the head of the mystical body, all the senses are to be found, while the saints only possess the sense of touch. The Lombard's comments stimulated discussion of the topic among later scholastic commentators. William's use of Origen recalls the venerable tradition of spiritual and ascetical theology, of which the doctrine of the spiritual senses is a part, that finds its earliest roots in Origen and other patristic figures, including Gregory of Nyssa, Augustine, Evagrius, Gregory the Great, and Cassian. After the patristic period, the doctrine of the spiritual senses emerged again with vigor in the twelfth century (with such figures as Bernard of Clairvaux, William of St.-Thierry, and Alcher of Clairvaux) and especially in the thirteenth century within the scholastic milieu. Rahner, "The 'Spiritual Senses' in the Middle Ages," pp. 104–6.

Whence: *I will listen to what the Lord God is saying to me* (Ps 84:9), and with spiritual smell [we will delight] in the good odor of God, and with spiritual touch in the pleasantness of God.[23]

Elsewhere, he offers a similar description of the spiritual senses and their objects:

We will delight in the beauty and symphony and aroma and sweetness and attractiveness of God. But in God these are none other than delectable things; and all these pertain to all the spiritual senses.[24]

Several initial observations are warranted regarding these passages: First, William affirms the presence of spiritual senses in the soul that are analogous to the five senses of the body. He does not, however, specify what precisely they are. Are they faculties, powers, or simply acts of the soul? What is clear is that the "inner man" experiences fruition through them: the blessed will delight in God through spiritual sight *(visus)*, hearing *(auditus)*, smell *(odoratus)*, taste *(gustus)*, and touch *(tactus)*. Second, his doctrine of the spiritual senses involves assumptions about their divine Object. The divine nature is characterized by various qualities which correspond to the spiritual senses and allow them to perceive it, namely, fullness *(plenitudine)*, beauty *(pulchritudo)*, symphony *(simphonia)*, good aroma *(bono odore)*, pleasantness *(suavitas)*, and sweetness *(dulcedo)*. What might be termed the *delectabilia divina* are central to his doctrine of the spiritual senses. Between the two passages, lastly, a certain instability in the objects of the spiritual senses is apparent, along with some fluidity in the relationships. William seems more concerned with the whole *sensorium* in its relationship to the whole of *delectabilia divina* than with any particular spiritual sense and its object.

---

23. SA IV 18.3.3.2.2: 505,8ff. *Ecce in hac auctoritate distinguuntur quinque sensus spirituales quibus fruimur Deo. Visu spirituali delectamur in plenitudine Dei, et auditu spirituali delectatmur in simphonia Dei. Unde: Audiam quid loquatuur in me Dominus Deus, et odoratu spirituali in bono odore Dei, et tactu spirituali in suavitate Dei.* (Note: Choosing an appropriate translation for the Latin *suavitas* is complicated by the fact that at times William associates it with spiritual touch, as here, while elsewhere he aligns it with spiritual taste. In the latter context, "sweetness" seems apt, while in the former, "pleasantness" or "suavity" will be used.)

24. SA IV 18.3.3.2.2: 506,39. *Item delectamur in pulcritudine Dei et simphonia et odore et dulcedine et suavitate. Sed in Deo non sunt alia delectabilia; et hec omnia pertinent ad omnes sensus spirituales.*

Having introduced the spiritual senses, William proceeds to give an account of how precisely the experience of fruition through them relates to the other two endowments, *cognitio* and *dilectio*. Are the spiritual senses properly acts of the former or the latter? William poses the question in the following way: are the spiritual senses acts of charity *(caritas)*, and so aligned with *dilectio* and the concupiscible power? His negative answer begins to clarify his understanding of how the spiritual senses function.

In support of the position he opposes—that fruition through the spiritual senses properly pertains to charity—William lists four arguments. The first appeals to Paul's enumeration of the fruit of the spirit in the Epistle to the Galatians, which begins with charity. If "charity is a fruit; then by charity we have fruition of God."[25] The second asserts that charity effects fruition or delight by uniting the soul to God. "For charity tends toward this, that we are united to God. But delight is the union of the fitting with the fitting *(convenientis cum convenienti)*; therefore since charity joins us to the highest good . . . , the highest delight is in charity. Therefore, by charity we have fruition of God."[26] Crediting Pliny with the aphorism "Nothing is sweeter than love," the third argues that "charity is the sweetest. . . . Therefore, since delight is in sweetness, there is delight in charity; . . . hence, charity has fruition of God."[27] The fourth invokes an Augustinian definition of fruition:[28] "'to delight is to adhere in love to something for its own sake'; therefore, fruition is in desire alone; therefore [it is] in charity alone."[29] All of these arguments seek to associate delight with the desire of charity.

In response, William produces a cataract of arguments, each of which attempts to drive a wedge between desire and delight by appealing to a particular feature of physical sense perception. He suggests that delight in physical things occurs through actual sensation, not through the desire for such delight: "with the physical senses alone do we delight in physically delectable things *(in delectabili corporali)*." For example: "we are not delighted by desiring food, but by eating it."[30] He then suggests a

25. SA IV 18.3.3.2.2: 505,15.
26. SA IV 18.3.3.2.2: 505,18f.
27. SA IV 18.3.3.2.2: 505,23f.
28. Cf. *De doctrina Christiana* I. 4. IV.
29. SA IV 18.3.3.2.2: 505–6,28ff.
30. SA IV 18.3.3.2.2: 506,35f.

parallel in this regard between physical and spiritual sensation: "The desire for physically delectable things does not possess delight, but moves the corporal senses to the act of delighting; therefore the desire for spiritually delectable things does not have delight, but moves the spiritual senses to the act of delighting spiritually."[31] William thus distinguishes between the desire for physically delectable things and the experience of possessing and enjoying them. In the physical context, delight occurs only in the act of sense perception, not in the desire for what is perceived. Accordingly, he argues, spiritual delight occurs only through the spiritual senses: "only with the spiritual senses do we delight in spiritually delectable things; therefore not by charity."[32] In short, charity *per se* does not possess delight.

In this regard, William also emphasizes the incompleteness and uncertainty of desire. He suggests that desire is not in and of itself capable of satisfying its own hunger: "when someone desires something, if he believes that he will possess it, he is delighted; but if he believes that he will not possess it, he is saddened." So, "in certain circumstances love *(amor)* has delectation and in certain circumstances it has sadness" and so, "with respect to itself, it has neither delectation nor sadness."[33] Quoting Augustine—"love is a certain sickness"—William further observes that unrequited love is often associated with misery and madness. Hence, "since some [kinds of] love have anguish, of itself love does not have delectation."[34] Accordingly, he concludes, "by charity *per se* we are neither delighted by God nor do we have fruition of God."[35] Thus, love's desire seeks, hungers, yearns, but of itself does not possess or enjoy, its object.

The crux of the matter, as William conceives of it, is whether charity has the characteristic of sense perception, since, as noted above, delight

---

31. SA IV 18.3.3.2.2: 506,43ff. *Item, desiderium delectandi corporaliter non habet delecationem, sed movet sensus corporales ad delectandum; ergo desiderium delectandi spiritualiter non habet delectationem, sed movet sensus spirituales ad delectandum spiritualiter.*

32. SA IV 18.3.3.2.2: 506,37. *Solis sensibus spiritualibus delectamur in delectabili spirituali; non ergo caritate.*

33. SA IV 18.3.3.2.2: 506,51.

34. SA IV 18.3.3.2.2: 507,60ff.

35. SA IV 18.3.3.2.2: 506,54. *Ergo caritate secundum se nec delectamur in Deo nec fruimur in ipso.*

is strictly speaking a function of sensation: "charity is either a sense or it is not." For William, it is not. And here he reveals a crucial assumption: "to sense *(sentire)* is to perceive *(percipere)*, and to perceive is to cognize *(cognoscere)*." But "*cognitio* is not in charity, since only in the intellect is there knowledge of spiritual things." Hence, charity is not a sense. Delight or fruition, accordingly, cannot properly be associated with it, for "there is only delight in things pertaining to the senses."[36] In sum, William contends that delight is a function of sensation, which is itself an act of the intellect. Hence, charity desires delight, but cannot experience it through its characteristic act.

Having rejected any intrinsic or essential relationship between charity and spiritual sensation, William offers his own position: "We say that by the spiritual senses alone and by faith alone we have fruition of God formally and properly. Thus, charity does not delight in God nor does it have fruition of God except by faith, and in the future it will only have fruition of God by vision."[37] Though William's language is terse, the reference to faith implies the activity of the soul's rational power and its perfection in the knowledge of God, now by faith and in the future by vision. Since fruition is essentially a delight in the *delectabilia divina* and delight pertains properly to perception and sensation, William is led to associate fruition with cognition, since, as noted above, sensation and perception pertain to cognition. Because it occurs through the spiritual senses, beatific delight pertains properly, in the manner of a formal cause, to faith/vision rather than to charity. The role of charity, pertaining to the concupiscible power, is not incidental though; rather it plays a crucial and necessary role: "charity moves faith to the act of having fruition of God. So, charity always has delight, since it is never without faith and hope. Hence, it always moves [faith/vision] to the act of delighting and having fruition, since 'where love is, there are the eyes.'"[38]

---

36. SA IV 18.3.3.2.2: 507,67. *Item, caritas aut est sensus, aut non. Si est sensus, contra. Sentire est percipere, et percipere cognoscere. Sed cognitio non est in caritate, quia in solo intellectu est cognitio spiritualium. Ergo caritas non est sensus; sed delectatio non est nisi in convenientis consensu; ergo caritate non delectamur in Deo, nec fruimur ipso.*

37. SA IV 18.3.3.2.2: 507,72ff. *Unde dicimus quod solis sensibus spiritualibus sive sola fide fruimur Deo formaliter et proprie. Unde caritas modo non delectatur in Deo nec fruitur nisi per fidem, nec in futuro fruetur nisis per visionem.*

38. SA IV 18.3.3.2.2: 507,75ff.

Charity moves faith/vision to the act of delight through its desire for delight. Thus, charity can be called the efficient cause of fruition's delight, since it "moves faith to the act of delighting" and the desire of charity "conserves and augments fruition";[39] "charity moves toward that conjunction [which occurs in the intellect through *cognitio*], and makes it and holds it in existence"; "charity has sweetness and delight; but not from itself, rather from its adjunct, namely *cognitio*."[40] As an efficient cause charity desires, pursues, and brings about fruition's delight, and maintains and augments it.[41] William gives the example of food: "Only that food eaten with desire is eaten with delight."[42] The actual experience of delight in God, however, occurs through the spiritual senses—now by faith, and in the future by vision. This is its proper and formal cause.

William next turns to an obvious question regarding his teaching on this matter: the number of the spiritual senses. Given the descriptions of the spiritual senses above and the analogy with physical sensation, it seems that there must be five discrete spiritual senses in the soul. Is this the case?

William offers a series of arguments in favor of this plurality thesis. Quoting Augustine—"[It would be] strange, if corporal light has eyes which it illuminates, and spiritual light did not have eyes which it illumi-

---

39. SA IV 18.3.3.2.2: 507,80. *Caritate fruimur Deo effective, quia ipsa movet fidem ad fruendum et delectandum, per caritatem etiam conservatur fruitio et delectatio in Deo et augmentatur.*

40. SA IV 18.3.3.2.2: 508,85ff. *Dicimus quod caritas coniungit nos Deo. Sed non est ipsa coniunctio, quia ipsa coniunctio convenientis cum conveniente est in cognitione, quia solus intellectus est ymago Dei. Unde proprie loquendo in coniunctione ymaginis ad illud cuius est ymago est fruitio. Sed verum est quod caritas movet ad illam coniunctionem, et facit illam et tenet illam in esse. Unde totum attributur ei, scilicet frui sive delectari. . . . Concedimus enim quod caritas dulcedinem et delectationem habet; sed non ex se, set ex adiunctio, scilicet ex cognitione.* William employs the distinction between formal and efficient causality in order to harmonize his own teaching with Augustine's well-known definition of fruition from *De doctrina Christiana*. He argues that Augustine's statement "to have fruition is to adhere in love, etc." must be understood efficiently, not formally: "For through love we have fruition efficiently, as was said; but through vision and contemplation we have fruition formally."

41. William's language here is noteworthy. The distinction between various kinds of causality, of Aristotelian inspiration if not of actual dependence, is typical of William; and it is indicative of the emerging Aristotelian influence.

42. SA IV 18.3.3.2.2: 507,82.

nates"⁴³—a representative argument infers: If spiritual light has eyes which it illuminates, then "in the same way spiritual sweetness has taste which it delights, and spiritual suavity has touch which it soothes; therefore there are many spiritual senses and not only one."⁴⁴ In the main, these arguments posit a basic similarity between physical and spiritual sensation: if diverse kinds of physical objects require diverse physical senses, there ought also to be diverse spiritual senses corresponding to diverse spiritual objects.

But William knows of other perspectives opposed to this one, views that he ultimately finds convincing. Citing a remark from Cassiodorus' *De anima* regarding the soul's use of the senses in the next life,⁴⁵ William surmises that [the soul] will then know fully, "with one spiritual sense."⁴⁶ He also appeals to Augustine, citing first *On Free Will*,⁴⁷ where the bishop suggests that there must be an interior sense which perceives singularly and as a whole an object which appears variously to the individual senses.⁴⁸ Augustine's remark from the *Tractates on the Gospel of John*⁴⁹—"believe and you have eaten"—is interpreted similarly: "we eat by faith; therefore we taste by faith, and we see by faith. . . . Therefore, spiritual vision and hearing and tasting are the same in essence." William then concludes: "there is, therefore, only one spiritual sense."⁵⁰

---

43. *Soliloquia* I, c.8, n.15 (PL 32.877).

44. SA IV 18.3.3.2.3: 510,48ff. Another argument is taken from *De spiritu et anima*, c.9, *ad sensum:* "Likewise, Augustine (rather *De spiritu et anima*, c.9 [PL 40.784–5] *ad sensum*) said: 'prudence clarifies spiritual vision, foolishness darkens it; the hearing is offended by falsehoods, it is soothed by the truth; regardless of its place, equity is fragrant to it, inequity is foul; vanity decays, virtue grows fertile.' Therefore, since there are diverse objects assigned to these, there ought to be diverse spiritual senses in essence" (SA IV 18.3.3.2.3: 510,54f).

45. *De anima*, c.2 (PL 70.1286): *Vivit anima post huius vite ammissionem; videt, audit, tangit et aliis sensibus efficacius valet; non autem ex partibus hic intelligens, sed tota cognoscens.*

46. SA IV 18.3.3.2.3: 509,30.

47. Apparently via the Lombard's *Gloss* (*Glossa Lombardiana, in Ephes.* 1:17 [PL 192.176D]; from Augustine, *De libero arbitrio*, II, c.3, n.8 [PL 32.1244]).

48. SA IV 18.3.3.2.3: 509,33. William finds a similar assertion in the *De spiritu et anima* c.9 (PL 40.784–5): "when the intellect understands through itself *(per se)*, it sees; when it understands from something else *(ab alio)*, it hears."

49. *In Johannes evangelium*, tr. 25, n. 12 (PL 35.1602).

50. SA IV 18.3.3.2.3: 509–10,36ff.

But there are still more weighty objections to the plurality thesis. If there are five essentially distinct spiritual senses, each should have a corresponding virtue. The sphere of physical sense perception suggests this. Each of the physical senses has an associated vice: excessive gustatory delight is called gluttony and excessive tactile delight is luxury. This implies the presence of a corresponding virtue. Conversely, if there were multiple spiritual senses, there would need to be a different virtue for each spiritual sense.[51] Since William assumes, however, that it is the theological virtues which perfect the soul's endowments and their corresponding powers, this would require more than three theological virtues, an implication that he finds untenable.

This comparison between physical and spiritual sensation allows William to develop his own position. He readily grants that the five physical senses differ essentially because individually they have different objects. In the spiritual context, though, he argues that "there is one simple and invariable Object of those five spiritual senses, namely God; therefore, the spiritual senses are one in essence, since even the physical senses are distinguished according to their objects."[52] It is precisely the single divine Object which implies a single spiritual sense. (How William reconciles this single Object with its diverse *delectabilia* will be seen below.)

Most significantly, however, William argues for the essential singularity of the spiritual senses from his conception of the nature of human knowing. Again, he associates to the point of identity the three acts of beatific knowing, this time adding the adverb "spiritually": "to sense spiritually is to perceive spiritually, is to cognize spiritually." Moreover, he asserts that "all spiritual *cognitio* is in the intellect." Accordingly, given this intimate relation between sensation, perception, and cognition, along with their "location" in the intellect, he concludes that "every spiritual sense is in the intellect," and "all spiritual sensing is understanding." Therefore, since "it is agreed that the intellect is one, there is only one

---

51. SA IV 18.3.3.2.3: 508–9,1ff.
52. SA IV 18.3.3.2.3: 509,23. *Unicum <<obiectum>> est simplex et invariable illorum quinque sensuum spiritualium, scilicet Deus; ergo unus est sensus spiritualis in essentia, quia secundum obiectum distinguuntur etiam sensus corporales.*

spiritual sense."⁵³ He then summarizes his position: "There is only one spiritual sense, namely the intellect, and only one virtue which perfects the spiritual sense, namely faith."⁵⁴ In short, William posits a singular spiritual sense, a capacity of the intellect, with a singular Object, namely God, and a single virtue that perfects it, namely, faith/vision.

After summarizing, William offers a further clarification. Besides the one just noted, an even more crucial difference exists between spiritual and physical sense perception: "corporal sense is a determinate nature and it is not able to know all things, but only determinate things." By contrast, he continues, "the spiritual sense, namely the intellect, is not a determinate nature, since it is the image of God. Hence, since God knows all things in act, the intellect is able to know all things."⁵⁵ William here freights the traditional notion of the *imago Dei* with Aristotelian assumptions concerning the nature of the soul and its noetic capacities. For Aristotle, the soul is essentially indeterminate in nature and thus capable *in potentia* of knowing all things. By contrast, each physical sense has a limited act and object. By thus construing spiritual sensation as an act of the intellect, William in effect releases spiritual sensation from the constrictions placed upon its physical analogue.

William then brings the foregoing to bear in order to justify his description of a singular spiritual sense with a singular Object, yet with multiple sensations and multiple *delectabilia*. His reply to an objection concerning a singular object of the spiritual senses grants the objection's premise, namely, that there are diverse objects of the spiritual senses. This, *prima facie*, seems to contradict his earlier statement that God is

---

53. SA IV 18.3.3.2.3: 510,43ff. *Item, sentire spiritualiter est percipere spiritualiter, est cognoscere spiritualiter. Sed omnis cognitio spiritualis est in intellectu; ergo omne sentire spirituale in intellectu est; ergo omnis sensus spiritualis est intellectus. Et constat quod non est nisi unus intellectus; ergo non est nisi unus sensus spiritualis.*

54. SA IV 18.3.3.2.3: 510,59. *Unus solus sensus spiritualis, scilicet intellectus, et una sola virtus perficit sensum spiritualem, scilicet fides.*

55. SA IV 18.3.3.2.3: 511,75. *Dicimus quod non est simile de sensu corporali et sensu spirituali, quia sensus corporalis natura determinata est, <<nec>> potest omnia cognoscere, sed aliquod determinatum; sed sensus spiritualis, scilicet intellectus, non est determinata natura, cum sit ymago Dei. Unde, cum Deus actu cognoscat omnia, intellectus potest cognoscere omnia.* The Aristotelian cast to this conception of the *imago Dei*, apparently taken straight from the *De anima*, is noteworthy. As an *imago Dei*, the soul's noetic capacities mirror *in potentia* those which are always *in actu* in its divine Exemplar.

the single Object of the singular spiritual sense. In rejecting the conclusion, however, he eludes the contradiction with an important distinction, namely, that between a material and a formal object. William appeals to the example of the intellect acting in faith: "There is one faith, even though it has many objects, such as hell, eternal life, and many other things. And this is the case since there is one formal object *(ratio)* of all things to be believed." Similarly, "since there is one formal object *(ratio)* of sensible delighting in spiritual things, the spiritual sense is one, even though it has many objects."[56] By this distinction between formal and material objects, William explicitly addresses the objection and implicitly the apparent contradiction.[57] In the process, he sets up an intriguing parallel between theological knowing and knowing through the spiritual senses. Just as faith has a single knowledge of diverse doctrines, so spiritual sensation is a single perception of diverse *delectabilia*. Formally, there is indeed only one Object of the spiritual sense, namely God; materially, however, there are various objects of *cognoscere*, *percipere*, and *sentire*. William thus allows a logical distinction *(secundum rationem)* between five different spiritual senses, while insisting that, strictly speaking, there is only one spiritual sense in essence *(in essentia)*, namely, the intellect.[58] In spiritual sensation, the essential singularity of subject and object does not preclude a multiplicity of sensations and delights.

William concludes his discussion of this question with a lapidary summary of beatific knowing through the spiritual senses, which is illustrious of its basic nature as described thus far:

By faith we see *(videmus)* spiritually. By faith we hear *(audimus)* what Jesus says. For *faith comes by hearing* (Rom 10:17). By faith we perceive scents *(odoramus)* spiritually. For by faith we cognize *(cognoscere)* that the Son of God was made man for us, that he wept for us and was tormented for us, that he sorrowed, that he suffered. And when we recall the benefits of this kind, we perceive *(odora-*

---

56. SA IV 18.3.3.2.3: 511,88ff.

57. The notion of a formal object *(ratio)* recalls scholastic discussions, contemporary and subsequent to William, concerning the scientific nature of theology, whose formal object, according to Aquinas, for example, is God and all things under the *ratio* of their relation to God.

58. SA IV 18.3.3.2.3: 509,18ff.

mus) the good odor of Christ *(bonum odorem Christi)* as an aromatic perfume flowing from him,[59] and *we will run after you to the scent of your ointments* (Cant 1:3). When by faith we meditate upon these things which we know, as if by chewing *(masticando),* we taste *(gustamus)* the sweetness of God *(dulcedinem Dei),* and this is by faith. By faith we touch *(tangimus)* the suavity of God *(suavitatem Dei);* for by faith we cognize *(cognoscere)* that in God with respect to himself, there is no bitterness, since *this work is foreign* to him, namely, to punish, as Isaiah says (cf. Is 28:21).[60]

This passage reveals not only the "manifold singularity" of beatific knowing, but also the link between *cognoscere* and *sentire.* The manifold material objects of faith's knowledge are at the same time the manifold material objects of spiritual sensation. Spiritual hearing, for example, is the knowledge of Jesus' teaching; cognition of doctrines about God (e.g., that the Son of God became incarnate and suffered) is the smell of the good aroma of Christ as well as a chewing and tasting of the divine sweetness; to cognize that God is merciful is to touch the suavity of God. In effect, beatific knowing encompasses two modes: *cognoscere* of theological affirmations and *sentire* of manifold *delectabilia divina.* The formal singularity emerges in that both cognition and sensation are acts of the intellect acting in faith and having thus a singular *ratio;* yet this singularity includes a material diversity of objects and experiences.

Hence, while earlier in the tractate William distinguished between the knowledge of faith and the knowledge of the spiritual senses in order to compare them, here he integrates them: spiritual sensation is part of the knowledge of faith. The full meaning of William's doctrine of beatific knowing (constituted by the triad *sentire, percipere, cognoscere*) now begins to emerge. Beatific knowledge of God is essentially an intellectual act, with a single perfecting virtue, and a single divine Object. Yet it is also an act of spiritual perception through the spiritual senses. In some sense, for William, the intellect is a spiritual sense. This is the meaning of his assertion that all spiritual sensation is in the intellect and is understanding.

If, then, there is essentially only one spiritual sense, why speak in the

---

59. See *Glossa ordinaria* on 2 Cor 2:15, Lyranus VI, 64r; from Augustine, *Enarratio in psalmum* 37, n.9 (PL 36.401).

60. SA IV 18.3.3.2.3: 510,60ff.

plural of spiritual senses at all? This is the final question that William addresses. He begins by introducing a basic assumption: if in essence there is only one spiritual sense, discourse about five different spiritual senses must assume some other distinction, either between their acts or their delights. Otherwise, "if there is a singular delight *(unica delectatio)* of the spiritual senses, and a singular act *(unica operatio)*, there would be no reason to speak of five, since there would be unity in essence, in act, and in delight."[61] How, then, to maintain that there is essentially only one spiritual sense, but that there are also genuinely distinct spiritual sense acts and delights?

This threefold distinction between essence, act, and delight, however, seems to introduce new difficulties for the singularity thesis. For it seems that distinct acts of spiritual sensation imply essential differences. Since by faith it is possible to see the beauty of God without, for example, tasting it, seeing and tasting are therefore essentially different.[62] Again, the diversity of the *delectabilia divina* (e.g., truth, goodness, beauty, sweetness), each having a different formal modality *(ratio)* that corresponds to separate acts in the soul (e.g., believing, loving, seeing, tasting), seems to suggest essential differences.[63]

Similarly, distinct delights seem to imply distinct spiritual senses. If the "bread of heaven," for example, contains within itself manifold delights, there must be a corresponding plurality of acts in which there is delight. But a plurality of acts implies a plurality of habits, which in turn

---

61. SA IV 18.3.3.2.4: 512,5.

62. SA IV 18.3.3.2.4: 512,9f. "Since we see the beauty of God by faith, it is not necessary that we meditate on his precepts and his goodness toward us gathered from them. But to meditate on these kinds of things is to taste spiritually; therefore when we see spiritually, it is not necessary to taste spiritually; therefore to see spiritually is not to taste spiritually; therefore the spiritual senses have diverse operations according to their species *(secundum speciem)*."

63. SA IV 18.3.3.2.4: 512,15. "Again, just as the highest truth and the highest good are the same in essence but differ formally *(ratione)*, so the highest beauty, the highest truth, the highest sweetness, the highest suavity are the same in essence, but differ formally *(ratione)*. Therefore, just as there is one movement toward the first truth, in as much as it is the first truth, namely, to believe, another [movement] toward the highest goodness, in as much as it is the highest goodness, namely, to desire, so there is another [movement] toward the first beauty, in as much as it is the first beauty, another [movement] toward the first sweetness, in as much as it is the first sweetness. Therefore to see spiritually is not to taste spiritually."

implies a plurality of virtues. But virtues—for example, faith, hope, and love—are indeed essentially distinguished according to their diverse proximate ends.[64] A similar objection utilizes an axiom with which William agrees—"there is no delectation without perception, and no perception without sense"—to argue for a conclusion that he opposes: namely that, since there are essentially distinct virtues which yield delight (e.g., faith, prudence, counsel), these must also be essentially distinct spiritual senses.[65]

Against all these objections, William simply invokes a terse statement from Augustine's *On Free Will* to reassert the essential unity of the spiritual senses: "'with the intellect it is the same thing to see what one hears, and to smell what one tastes.' Therefore, the spiritual senses do not have essentially diverse operations."[66]

The *aporia* thus created, William begins his solution by distinguishing between two contexts of activity for the spiritual senses: *in patria* and *in via*. On the one hand, he concedes that in the next life "vision will be the whole reward" and there the singular spiritual sense *(sensus spiritualis)* will have a singular act and a singular delight:

For by seeing God we will hear spiritually, since by seeing we will have cognition *(cognitio);* and this is to hear by seeing *(audire videndo)*. We will assemble the goods given to us by God and this will be to perceive the odor of God by seeing *(odorari videndo)*. We will know the internal *rationes* of God; and this will be to taste *(gustare)* spiritually. Likewise, by seeing God we will be inflamed by his love, of which it is said: *our God is a consuming fire* (Heb 12:29); and this will be

---

64. SA IV 18.3.3.2.4: 512,24ff. "Again, in the book of Wisdom (16:20): *he gave them bread from heaven prepared without labor, having in it all that is delicious, and the sweetness of every taste*. Therefore in the bread of heaven there are many delectations; therefore there are many operations by which we delight in the bread of heaven. But if this [is so], since diverse habits are distinguished according to diverse operations in species, there are therefore diverse habits; therefore there are diverse spiritual senses in habit with respect to those diverse operations, since faith, hope, and charity have the same end, but they are distinguished according to diverse spiritual movements; and so the spiritual senses are diverse in essence."

65. SA IV 18.3.3.2.4: 513,33f. "Again, by faith we cognize God and we delight similarly in the understanding by the gifts of prudence and counsel. But there is no delectation without perception, and no perception without sense; therefore by either of those two virtues we sense *(sentimus)* spiritual delights; therefore either one of them is a spiritual sense; and so the spiritual senses are diverse in essence."

66. SA IV 18.3.3.2.4: 513,53f.

to touch *(tangere)* him. . . .⁶⁷ And, just as all natures exist in their own way in God, namely power, goodness, sweetness and other similar things, so also will that vision have in itself every delectable without multiplication of movements and delectations.⁶⁸

In this description, William subsumes under the term *visio* all other forms of spiritual sensation. The single, unified act of vision and its delectation contains the experience of every *delectamentum* associated with the individual spiritual senses. Accordingly, his description of the spiritual senses *in patria* has a synaesthetic quality: the blessed will "hear by seeing," "smell by seeing," and so forth. It is apparently this synaesthetic quality that distinguishes the activity of the spiritual senses in the two states of life.

In this life, on the other hand, William argues that the spiritual senses function differently: "in this present life, however, the spiritual sense has many acts,"⁶⁹ for "the spiritual sense, even though it is one in essence, nevertheless has diverse acts and diverse delectations."⁷⁰ Here, he affirms the essential unity of the spiritual sense, but allows for a variety of acts and delectations. Returning to the objections—which had argued variously that a diversity of acts or delights implies essential difference in the spiritual senses—he takes up his rebuttal.

William begins by proposing yet another comparison with physical sensation, taken in this case from Aristotle's *De anima*, Book III.⁷¹ With the spiritual senses, there is a diversity of acts in the same way that "to see white and to see black are diverse visions, and just as touch, though it is one sense, nevertheless has to know many contrary things such as heat, cold, dryness, lightness, heaviness, and the like."⁷² He then observes that "just as the interior sense, as Augustine said in his book *On Free Will*—which interior sense Aristotle called the common sense—is held

---

67. Here, William quotes the same passage from Cassiodorus's *De anima* cited in note 45 above.
68. SA IV 18.3.3.2.4: 513–14,56ff.
69. SA IV 18.3.3.2.4: 514,68.
70. SA IV 18.3.3.2.4: 514,70. *Dicimus quod sensus spiritualis, licet sit unus in essentia, habet tamen diversas operationes et diversas delecationes.*
71. *De anima* III, 425a 27.
72. SA IV 18.3.3.2.4: 514,72.

to know every sensation, so the spiritual sense, though it is one, is held to cognize *(cognoscere)* every spiritual sensation."[73] This reference to the "common sense" discloses a primary influence informing William's doctrine of the spiritual senses—the Aristotelian notion of the so-called "interior senses." Though he does not take up the whole apparatus of the Aristotelian psychology of sense perception, on this particular point he seems to have modeled his conception of the spiritual sense on the Aristotelian concept of the internal senses (transmitted to him through the Stagirite's medieval Arabic readers and commentators). William has this analogy in mind as he argues: "the spiritual senses, thus, differ from each other in their mode of acting and in their mode of delighting. For they are understood on analogy with the corporal senses."[74] William's notion of a singular spiritual sense, namely the intellect, which cognizes all spiritual realities through the diverse acts of the spiritual senses, is formally similar to the Aristotelian notion of a single, inner "common sense," which acts through various external senses.[75]

Having introduced this Aristotelian analogy, William brings it to bear on his description of the manifold experience of the spiritual senses *in via*:

---

73. SA IV 18.3.3.2.4: 514,75f. *Et sicut ensus interior, ut dicit Augustinus in libro de libero arbitrio—quem sensum interiorem vocat Aristoteles sensum communem—omnia sensata spiritualia habet cognoscere.*

74. SA IV 18.3.3.2.4: 515,91. *Dicimus ergo quod sensus spirituales ab invicem differunt in modo operandi et modo delectandi. Sumuntur enim ad proportionem sensuum corporalium.*

75. This aspect of William's theology will be explored in greater detail in a subsequent chapter. For now, it must suffice to make several brief observations. The Aristotelian-Arabic doctrine of sense perception involves not only the five physical, external senses, but also several distinguishable "inner senses," the number of which varies from commentator to commentator, and even with the same commentator. The argument for the existence of these inner senses emerges from the observation that the five external senses can only perceive the sensory *qualia* associated with external objects which are proper to their natures. In order, therefore, to account for the fact that humans experience the various sensory qualities of external objects in a unified way, there must be some "interior sense" which unites these disparate sensory stimuli into a single, unified image or form. This capacity is the so-called "common sense." Once perceived by the common sense, the intelligible image or species can be operated upon by the other inner senses. It can be stored in the imagination; considered and evaluated by the cogitative-estimative powers; and finally stored in memory.

each spiritual sense whatsoever has many acts, as is clear in spiritual sight: we see the goodness of God, the majesty of God and the other exemplary virtues which are in God, and these are diverse visions. With the same sense [i.e., the *sensus communis*], we both hear spiritually and taste spiritually, etc. For when we cognize the goodness, the majesty, the omnipotence of God and so the other [aspects of God] from someone else, then we hear spiritually what Jesus said; we are able to cognize the same thing through ourselves, and this is to see spiritually. Again, when we cognize that from these things goodness is poured out upon creatures, we perceive the odor *(odoramur)* of God spiritually; and when we meditate on this, we chew *(masticamus)* spiritually; and when we are inflamed by these thoughts toward the love of God, then we touch *(tangimus)* God spiritually. For we touch the heat *(calorem)* of God. So also, when we sense ourselves lifted above ourselves, we touch the smoothness *(levitatem)* of God.[76]

In this passage, William depicts a singular spiritual "common sense" cognizing divine things (e.g., the divine goodness, majesty, omnipotence) through various spiritual senses, which perceive them as spiritual odor, heat, and smoothness. The analogy with the Aristotelian notion of the "common sense" provides a model for conceiving of an essentially singular spiritual sense, which nonetheless has diverse spiritual sensations.

In various ways, finally, the remaining objections had critiqued the notion that there could be a plurality of acts or delights without an essential plurality of senses. For diverse acts imply diverse virtues, which in turn imply essentially diverse senses. The argument can be stated helpfully as a question: How can a single power of the soul, with a single virtue which perfects it, nonetheless have diverse acts and delectations? William's answer is crucial. He makes a comparison with his conception of faith. "For just as it was said in the question on faith, even though there are diverse things to be believed *(credentia)* and diverse believable things *(credulitates)*, nevertheless there is one faith, since the formal object *(ratio credendi)* of believing is the same." In the same way, "even though there are diverse acts of the spiritual senses, there is, nevertheless, one virtue and one habit, since there is one formal object of perceiving *(ratio percipiendi)*, namely, through faith."[77] As before, William again

---

76. SA IV 18.3.3.2.4: 514,78ff.
77. SA IV 18.3.3.2.4: 515,93ff. *Sicut enim dictum est in questione de fide, licet sint diversa credentia et diverse credulitas, tamen una est fides, quia eadem est ratio credendi. Similiter,*

posits a parallel between the material and formal aspects of faith and of the spiritual sense. Despite the various things to be believed and the correspondingly diverse acts of belief, faith remains singular and unified. The case is similar with the spiritual sense. Materially, it has diverse sense objects, diverse acts of spiritual sensation, and diverse forms of spiritual delectation. Yet, formally there remains a singular spiritual sense, the intellect, and a single perfecting virtue, faith. It is apparent too that William sees more than a parallel here. In actuality, both the virtue of faith and the spiritual senses pertain to the intellect. As will be evident below, then, they form part of the same experience of the knowledge of God.

William makes one last point here that must not be neglected. One of the above-noted objections had argued that the virtues of faith, wisdom, understanding, and prudence, for example, are all senses of some kind and yet they are different virtues. William's noteworthy response grants the major premise, but refutes the minor premise and thus the conclusion: "Wisdom and understanding are senses *(sensus)*; but they are not a different sense from faith. For it is the same thing to cognize by faith, by wisdom, and by understanding. But by faith we cognize *that (quia)* something is the case, but through wisdom and understanding [we cognize] *the reason why (propter quid)*."[78] For William, then, in some important way, not simply the knowledge of faith, but also that of understanding and wisdom, are forms of spiritual sensation, or at least they share a common "sense-like" character.

William's assertions in this final discussion merit close attention. Essentially, there is only a singular spiritual sense, having a single habit, virtue, and perfection. Yet this singularity does not preclude the presence of diverse spiritual senses or at least a genuine diversity of acts of spiritual sensation. Particularly *in via*, the spiritual sense has various acts, various objects, and various delights. William's analogy with the Aristotelian "common sense" is helpful, serving as a model for conceiving of the

---

licet sint diverse operationes sensus spiritualis, unica tamen est virtus, et unicus habitus, quia unica est ratio percipiendi, scilicet per fidem.

78. SA IV 18.3.3.2.4: 515,100. *Dicimus quod sapientia et intellectus sensus sunt; sed non sunt alius sensus quam fides. Idem enim cognoscitur per fidem, sapientiam et intellectum. Sed per fidem cognoscimus quia est, per sapientiam autem et intellectum propter quid est.*

"unified diversity" of the spiritual sense(s). Of greater significance, though, is the use of the distinction between formal unity and material diversity in the comparison between the spiritual sense(s) and faith. Not only does it illuminate the unity of the diverse acts of the spiritual senses, but it also demonstrates the important link between the knowledge of faith and that of spiritual sensation.

Conclusion

The inductive labor of the foregoing provides now the basis for some preliminary conclusions. These more synthetic remarks will introduce the framework for the rest of this study, which, it is hoped, will facilitate a fuller appreciation of William of Auxerre's unique account of human knowledge of God. They are organized around the following three themes: the object, the subject, and the nature/acts of the spiritual senses.

At the outset of his discussion of beatitude, William designated the object of beatific knowledge to be Christ in both natures: humanity for the physical senses, divinity for the spiritual senses. With respect to the divine nature, he stressed the singularity of the object *in se*, its formal unity, while materially and in effect allowing diverse manifestations. Here, the notion of the *delectabilia divina* emerged. Generally, this referred to the manifestations of the divine nature perceptible by the spiritual senses. Though William is not especially concerned with any one pair and while some variation exists between descriptions, the following alignments obtain: (1) for vision, beauty *(pulcritudo)* and fullness *(plenitudo)*; (2) for audition, melody *(melodia)* and symphony *(simphonia)*; (3) for olfaction, odor *(odor)*; (4) for taste, sweetness *(dulcedo)* and attractiveness *(suavitas)*; (5) for touch, suavity *(suavitas)*, heat *(calor)*, and smoothness *(levitas)*.

Foundationally, the subject of beatitude is the ecclesial community, the mystical bride of Christ. Only as a member of Christ's body, the church, do individual souls receive the wedding gifts *(dotes)* from the Bridegroom. William's descriptions of beatific knowledge through the spiritual senses typically use the first-person plural, such as: "we see, we taste, we touch." With respect to the individual, the subject of the spiritual senses *in patria* is the Pauline "inner man" or *homo spiritualis*. More precisely, the intellect or rational power, the recipient of the endowment, *cognitio*, is the proper subject of the acts of the spiritual senses. Here, it is helpful to recall how William, providing an Aristotelian nuance to the soul's *imago Dei*, emphasizes its essentially indeterminate nature. It is capable *in potentia* of knowing all things. In this way, the intellect functions as the *"sensus communis"* of the spiritual senses. Despite the priority of *cognitio*, though, William allots a crucial role to *dilectio*, and both require their respective virtues of faith and charity.

What precisely are the spiritual senses? Powers or faculties of the soul? How many are there? Though William does not address the question fully, his position can be traced with adequate clarity. Strictly speaking, there is only one spiritual sense, namely, the intellect, the rational part of the soul. It is *the* "organ" of spiritual sensation. Regarding spiritual senses in the plural, these are best conceived of as diverse acts of perception or sensation on the part of the intellect, through which it delights in God. Though formally and essentially one, the spiritual sense has diverse acts and delights, just as its divine Object is formally one, but is nonetheless manifest in manifold *delectabilia*.

Emerging from the soul's first two endowments, *cognitio* and *dilectio*, is the third, *fruitio*, fruition or delight, which is their consummation. For William, both *in patria* and *in via*, delight *(delectatio)* is a perduring theme in his analysis of human knowledge of God (reminiscent of earlier theologies of a monastic orientation). In both contexts, it is a sine qua non of true knowledge of God. It must be stressed, though, that for William delight—and this is true in both physical and spiritual spheres—is fundamentally a function of sensation. Accordingly, it is precisely the spiritual senses and their acts which effect the soul's experience of fruition or delight and thus facilitate the consummation of the knowledge of God. Moreover, since spiritual delight is a function of spiritual sensation, and since as just noted spiritual sensation is fundamentally an act of the intellect, William's doctrine of the spiritual senses introduces an affective element into the essentially intellectual act of knowing God. This presumably accounts for his relegation of love *(dilectio)*, typically the sphere of affectivity, to the diminished role of desiring the delight experienced by the intellect.

Finally, and perhaps most importantly, William's account of beatitude through the spiritual senses raises the issue of the relationship between intellection and sensation. In the foregoing, he closely associated three distinct intellectual acts: *cognoscere, percipere,* and *sentire* in his descriptions of beatitude. *Sentire* and *percipere* pertain to spiritual sensation and the acts of the spiritual senses. *Cognoscere* is a conceptual, noetic act of the endowment *cognitio*. Beatitude is formally and properly a cognitive act; yet it also entails spiritual perception and sensation of the *delectabilia divina*. How precisely does William conceive of the relationship between the members of this triad? An answer begins to emerge from his descriptions of fruition through the spiritual senses, cited above.

At times, William's descriptions of beatitude include only acts of spiritual perception: "We will delight in the beauty, symphony, aroma, sweetness, and attractiveness of God."[79] Typically, however, his descriptions combine acts of spiritual *percipere* and intellectual *cognoscere*, as here, in a passage also cited above:

> By faith we see *(videmus)* spiritually. By faith we hear *(audimus)* what Jesus says. For *faith comes by hearing* (Rom 10:17). By faith we perceive scents *(odoramus)* spiritually. For by faith we cognize *(cognoscere)* that the Son of God was made man for us, that he wept for us and was tormented for us, that he sorrowed, that he suffered. And when we recall the benefits of this kind, we perceive *(odoramus)* the good odor of Christ *(bonum odorem Christi)* as an aromatic perfume flowing from him, and *we will run after you to the scent of your ointments* (Cant 1:3). When by faith we meditate upon these things which we know, as if by chewing *(masticando)*, we taste *(gustamus)* the sweetness of God *(dulcedinem Dei)*, and this is by faith. By faith we touch *(tangimus)* the suavity of God *(suavitatem Dei)*; for by faith we cognize *(cognoscere)* that in God with respect to himself, there is no bitterness, since *this work is foreign* to him, namely, to punish, as Isaiah says (cf. Is 28:21).[80]

There is then a "bivalence" in William's account of beatitude. It pertains both to cognitive understanding of and reflection on theological doctrines (e.g., the significance of the Incarnation, the attributes of the divine nature), as well as to perception or sensation of the *delectabilia divina* (e.g., beauty, odor, suavity).

79. SA IV 18.3.3.2.2: 506,39.
80. SA IV 18.3.3.2.3: 510,60ff.

A careful review of these descriptions suggests that William views spiritual sensation as a fruit plucked from a conceptual or, more precisely, a doctrinal branch. Typically, theological affirmation precedes spiritual sensation. Of greater significance, though, in some crucial way theological *cognoscere* mediates and informs spiritual sensation, while, conversely, spiritual *sentire* subsumes within itself the prior doctrinal cognition. In the passage above, for example, perception of spiritual scents comes from the cognition of Christ's incarnation, torment, sorrow, and suffering; from this recollection comes the good odor of Christ as an aromatic perfume; meditation on that "which we know," as a form of spiritual chewing, yields a taste of the divine nature; and, finally, an understanding of God's mercy gives way to touching the divine suavity. Other examples could be adduced, but perhaps this is the clearest:

> When we cognize *(cognoscere)* the goodness, the majesty, the omnipotence of God and so the other [aspects of God] from someone else, then we hear spiritually what Jesus says; we are able to cognize the same thing through ourselves, and this is to see spiritually. When we cognize that from these things goodness is poured out upon creatures, we perceive the odor *(odoramur)* of God spiritually; and when we meditate on this, we chew *(masticamus)* spiritually; and when we are inflamed by these thoughts toward the love of God, then we touch *(tangimus)* God spiritually. For we touch the heat *(calorem)* of God. So also, when we sense ourselves lifted above ourselves, we touch the smoothness *(levitatem)* of God.[81]

Here, theological cognition of divine attributes and meditation on God's creative acts precedes and informs each act of spiritual sensation.

For William, then, doctrinal *noesis* leads—through cognition, recollection, meditation, and reflection—to spiritual *aesthesis*. Spiritual sensation, for its part, emerges from, is mediated and structured by, doctrinal affirmation. To know God is to understand the meaning of the Incarnation, to grasp conceptually the internal *rationes* of God, to cognize the divine attributes; it is also to see, hear, smell, taste, and touch the divine *pulchritudo, simphonia, odor, dulcedo, suavitas Dei*. William accommodates both through the language and categories of his spiritual *sensorium*. The *intellectus fidei* can be described as gustatory savoring or olfac-

---

81. SA IV 18.3.3.2.4: 514,78ff.

tive appreciation of the truths of revelation; the *intellectus Dei* can be described as tasting the divine sweetness or touching the divine suavity. Beatific knowledge of God is a form of knowing that embraces theological concept and spiritual percept. In light of this integration, the term "spiritual apprehension" presents itself as an apt term for this constellation of ideas. Henceforth in this study, accordingly, the term will be used to refer to the knowledge that embraces *cognoscere, percipere,* and *sentire*.

Lastly, William's treatment of beatitude suggests that there is a crucial relationship between spiritual apprehension *in via* and *in patria*. There is both continuity and difference between the two states of life with regard to the spiritual senses. William understands the final state of life to be consummation of something begun in this life, albeit inchoatively and in a preambulatory way: "in the present time, the spiritual sight only apprehends *(cognoscere)* spiritual things in a preambulatory sense *(sensu preambulo)*." The goal, in the next life, is the unified, synaesthetic act of spiritual vision (for *"in patria* vision will be the whole reward") wherein the soul will taste "by seeing," touch "by seeing," hear "by seeing," etc. Gradually, human persons move from a diversity of spiritual sense-acts and delights to a single, synaesthetic *visio Dei*.

This link between these two states of life suggests that other aspects of William's theology can be fruitfully explored from this perspective. His teaching on the spiritual senses assumes many other aspects of his thought, and a proper appreciation of this doctrine requires that they be explored from this perspective.

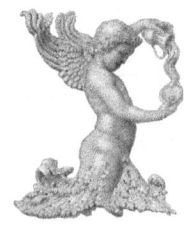# PART II
THE OBJECTS OF SPIRITUAL APPREHENSION

CHAPTER 3

THE MANIFOLD EFFECTS OF THE METAPHYSICAL GOOD

AS ARGUED ABOVE, William envisions knowledge of God *in patria* as an apprehension of the manifold *delectabilia divina* through the soul's spiritual senses. In addition, his conception of beatitude is not unrelated to the knowledge of God possible *in via*. In fact, the apprehension of God *in patria* is the culmination—literally, the fruition—of the knowledge of God begun *in via*. As such, it is the perfection of a kind of knowing that can be generalized to include other preliminary forms: knowledge of God, both in this life and the next, is the apprehension *(cognoscere, percipere, sentire)* of uncreated goodness within its created effects.

In his discussion of beatitude, William summarized the operation of the spiritual senses *in via*, referring explicitly to this theme:

> Each spiritual sense whatsoever has many operations . . . we see the goodness of God, the majesty of God, and the other exemplary virtues which are in God, and these are diverse visions. . . . Likewise, when we apprehend that from these things goodness is poured out upon creatures, we perceive the odor of God spiritually; and when we meditate on this, we chew spiritually; and when we are inflamed toward the love of God by these things, then we touch God spiritually.[1]

He suggests here that God's goodness can be both heard through spiritual hearing and glimpsed through spiritual sight. Likewise, the realization

---

1. SA IV 18.3.3.2.4: 514,78ff.

that uncreated goodness has been poured out upon creatures is compared progressively to smell, to taste, and, finally, to ecstatic touch. William's references to the good as the primary object of spiritual apprehension are not casual. Rather, they reflect a fundamental assumption in his theology which bears directly on the possibility of spiritual apprehension. Accordingly, this chapter will sketch the outline of William's theological metaphysics of the good. In the passage above, three aspects of the good emerge: (1) the goodness which is an attribute of the divine nature; (2) that same goodness as it "flows" out into created realities; (3) the possibility that the divine goodness can be apprehended within its created effects through the spiritual senses.

"On the Nature of the Good"

Students of scholastic theology and philosophy have long noted the presence of a short chapter in Book III of William's *Summa Aurea* entitled "On the Nature of the Good." Book III itself begins with a discussion of his Christology (Tractates 1–9), before engaging in a lengthy discussion of the virtues that constitutes the remainder of the book. William's discussion of the moral life begins with Tractate 10, which he rather vaguely entitles "Preambulatory Questions on the Virtues," the first three chapters of which consider such themes as the relationship between justification, grace, merit, and good works. Chapter 4, "On the Nature of the Good," treats a completely different issue, and thus in one sense appears out of place in this tractate. Indeed, it has been seen as a separate self-contained treatise.[2]

The historical importance of William's treatise on the good for the development of the medieval theory of the transcendentals was noted long ago by Dom Henri Pouillon,[3] and has been confirmed by more re-

---

2. Chapter 4 is divided as follows: Question 1—What the good is, what goodness is, and whether all things are called good from the first good; Question 2—What the difference is between *esse* and *bonum esse*; Question 3—What the difference is between the good and the true; Question 4—On the contrast between good and evil; Question 5—On the good and the bad generally.

3. Henri Pouillon, "Le premier traité des propriétés transcendentals, La 'Summa de bono' du Chancellier Phillipe," *Revue néoscolastique de philosophie* 42 (1939): pp. 40–77. Pouillon points out Philip the Chancellor's significance in the development of the medieval theory of the transcendentals. He also showed how the seeds of Philip's conception

cent scholars.[4] William seems to be the first to gather together in a single place the set of issues and questions that became the standard core of subsequent scholastic discussions, from Philip the Chancellor to Thomas Aquinas.[5] In his classic article Pouillon argued that *"dans la Somme de Guillaume d'Auxerre on trouve un embryon de traité."*[6] Since then William's reflections on the nature of the good have been seen as the embryonic beginning of the medieval doctrine of the transcendentals, part of its "earliest systematic formulation," along with Philip the Chancellor's. Accordingly, "there is some justification for considering William's *Summa*, probably written no more than a decade before Philip composed his *Summa de bono*, a rival candidate for the designation 'first treatise on the transcendentals.'"[7] Yet, while scholars have noted the significance of this treatise for scholastic reflections on the transcendentals, they have not appreciated its importance for William's doctrine of the spiritual senses. It should be noted, further, that the failure to consider how this treatise and its contents inform the whole of the *Summa Aurea* has resulted in a less than full appreciation of William's thought in this matter. For example, scholars have contrasted Philip's use of the concept of the good as the organizing principle of the whole *Summa de bono* with the apparently unintegrated, dropped-out-of-nowhere, appearance of the concept in the middle of the *Summa Aurea*. In fact, a more com-

---

of the good as well as the embryonic plan of his *Summa de bono* are found in William's treatise on the good.

4. Cf. Scott MacDonald, "Goodness as a Transcendental: The Early Thirteenth-Century Recovery of an Aristotelian Idea," *Topoi* 11 (1992): pp. 173–86; Jan A. Aertsen, *Medieval Philosophy and the Transcendentals* (Leiden: Brill, 1996), pp. 25–26.

5. MacDonald, "Goodness as Transcendental," p. 174. MacDonald argues that William's discussion "is in essence a self-contained treatise on the nature of the good." Accordingly, he suggests that "although William raises these issues within his discussion of the moral and theological virtues, he sets them out in such a way that they constitute a distinct, independent discussion that is in principle detachable from its particular context" (p. 174). This is perhaps true, but it creates the erroneous impression that William's reflections on the good are not well integrated into the rest of the work. As will be evident, precisely the opposite is the case. This approach to William's contribution to the development of medieval scholastic theology is symptomatic of a broader tendency to treat his thought as an inchoate seedbed of doctrines which blossom in the soil of later thinkers. This narrow approach obscures the unity and integrity of William's thought.

6. Pouillon, "Le premier traité," p. 72.

7. MacDonald, "Goodness as Transcendental," p. 173.

prehensive reading of the *Summa Aurea* reveals that the concept of the good is central to William's thought and shapes both the content and the organization of his *Summa*.[8]

Essential and Participatory Goodness

William's analysis of the good begins with a fundamental distinction between uncreated and created goodness, introduced at the outset of Question 1. He construes this distinction in terms of essential and participatory goodness: "one kind of good is good in essence *(bonum in essentia)*, another is good through participation *(per participationem)*."[9] Essential goodness "is that whose essence is its goodness, that is, that which is good in itself; and in this sense only God is good."[10] Participatory goodness, by contrast, "pertains to all creatures whatsoever, in that each possesses a particular goodness with respect to something of the divine goodness; and in a certain remote way imitates and represents the divine goodness."[11] While God's essence is God's goodness—God is good *se ipso*—all other things can be called good in so far as they derivatively possess and reflect aspects of the divine goodness. This distinction between essential (uncreated) and participatory (created) goodness is the most basic division of the good in William's theology and it governs all else.[12]

William then introduces a threefold subdivision of participatory goodness:[13] the good of nature *(bonum naturae)*, the generic good *(bonum in genere)*, and the good of grace *(bonum gratiae)*.[14] Accordingly, the

---

8. This, of course, is not meant to gloss over the striking differences in both content and form between William's and Philip's consideration of the good.

9. Boethius, *De Hebdomadibus* (PL 64.1313A). Principe notes that the entire discussion in Question 1 is patently inspired by, at least in its statement of the problem and the general outline of its solution, the *De Hebdomadibus* of Boethius (*Hypostatic Union*, p. 27).

10. SA III 10.4.1: 143,3ff.

11. SA III 10.4.1: 143,7.

12. In the remainder of the treatise, William does not explicitly focus on the essential good; it is, however, considered extensively in the opening treatises of the *Summa Aurea*, where William considers the nature of God.

13. This threefold division seems to come from Stephen Langton, *Quaestiones* 147va; text in Lottin, *Psychologie et morale*, vol. 2, p. 425, n. 3.

14. SA III 10.4.1: 143–44,10. *Et secundum hoc multipliciter dicitur bonum: scilicet bonum nature, bonum in genere, bonum gratie.* Pouillon refers to these as "ontologique, morale, et surnaturelle" ("Le premier traité," p. 47).

complete division for William is fourfold: the essential good (God alone) and the participatory good: either of nature, in general, or of grace. The rest of the treatise considers these three types of participatory goodness—natural (Qq. 1b–3), general (Q. 5, a. 1), and graced (Q. 5, aa. 2–4)—in their relationship with the essential good. The third type of participatory goodness, that of grace, is treated mostly by way of definition—the good of grace consists in the virtues and their acts[15]—and in some preliminary ways in the final articles of Question 5. In reality, however, this third type is the primary focus of the rest of Book III (on the theological and cardinal virtues, the gifts of the Spirit, and the beatitudes) and Book IV (on the sacraments). Moreover, the second type, the good in general, pertains primarily to the virtues. In effect, then, William operates with a three-part division of the good: essential goodness, on the one hand, and natural and graced participatory goodness, on the other.

Concerning the Good of Nature (bonum natura)

In Questions 1 and 2, William analyzes the category of *bonum naturae*. It is clear as he proceeds that his concern is not with physics or nature but with ontology. By *natura* William means simply all created reality. The burden of Question 1 is to argue that all created things derive their goodness from participation in the *summum bonum*, that they are good from the first, uncreated goodness *(a prima bonitate increata)*.[16]

William's view of the good *(bonum)* is clarified as he compares it to being *(esse)*,[17] which he considers to be twofold in created things. The

---

15. SA III 10.4.4: 153,7. "In the third mode the good is called the *bonum gratiae*, in as much as the virtues and the works of virtue are goods."

16. SA III 10.4.1: 144,12.

17. Principe observes that in the main William's philosophical assumptions concerning created *esse* can be described generally as "essentialist," in the sense that for him "being or *esse* means to be an essence, to be drawn from a state of non-formation to one of formation, to be determined and constituted by a form" (*Hypostatic Union*, p. 23). He observes: "Although William considers the existing world about him and is aware of the fact that things exist and have their existence from God, in his logico-metaphysical analysis of the constitution of created beings and of God himself their existence is presupposed rather than expressly envisaged. His philosophical and theological investigations analyze existing beings in terms of their intelligibility" (p. 31). William tends to identify the form-giving *esse* with the essence or nature and thus develops even more explicitly than

statement "Socrates is" implies a twofold *esse*, namely, the created *esse* which is in Socrates and an uncreated *esse*. The created *esse* is predicated of Socrates as that in which he is *(in quo est)*, but the uncreated *esse* is predicated as that from which it is *(a quo est)*.[18] For William, the latter is of course God.[19] Similarly, created things entail both created and uncreated goodness. "When it is said: 'whatsoever is, is good,' in as much as it is understood of substances, a twofold good is thus posited, namely the created and uncreated good."[20] This parallel between *esse* and *bonum* is instructive. Just as every existing thing entails both created and uncreated *esse*, so also it entails created and uncreated *bonum*. Moreover, the language used for *esse* can also be used for *bonum*. Created *bonum* is that which belongs to something good or in which it is *(in quo est)*, while uncreated *bonum* is that by which it is *(a quo est)* good.

Boethius a doctrine of real being in terms of intelligible forms (p. 24) or its intelligible structure (p. 25).

18. SA III 10.4.1: 147,99ff. These terms and concepts are reminiscent of Boethius's distinction in the *De Hebdomadibus* between the *quod est* and the *esse* or *quo est* of creatures. Advisedly, these could be translated "that which it is" and "that by which it is" respectively, though the exact meaning of these terms in Boethius and later medieval thinkers is controverted and must be determined for individual authors. William's terminology of *in quo est* and *a quo est* also reflects the thought of Avicenna and Al Ghazali, though William has not completely assimilated the content of their thought. For the Arabs, the duality distinguished in every creature is, on the one hand, an essence which appears in the creature, and, on the other, an existence which resides in the creature, though the creature has received this from another. William, however, discerns simply a single created existence, which resides in the creature, and the uncreated existence of God, from whom the created existence has come. According to Duhem, William here has created a *mélange* of the thought of Avicenna and Eriugena, while at the same time building upon the foundation laid by Boethius. See Pierre Duhem, *La crue de l'Aristotélisme*, part 3, in vol. 5 of *Le systèm du monde: Histoire de doctrines cosmologique de Platon à Copernic* [Paris: Hermann et Fils, 1917], p. 299.

19. The notion that the *esse* of the creature is derived from the divine *esse* and is predicated of the creature with reference to that first *esse* locates William within the various medieval traditions of interpretations of Boethius. He stands in the line of interpreters which stems from Gilbert of Poitiers and passes through Alan of Lille, Simon of Tournai, and others. In Gilbert's words, God communicates *esse* to all beings other than himself by a certain "extrinsic participation" and that *esse* is said of creatures by a "certain extrinsic denomination from the essence of its Principle." Though William does not state the relationship in precisely these terms, his view appears basically the same. On the other hand, William appears somewhat more emphatic than these earlier authors in positing in the creature a true *esse* of its own, and this logically prior to its *esse aliquid* (Principe, *Hypostatic Union*, p. 30).

20. SA III 10.4.1: 147,112ff.

At this point, however, William introduces an important distinction between *esse* and *bonum*. While the uncreated *esse* predicated in any created thing is simply that from which *(a quo)* it derives its *esse*, the uncreated *bonum* has an additional relationship with created reality. William observes: "The created good [is predicated] as that which is in those substances, but the uncreated good as that *toward which (ad quam)* every created good is [oriented]."[21] The *bonum increata*, which is posited in created things, therefore, is not only that from which *(a quo)* every created thing receives its goodness, but also that "toward which" every created good is oriented.

This first difference between *bonum* and *esse* leads to a second. William grants that *esse* is not greater or lesser in things, but that goodness is. "Every good is deductive *(deductivum)* toward the first good or is somehow imitative *(imitativum)* of the first good, and this [deductivity or imitation] indeed does receive greater or lesser."[22] By contrast, *esse* does not receive greater or lesser. *Bonum*, thus, is an accidental quality, receiving and reflecting various degrees in things. Here, then, a graduated hierarchy of goodness within created reality is envisioned, wherein some things have a greater degree of goodness and, accordingly, are more conductive to the *summum bonum* than others. Within this hierarchy, as William observes, "all creatures cry out *(clamant)*: 'God made us,' and every thing desires that good with an appetite appropriate to it." He then concludes: "Since all things are from the highest good, they are therefore deductive *(deductiva)* toward and useful *(utilia)* [for arriving at] the highest good, and in their own way they have a desire for the highest good."[23] William thus posits a broader, more encompassing relationship between created and uncreated *bonum* than that between created and uncreated *esse*. Like *esse*, *bonum naturae* reflects *bonum increata* as its source; but unlike *esse* it also leads to *bonum increata* as its end.

This then is William's metaphysics of the good. The essential, uncre-

---

21. SA III 10.4.1: 147,114ff.
22. SA III 10.4.1: 149,24ff.
23. SA III 10.4.1: 148,129ff. Elsewhere William uses a different description: something is called good "in comparison with the first good and in this way it is inductive *(inductiva)* or useful *(utilia)* with respect to the first good" (SA III 10.4.1: 147,114ff.).

ated goodness of God is good *per se*, while all other created realities are good through participation in that divine goodness. To call a created thing good is always to posit a twofold goodness: the uncreated goodness as that from which it is good and the created goodness which belongs to it as a created *esse*. Moreover, uncreated good stands in a twofold relation to created things: as both source and end. The first good is both the *a quo* and the *ad quam* of created goodness. Created things not only flow out from the good, but also desire to return to the *summum bonum*. Moreover, as so many imitations of uncreated goodness they reflect, proclaim, lead back to, are conductive toward *(inductiva, deductiva)*, and are useful *(utilia)* for arriving at their source in varying degrees.[24] In sum, the essential good is both source and goal, beginning and end of the *bonum naturae*.

Clearly, epistemological as well as metaphysical dimensions are present in this account of the good. This is of particular interest to William. Since all things manifest the divine goodness, when correctly perceived, those beholding them are stirred, roused, persuasively induced and drawn towards the *summum bonum*. In short, for William, the *bonum natura* proclaims[25] the *bonum in essentia*. This is an essential assumption in his general notion of the knowledge of God.

---

24. Clearly, William is operating within a generally Neoplatonic metaphysical framework of self-diffusive goodness and the implied dynamic of procession and return. We say "generally Neoplatonic" since nowhere in this treatise on the metaphysics of the good does William explicitly refer to the Dionysian corpus, though he is clearly familiar with the corpus and cites it elsewhere. As is evident, the general ideas expressed here are also found in Boethius.

25. The echo of Augustine's *Confessions* (Book X.vi [8–9]) here is noteworthy in relation to the theme of the spiritual senses. The context is Augustine's well-known dialogue with his Maker: "But when I love you, what do I love?" His own reply to the question includes the notion of the spiritual senses: "It is not physical beauty nor temporal glory nor the brightness of light dear to earthly eyes, nor the sweet melodies of all kinds of songs, nor the gentle odour of flowers and ointments and perfumes, nor manna or honey, nor limbs welcoming the embraces of the flesh; it is not these I love when I love my God. Yet there is a light I love, and a food, and a kind of embrace when I love my God—a light, voice, odour, food, embrace of my inner man, where my soul is floodlit by light which space cannot contain, where there is sound that time cannot seize, where there is a perfume which no breeze disperses, where there is a taste for food no amount of eating can lessen, and where there is a bond of union that no satiety can part. That is what I love when I love my God." He then turns to the creation around him with further questions: "And what is the object of my love?" In turn all the things in his external environment

The Relation between the Good and the True

It is this epistemological aspect which William considers more fully as he proceeds to the question: "What the difference is between the Good *(bonum)* and the True *(verum)*." This question is crucial and merits close attention, as it reveals his abiding concern with theological apprehension and also gives an explicit indication of the role of the spiritual senses within his thought. In later chapters, the question will form the starting point for a detailed analysis of the function of the spiritual senses in the knowledge of God.

William situates the question of the difference between the good and the true within the framework of essential and participated goodness, wherein created things reflect and desire the first good in a manner consistent with their natures. This is apparent as he offers a further (Boethian) definition for the good: "the good is that which all things desire."[26] He then introduces a problem which dominates the entire question: Granted that the *prima bonitas* is the desired end of rational creatures, how precisely is it related to the *prima veritas*, and how exactly do rational creatures relate to both?[27] Whereas above William developed his thought in relation to *esse*, now the comparison is with *veritas*, shifting the emphasis more sharply from being to knowing.

The dilemma emerges thus: Since the good is that which is desired by all, it follows that "the good is the same thing as the calming of desire or that which *in se* quiets desire. But all agree that our understanding *(intellectus)* rests in the first truth or in the first light, as the affection *(affectus)* [rests] in the first good."[28] From this perspective, the true and the good are distinct: the former as the object of understanding's knowledge, the latter as the object of love's affection.

"cried out with a loud voice *(exclamaverunt voce magna)*: [God] made us *(ipse fecit nos)*." Augustine, *Confessions*, translated with an introduction and notes by Henry Chadwick (Oxford: Oxford University Press, 1991), p. 183.

26. Boethius, *De consolatione philosophiae*, III pr. 2 (PL 63.724; CSEL 67.47; CCL 94.38–39).

27. SA III 10.4.3: 150,4ff. "But since 'nothing is loved *(diligitur)* or desired *(desideratur)* unless it is known *(cognitum)*' as Augustine said, it follows that the good, which is loved *per se*, and naturally, is that which is known *per se* naturally."

28. SA III 10.4.3: 150,9ff.

William, however, finds this initial position untenable. Citing Aristotle, he argues: "that of which there is rest *(quies)*, is that whose movement *(motus)* is toward rest." But a movement toward rest pertains to desire. It would seem then that the intellect, which (as agreed) rests in the first truth, desires so to rest. The desire for the first truth would then be a desire of the intellect, since it desires to rest there. But that which quiets desire (as also agreed) is the good. It seems, accordingly, that the intellect's desire to rest in the first truth is a desire for the first or highest good. But, the love of the highest good is nothing other than charity, which is not in the rational power but in the concupiscible power. From this perspective, then, the true and the good seem to be identical and to be the object of charity's affection rather than faith's intellection.[29]

Another argument pursues the point, while introducing another subdivision of the good to which William frequently returns. Here, the good is spoken of triply: "the delectable good *(bonum delectabile)*, such as God; the beautiful good *(bonum honestum)*, such as virtues and works of virtue; [and] the useful good *(bonum utile)* such as tribulations of the world and all those things which are useful for the possession of the highest good."[30] This division has a classical and patristic pedigree,[31] and for William it sits comfortably aside the earlier division between essential and participatory goodness.[32] This triad is significant, though, be-

---

29. SA III 10.4.3: 150–51,14–26. "Likewise, it is agreed that 'that of which there is rest *(quies)*, is that whose *motus* is toward rest [Aristotle, *Physica*, c. 6, 8]. But the *motus* toward rest is of desire; that which rests in the first truth is that which desires the first truth. But it is agreed that rest in the first truth is of nothing except of the desire of the intellect; thus the desire for the first truth, in as much as it is the first truth, is the desire of the intellect; thus the first truth in as much as it is the first truth is the quieter of desire; thus, in as much as it is the first truth, it is good; thus the love of the first truth in as much as it is the first truth is the love of the first or highest good; but the love of the highest good is nothing other than charity; therefore the love of the first truth in as much as it is the first truth, is in the concupiscible power; thus the desire for the first truth, in as much as it is the first truth, is in the concupiscible power, not therefore in the *intellectus*, which was yet proved before."

30. SA III 10.4.3: 151,27.

31. Cicero, *De officiis*, II, c.3; Ambrose, *De officiis*, I. c.9 (PL 16.31–32); Augustine, *De div. quest. 83*, q. 30 (PL 40.19).

32. William will sometimes substitute the notion of *bonum conferens* or *expediens* for the *bonum utile*. In either case, he also frequently associates the *bonum delectabile* with final causality and the *bonum utile, conferens,* or *expediens* with efficient causality.

cause it introduces the notion of delectability into the discussion. The objection then argues that since the understanding delights in the first truth, the first truth is thus delectable. But since the delectable is a sub-category of the good—following Aristotle, the good is "that whose apprehension is delight"[33]—the love of the first truth would be the love of the delectable, and thus highest, good. But again, this would be the same thing as charity.[34]

Before proceeding to his solution, William introduces one last alternative. Within the concept of the love of the good, two different meanings might be distinguished. One could mean the love by which someone desires to have *apprehension* of the good. If so, this would be the love of the truth in the intellect, and pertain to faith. One could, alternatively, mean the love by which someone desires to have fruition *of the good itself*. This would be the love of the good in the concupiscible power and pertain to charity. Without explicitly saying so, William is employing a distinction which later scholastics will make explicit: namely, the distinction between the *finis quo* of fruition (the end *by which* there is fruition), the apprehension of the good, and the *finis in quo* of fruition (the end *in which* there is fruition), the good itself. While William ultimately rejects this proposal, he agrees with the distinction between two types of ends.

Accordingly, he rejects the distinction, not between the *finis quo* and the *finis in quo* of fruition, but rather the association of these two components of fruition with the two different parts of the soul and their respective virtues. William argues that the preceding distinction amounts to nothing, since "the understanding delights in the first truth through faith; thus, its desire is to delight in the first truth; thus the love *(amor)* of the first truth is the love by which the understanding desires to delight in the first truth and so in the first good."[35] Both the desire for apprehension of the truth and the desire for the truth itself are in the understanding. He emphasizes the point in another rejoinder: "If there were one

---

33. "*bonum est cuius apprehensio est delectatio*" (Aristotle, *Ethica Nicom.*, VIII c.2; 1155b, 19–21).
34. SA III 10.4.3: 151,30.
35. SA III 10.4.3: 151,41.

love *(amor)* by which the soul desired to delight in the highest good, and another by which it desired to delight in the apprehension of the highest good, then similarly there would be one love by which the soul desired to delight in the highest good and another love by which it desired to delight in love of the highest good." For William, such a scenario is false: "for in the same way that I love the first good, I love its charity and I have fruition in its love; similarly in the same love by which I love the first truth, I love its apprehension."[36] The separation of the desire of a power for its proper end from the desire for the means by which that end is achieved cannot stand.

Having then created the *aporia*—how are the good and the true related, and how do rational creatures relate to them?—William proceeds to his solution. He begins by distinguishing between the highest good's two modes of delectability: "the first good—that is the first delectable which is God—is delectable in two ways."[37] In the first way, "in as much as God is the illuminating light, God is delectable to the intellect through the mode of sight *(visus)* or through the mode of apprehension *(cognitio)*; and such delectable love, as was said, is of the substance of faith."[38] In the second way, "God is delectable in as much as God sweetly delights *(suavis delectans)* or sensuously pleases *(delicians)* the affection *(affectus)* or the concupiscible power through the mode of touch *(tactus)*. Thus, the love of the highest good is charity."[39] And so, William argues: "the true and the good are the same thing, but it is called *verum* in as much as it is the end of the intellect or of speculation; while it is called *bonum* in as much as it is the end of desire and of action." Citing Aristotle's *De anima*,[40] he concludes: "the good and the true are the same; but it is called the truth in as much as it is without action, the good in as much as it is with action."[41] William's solution here is to identify the good and the true under the concept of delectability: the first good is also the first delectable. Goodness and truth are the two primary modalities by which God is encountered delectably by rational creatures. This identity is the foundation of his concept of the *delectabilia divina*, which figured

36. SA III 10.4.3: 151,45.
38. SA III 10.4.3: 151–52,53ff.
40. Aristotle, *De anima*, III 431b, 10–11.
37. SA III 10.4.3: 151,52.
39. SA III 10.4.3: 152,56ff.
41. SA III 10.4.3: 153,86ff.

prominently in his description of beatitude. The *delectabilia divina* are a function of the fact that as the first good, God is also the first delectable for the two primary human modes of experience, through which the *delectabilia* are encountered by the human person: the mode of apprehension and the mode of affection. These two modes are associated with the rational and concupiscible powers of the soul, their proper acts (understanding, speculation and affection, desire, action), and their perfecting virtues (faith and charity). Finally, as in the treatise on beatitude, William employs the doctrine of the spiritual senses in order to explicate these two modes of relating to the highest good. Faith is associated with spiritual sight, charity with spiritual touch.[42]

Having introduced the doctrine of the spiritual senses at this juncture, two interrelated issues arise with respect to William's association of charity with touch. First, what of the other spiritual senses? For one might suppose that, "if there is one virtue which delights the soul in God through the mode of *spiritualis visus*, namely faith, and another which delights the soul in God through the mode of spiritual touch *(tactus spiritualis)*, namely charity, similarly, there should be one virtue which delights the soul in God through the mode of spiritual hearing *(auditus spiritualis)*, another through the mode of smell *(olfactus)*, another through the mode of taste *(gustus)*; and so in conjunction with the five spiritual senses there would be five theological virtues."[43] Behind this objection, though, is a larger issue which William appears to realize without saying so explicitly. He seems, prima facie, to contradict himself here. The notion that charity delights in the highest good through the

---

42. William's solution here combines various parts of the initial objections. With the first objection, he grants the true as the object of understanding and the good as the object of affection. He rejects, however, a real distinction between these two objects. With the second objection, he grants the unity of object, but rejects the notion of a singular relationship to it on the part of the affection in the soul's concupiscible power. With the third objection, he grants the notion of the first delectable, but again rejects its singular relation to charity. Finally, with the fourth objection, he grants the distinction between the end by which *(finis quo)* and the end in which *(finis in quo)*, but rejects a strict alignment of the former with the rational power and the latter the concupiscible power. Rather, each power relates to a different modality of the first delectable as its proper end (in this way the ends are distinguished) but each relates to its proper end in both ways: as end in which and end by which.

43. SA III 10.4.3: 152,64ff.

mode of touch seems at odds with his statements in the treatise on beatitude, where he explicitly argued that charity is not a sense and strictly speaking has no experience of delight, but only the desire for it. Here, however, William has not only aligned charity with the spiritual sense of touch, but also suggested that "just as there is greater delight *in tactu* than in the other senses, so there is greater delight in charity than in the other virtues."[44]

Concern for this larger issue governs William's response to both objections. He begins by clarifying his understanding of desire or love *(amor)* with respect to the virtues. Each virtue has a desire which is proper to it: desire for apprehension of the highest good as truth pertains to faith; desire for the highest good as good pertains to charity.[45] He then adverts to the distinction between desire and delight, which figured so prominently in his teaching on beatitude, by arguing that "we do not say that the delight which is according to spiritual touch *is* charity, rather it is the *end of the movement (motus)* of charity. Similarly, the delight which is in spiritual taste or smell is not charity, but the end of the movement of charity; spiritual sight is to be understood similarly."[46] Properly speaking, charity does not experience delight, but rather desires it; while faith alone experiences the delight which charity desires. William concludes then with an important clarification. "We say that the desire for apprehending God is the understanding of faith; but the desire for delighting in God either in the mode of sight or smell or taste or touch is of charity. For this is the desire for the good in as much as it is the good, that is, the delectable, in as much as it is delectable."[47] While there is a desire on the part of the understanding for its proper end, this is simply due to the nature of a power or virtue, which naturally desires its proper end. Charity too, in this sense, has a specific (literally, pertaining to its species) desire which pertains to it. This is a kind of generic desire. On the other hand, in a theologically significant sense, charity is the desire for delight in God, not simply in its generic desire as a specific virtue, but for the delight which emerges through the encounter of all

44. SA III 10.4.3: 152,59.
46. SA III 10.4.3: 152,73ff.
45. SA III 10.4.3: 152,71.
47. SA III 10.4.3: 152,77ff.

the spiritual senses with their divine objects, which are themselves properly seen in conjunction with faith and understanding. As in the treatise on beatitude, William appeals to the experience of the physical senses to confirm his point. In the physical sphere, "the desire for delight in sensibly delectable things is in the concupiscible power; but the delectation which is the end of that desire is in the senses."[48] So, the desire for delight corresponds to the desire of the concupiscible power for the good as good, while the experience of delight corresponds to the actual apprehension of the good as true, which William here construes as a kind of spiritual sense experience.

Ambiguity remains, however, concerning William's position on the relative roles of faith and charity in the soul's encounter with the first delectable. At times he seems to segregate strictly charity's desire for delight from the delight itself of faith. Yet, ultimately, he struggles to avoid attributing some experience of delight to charity. In some way, charity "touches" its object, is thus a kind of sense, and therefore can even be granted an experience of delight which is greater than that of the other virtues. In some way, faith's spiritually sensuous delight appears to redound to charity. In short, the question lingers: can charity in some manner be called a spiritual sense?

To summarize thus far, several points should be stressed. The *summum bonum* is a singular delectable reality which has two modalities: as good and as true. These correspond to the rational and concupiscible powers of the soul, which in turn are perfected by the theological virtues of faith and charity. Charity, which William locates in the concupiscible power, desires to delight in the *summum bonum* in as much as it is good. Accordingly, charity is associated with desire and the movement which flows from it. Located in the understanding or rational power of the soul, faith desires to delight in the *summum bonum*, in as much as it is true. Its delight occurs in the apprehension of the good as the true, through the spiritual senses; yet in some way charity also experiences delight in the good as good.

---

48. SA III 10.4.3: 152–53, 83ff.

On the Good and Evil Generically

While the prior question considered the relation of the good and the true within the category of *bonum naturae,* William's analysis patently presumed the presence and proper functioning of the theological virtues, namely faith and charity. But the virtues, especially the theological virtues, fall under another category of the participatory good, namely, the *bonum gratiae.* It is this particular category, the *bonum gratiae,* to which William turns in the fifth and final question of his treatise on the good. Though the title of this question—"On the Good and Evil *in genere*"—suggests otherwise, in actuality William uses the notion of generic good as a point of entry into the discussion of the theological virtues. Although the notion of the *bonum in genere* has a broader applicability than the realm of the virtues, in the context of this treatise it is simply a way of further classifying the character of the *bonum gratiae.*

For present purposes, the interest of this question is that in it William again takes up the issue that dominated the prior discussion: the relationship between faith, charity, and the spiritual senses. At one point, he argues that without qualification *(simpliciter)* all the virtues are equally good, generally speaking *(in genere).*[49] Yet if a qualification be permitted, it can be said that: "in one way charity is better, since in a greater way it unites [us] with God and in a greater way causes [us] to delight in God, but this is . . . from the *ratio* of the end *(ex ratione finis),* since in the *affectus* of charity one is immediately drawn by the sweetness *(dulcedine)* or the suavity of God." At the same time, "the remaining virtues are not drawn by the final end except through other intermediate ends. Hence, it is clear that charity unites itself to God in a greater way than the other virtues, even than faith and hope, since the highest good moves faith and hope through the mode of estimation *(per modum aestimationis);* but charity moves through the mode of touch *(per modum tactus)* to God's suavity."[50] Rather than clarifying the issue, though, William's comment here further complicates it. The issue of immediacy was not raised explicitly in the prior discussion and its whole relevance will not be clear

49. SA III 10.4.5.2: 162,66.
50. SA III 10.4.5.2: 162,69ff.

until his explicit treatment of the individual virtues. Novel too in the discussion thus far is the use of the notion of estimation *(aestimatio)* to characterize faith's mode of apprehension in contrast to charity's mode of touch. It will be clear later on, however, that this term is quite significant. It will figure prominently in William's analysis of faith's relationship to the spiritual senses.[51] Moreover, it is a term whose technical domain is philosophical discussions on the so-called "interior senses" among those influenced by Aristotle and his Arabic commentators; William's use of it suggests that he is in some way familiar with and inspired by these philosophical traditions. For the present, though, it is sufficient to note that William's preferred manner of characterizing the experience of faith and charity is in terms of *aestimatio* and *tactus*, respectively.

Conclusion

This tractate, which constitutes William's "embryonic treatment of the transcendentals," is a compact summary of his theological metaphysics of the good. In the main, he posits a threefold division of the good: *bonum in essentia, bonum naturae,* and *bonum gratiae.*

William's treatise on the nature of the good is oriented toward theological and spiritual apprehension. This can be seen by summarizing the treatise in the following way. God alone is essentially *(in essentia* or *per se)* good. Created reality (the *bonum naturae*), by contrast, is good derivatively. This relationship between essential and participatory goodness is twofold: the *summum bonum* is not only source but also end of creatures. Conversely, creatures not only flow out from the divine goodness but also desire and tend toward it in a manner congruent with their natures. This dual relationship to uncreated goodness has a further implication: all created reality imitates, reflects, and leads back to its source and end. As a quality inhering in various ways and degrees within created reality, goodness is an intelligible and delectable expression of uncreated goodness. This participatory relationship to the divine goodness thus contains both a metaphysical and epistemological dimension: cre-

---

51. This will be discussed in Chapter 7.

ated reality not only is good from uncreated goodness but also manifests that goodness. With respect to human persons, endowed with desiring and apprehending capacities, all created reality, when rightly perceived, proclaims the highest good, and is thus conductive to it. In a general way, then, William's concept of the knowledge of God can be described as the apprehension of uncreated goodness within its created effects.

That created goodness can function thus in relation to its uncreated counterpart is made possible, however, through the *bonum gratiae*, namely, the theological virtues. Only through faith and charity, which correspond to the rational and appetitive powers of the soul, can the first good be experienced delectably as the good and the true. Charity's desire for the good as good comes to fruition in faith's delectable apprehension of the good as true. Conversely, faith's apprehension of the good as true results in charity's union with the good as good. Precisely at this juncture and perhaps in order to accommodate both of these modalities, William introduces the doctrine of the spiritual senses. Ultimately, this graced encounter with uncreated goodness occurs through the soul's "spiritually sensuous" capacities. God is apprehended as an illuminating light by spiritual sight *(visus)*; sensed as sweetly delighting or sensuously pleasing by spiritual touch *(tactus)*.

Thus, at the heart of William's metaphysics of the good stands his doctrine of the spiritual senses. Not confined to beatitude, not even restricted to rarefied moments of mystical experience, knowledge of God through the spiritual senses is the perfected culmination of the general process of theological perception and apprehension.

Much, however, concerning William's doctrine of knowledge of God through the spiritual senses remains to be clarified. For instance, how does the notion of essential goodness relate to other aspects of the divine nature? Also, how exactly do the spiritual senses relate to the powers or capacities of the soul? How are they integrated within William's theological anthropology? Moreover, the relationship of the spiritual senses to faith and charity remains ambiguous. How precisely do faith and charity relate to each other and to their respective objects? Is charity a *sensus* in some fashion? What is the significance of the notion of estimation in relation to faith? Where precisely is delight to be located in the experience of knowledge of God? Is it significant, moreover, that William here aligns faith and charity with the two extremes, as it were, of the physical senses: sight having the greatest distance between sensor and sensed, touch the least or even none. Does he envision a continuum of knowledge of God, like that found in the treatise on beatitude, in which the various spiritual senses are associated with different degrees and/or different forms of theological perception and apprehension? These and other issues will be taken up in the chapters that follow.

CHAPTER 4

THE TRINITY AS MANIFOLD DELECTABLE

IN HIS TREATISE ON BEATITUDE, a central feature of William's doctrine of the knowledge of God is the assumption that the spiritual sense(s) have multiple objects. He described these objects variously, as *pulchritudo, simphonia, odor, dulcedo,* and *suavitas,* among others, and referred to them collectively as *delectabilia divina.* Yet, he also emphasized the singularity of the divine object of knowledge: though encountered in manifold ways, God nevertheless remains in William's view a single object of spiritual perception. In that treatise, William offers no justification for this "manifold singularity." In his *ex professo* treatment of the divine nature in Book I of the *Summa Aurea,* though, he provides the looked-for rationale. More precisely, his doctrine of the Trinity allows him to conceive of the one God as delectable in a variety of modes.

William's trinitarian theology is closely linked with his metaphysics of the good, described earlier, and that link is especially evident in a particular principle that determines the relations between the divine persons *ad intra:* uncreated goodness flows *from* the Father, is manifest and perceived *in* the Son, and is perceived with delectation *through* the Holy Spirit. As Trinity, then, God enjoys the highest beatitude through the experience of delectable self-apprehension. This is the foundation of human beatitude, which participates in its divine counterpart.

After the Prologue, which introduces the methodological approach of the entire work,[1] Book I of the *Summa Aurea* considers various aspects

---

1. The Prologue and its implications for William's doctrine of the knowledge of God will be considered in detail in Chapter 9 below.

of the divine nature: God's existence and triune nature (Tractates 1–3); the divine names and properties (Tractates 4–8); other aspects of the divine nature—knowledge, providence, power, will, mercy, and justice (Tractates 9–13).

The Essential Good and the Trinity ad intra

In his treatise on the good, William simply asserted that God is essentially good. In the first three tractates of Book I, however, he articulates his view of the divine nature primarily from this perspective, considering the implications of essential goodness for God's existence and nature. First, he subsumes a basically Anselmian notion of $esse^2$ within *bonum*, which will be for him a more fundamental category, and then introduces a thesis which will henceforth be defended by scholastic theologians: the *summum bonum* is such that it cannot be understood not to exist.[3] Next, he argues for the simplicity and oneness of God from the assumption of God's essential goodness.[4] From these fundamental affirmations, William develops his full trinitarian doctrine.

Considering the generation of the Son, William structures the question around the relationship between divine power and will,[5] and ori-

2. See Jean Châtillon, "De Guillaume d'Auxerre à Saint Thomas d'Aquin: L'argument de Saint Anselme chez les premiers scolastiques du XIIIe siècle," in *D'Isidore de Séville à Saint Thomas d'Aquin: Etudes d'histoire et de théologie* (London: Variorum Reprints, 1985), pp. 209–31, p. 217ff: According to Châtillon, William appears to be the first early thirteenth-century scholastic master to discuss Anselm's argument from the *Proslogion* for God's existence. The *Summa Aurea* also contains, gathered together for the first time, a set of authorities and arguments which reappear thereafter in subsequent scholastic discussions, both with the very same number of defenses and the very rare adversaries of the Anselmian proof. Châtillon also argues that William truncates Anselm's method by excluding faith as the starting point. He sees William pursuing a purely philosophical proof, which presupposes that there is a complete correspondence between thinking and being and that humans possess something like innate knowledge of God's existence. Now, the proof is based on human reason alone: the denial of God's existence is self-contradictory. Châtillon further argues that, probably under William's influence, later figures like Richard Fishacre, the *Summa Halesiana*, Bonaventure, and Aquinas, adopted a similar approach.

3. Châtillon, "De Guillaume d'Auxerre à Saint Thomas d'Aquin," p. 217.

4. William here appeals to Augustine's statement in *De Trinitate*: God must be the good by which God is good, since otherwise the good would be prior to God.

5. William argues that four possible scenarios emerge: either the Father was willing and able to generate a Son equal to himself, or he was willing but unable, or was able but unwilling, or finally was neither willing nor able (SA I 3.1: 26,4ff).

ents his own thesis around the concept of the good.⁶ With respect to the divine will, he finds in the concept of the *summum bonum* the idea of the highest generosity *(summa liberalitas)*, to which he contrasts the highest avarice *(summa avaritia)*. If the highest avarice wills to communicate nothing of its goodness, the highest generosity by contrast must will to share all of its goodness. Since from eternity the Father is the highest generosity *(summa liberalitas)*, from eternity he therefore wills to communicate the fullness of his majesty *(maiestatis plenitudinem)*, implying that from eternity he willed to generate a Son equal to himself.⁷

William argues similarly regarding divine power. The concept of the *summa bonitas* also entails the idea of the highest fecundity *(summam fecunditatem)*.⁸ Since the power of God is most abundant *(potentia Dei*

---

6. Throughout these early tractates, William is indebted to Richard of St. Victor—though with significant differences. In his *De Trinitate,* Richard argued first that in God a plurality of persons exists, in order to then show that it must be a *Trinitas personarum* (*Trin.* III 2 and III 11). Regarding both the *pluralitas* and the *Trinitas* of the divine persons, Richard proceeds from three starting points: from the fullness of the good *(plenitudo bonitatis),* the fullness of felicity *(plenitudo felicitatis),* and the fullness of divine glory *(plenitudo divinae gloriae)* (*Trin.* III 2–5 and III 11–14). William modifies the essential structure of the argumentation in order to give it his own emphases; see Johannes Arnold, *Perfecta communicatio: die Trinitätstheologie Wilhelms vons Auxerre,* Beiträge zur Geschichte der Philosophie und Theologie des Mittelalters, vol. 42 (Münster: Aschendorff, 1995), pp. 114–15. While Richard introduces the names "Father," "Son," and "Holy Spirit" only after the logical derivation of the inner-divine references and as justified by the analogy of language, William presupposes these names. Also, the generation of the Son and the procession of the Spirit are presupposed as concrete theological issues by William (Arnold, *Perfecta communicatio,* p. 83). Generally speaking, Richard's influence on William is significant but not exclusive, nor perhaps even determinative. Relative to the Victorine, William is more clearly indebted to Neoplatonic thought, especially to that of Boethius and Pseudo-Dionysius. In the *Summa Aurea,* William uses Richard's argumentation, which he streamlines and condenses, as an alternative to the primary explanation of inner-divine emanation as the outflowing of the self-diffusive good (Arnold, *Perfecta communicatio,* pp. 117–18).

7. SA I 3.1: 26,8ff.

8. Richard of St. Victor introduces his third proof of the Trinity with a similar question regarding the power and will of the Father to generate a coequal Son. In this case, however, the *Summa Aurea* depends more on the *Sentences* of Lombard, who in contrast to the Victorine speaks expressly of God as Father. Also, in his choice of words, William reflects the *Sentences.* This is seems especially true regarding the terminology *(communicare, maiestas, plenitudo, reservare).* According to Arnold, the differences between Richard and William are quite remarkable in regard to the relative weight each gives to the two aspects of the problem, whether the Father could and willed to generate a Son. While William demonstrates the Father's *potentia* in several steps, Richard does so with only one

copiosissima), God can generate a Son equal to himself.⁹ Thus, in his demonstration of both God's will and power to generate a coequal Son, William has recourse to the concept of the good and the concomitant ideas of *liberalitas* and *fecunditas*.¹⁰

The concept of the good is central not only to the Father's generativity, but also to the nature of the Son thus generated. In Wisdom (7:26), the Son is called the mirror *(speculum)* and image *(imago)* of God the Father, "because in the Son is seen the *summa bonitas* and the *summa liberalitas* of God the Father, who wished to possess nothing which he did not communicate to the Son; but gave to him all the riches of his majesty, as [the Son] himself said in the Gospel: *all that is mine is yours and yours is mine* (Jn 17:10)." In the Son, "the essential goodness of God the Father most highly shines forth *(summe relucet)*. . . . Hence, the Gospel says: *whoever sees me, also sees the Father* (Jn 14:9)."¹¹ The Son then is the perfect and express representation of the Father's goodness.

After describing the Son from the perspective of the sense of sight—calling the Son the Father's image and mirror—William shifts to the sense of hearing, taking up the term *verbum*, again in relation to the Fa-

---

sentence; conversely, Richard discusses the Father's will in great detail and with extensive rhetorical expansion, while William is relatively terse (Arnold, *Perfecta communicatio*, p. 115).

9. SA I 3.1: 27,37ff.

10. William defends the idea of divine fecundity variously. Since human fathers can generate sons equal to themselves, how much more can God? (SA I 3.1: 26,19ff) Following the *Glossa interlinearis* on Psalm 109:3 (Lyranus IV, 107r), *from the womb before the day star I begot you*, he repeats the interpretation that the womb refers to the *fecunditas summi Dei* which, he adds, comes from God's *summa bonitas* or *liberalitas* (SA I 3.1: 27,34ff.). Citing the prophet Isaiah, *shall not I that make others to produce offspring, myself produce offspring, says the Lord?* (Is 66:9), he argues that the *fecunditas* of things indicates the *summa fecunditas* (SA I 3.1: 26,23ff). This particular argument, along with the reference to Isaiah, is not among Richard of St. Victor's arguments. He also refers to Pseudo-Dionysius's *On the Divine Names* (c. 1 [PG 3.590; PL 122.1115s]), where the super-essential *fecunditas* of God is mentioned (SA I 3.1: 27,28ff). The reference to Dionysius here concerning the fecundity of God also has no parallel in Richard's *De Trinitate*, nor does William's demonstration of the generation and procession as emanations from the first font of the highest goodness. This demonstration reflects the generally intensified interest in the theology of the Areopagite. Even if Neoplatonic influences on Richard's trinitarian theology are granted, they are not as pronounced as in William. Direct quotations of Pseudo-Dionysius, which are relatively frequent with William, are absent in Richard (Arnold, *Perfecta communicatio*, pp. 115–16).

11. SA I 3.1: 27,45ff.

ther's goodness: "For this reason [the Son] is called the *Verbum* of God the Father, since he perfectly speaks the goodness of his Father." Though the beauty and goodness of creation express the goodness and beauty of God "with a certain kind of voice," since they imitate their Creator "from a great distance," "they do not perfectly speak [the Father's] goodness. But the Son of God who is the image in every way like and equal to God, perfectly speaks the goodness of the Father."[12] In the Son, the essential goodness of the Father not only shines forth and thus becomes visible, but is also spoken and thus becomes audible.[13]

William thus describes the nature of both the Father and the Son in terms of the good. The Father is the *summum bonum* (also *summa bonitas* or *fons bonitatis*), which entails his *liberalitas* and *fecunditas*. Similarly, the Son is the *imago* and *speculum* in which the Father's goodness shines forth most supremely, and the *Verbum* which perfectly speaks that goodness.

Regarding the procession of the Holy Spirit, William proceeds similarly: the Holy Spirit proceeds from the Father's benevolence *(benignitatis)*, which stems from his goodness. William describes the Spirit's coming forth as "the most beautiful *(gratissima)* and most pleasing *(iocundissima)* emanation." Moreover, he emphasizes that the Spirit stems from the highest good, which is "the first, highest, and fullest font of every true pleasure and beatitude *(primus fons et summus et plenissimus omnis vere iocunditatis et beatitudinis).*"[14] The Spirit is thus called the highest gift and the highest love in a manner parallel to the Son's designations: "that which emanates through the mode of *benignitas* and *liberalitas*, is also called a gift . . . and that which proceeds from the highest *liberalitas* is the highest gift *(summum donum)* . . . and the first gift *(primum donum).*" And, "that which proceeds as the first gift from benevolence *(benignitas)* is love *(amor)*" and "that which proceeds from the highest font of goodness *(a summo fonte bonitatis)* first according to the

12. SA I 3.1: 27,53ff.
13. SA I 3.1: 28,61ff. William concludes that generation is the most perfect instance of the process by which something emanates from something else, because generation fully assimilates and adequates the generated to the generator. So, the Father, whom William here calls the *fons bonitatis*, generates a Son coequal, cosubstantial, and coeternal with himself.
14. SA I 3.2: 29,1ff.

mode of *benignitatis* is the highest love *(amor summus)*."[15] So, parallel to the derivation of highest self-communication from the good in relation to the Son, William here associates the highest delight and pleasure from the good with the Holy Spirit. Moreover, just as essential goodness was most liberal in relation to the Son, similarly it is most benevolent regarding the Holy Spirit.

Divine Beatitude

This foundational description of the divine persons in place, William turns to the intra-trinitarian life in general, with a discussion of the supreme beatitude enjoyed by and within God. Here, too, the concept of essential goodness is central; the beatitude which characterizes God's own life *in se* is a function of the good.

William here rehearses three forms of an argument for the necessity of three persons in God, all of which originated with Richard of St. Victor,[16] but which for William are made to reflect his basic assumption that in God is found the highest realization of the delights of love and knowledge. The structure of the argument also follows the Victorine's, yet William shortens it significantly, accentuating the concept of the good. First, he asserts that in the highest good, the highest beatitude *(summa beatitudo)* and the highest pleasure *(summa iocunditas)* have existed from eternity. William continues by arguing that nothing is more enjoyable *(gratiosius)*, nothing more pleasing *(iocundius)* than mutual charity *(mutua caritas)*.[17] From eternity then there must be mutual charity in the *summum bonum*. But mutual charity can only exist among a plurality of persons.[18] Second, William argues that the presence of mutual charity also proves the equality of the persons, since if one person loved

---

15. SA I 3.2: 29,11ff.

16. Here, especially, William's arguments are influenced by Richard of St. Victor, though William does not follow the Victorine in all details. William here borrows Richard's proof from the *plenitudo felicitatis* for the procession of the *pluralitas personarum* (Arnold, *Perfecta communicatio*, p. 116).

17. While Richard of St. Victor requires two steps to prove that nothing is more joyful than charity, William summarizes these thoughts in this terse aphorism: nothing is more joyful than mutual charity. Also, while Richard justifies his thesis by a reference to human nature and experience, William has recourse to Seneca, *Epist.* 6, *ad Lucilium* (Arnold, *Perfecta communicatio*, p. 116).

18. SA I 3.3: 30,2ff.

more than another such love would not be the most orderly or appropriate *(discretissima dilectio)*.[19] Third, the presence of mutual charity requires a third person to whom the lover and the beloved could communicate the delights of their goodness *(delicias bonitatis)* and the delights of love *(delicias dilectionis)*.[20] William summarizes: "among three persons, therefore, a complete communication is possible, namely, the communication of all riches and of the whole majesty and the communication of love."[21]

An objection allows William to round out his thought: if the two persons require a third in order to enjoy perfect beatitude, would not a fourth be required to complete the joy of the three? It is significant that William begins his response by alluding to the definition of beatitude which figured prominently in his treatment of the beatific vision: beatitude consists in apprehension and desire *(in cognitione et dilectione)*.[22] Apprehension by itself, William allows, is possible in a singular person, but there cannot be mutual charity except among at least two persons. The mutual charity among two persons, however, would not be the most generous unless they communicated the delights of their mutual charity with perfect communication. For this it is necessary, but also sufficient that there be a third divine person in God, perfecting the communica-

---

19. William here argues for the equality of the divine persons with reference to *ordo amoris*. In so doing, he borrows Richard of St. Victor's concept of "appropriate love" *(discretus amor)*, a love whose measure corresponds exactly to the worthiness of its object. Richard opposed appropriate love to disordered love or charity *(inordinatus amor* or *caritas inordinata)*. This concept goes back to the Song of Songs 2:4b (Vulgate): *Ordinavit in me caritatem*. The comments of the early church fathers concerning ordered love were taken up again in the twelfth century. Peter Lombard quotes Augustine with the expression *ordinata dilectio* (III *Sent.* 29,1) and combines—under the name of Ambrose—a paragraph from Origen's *Second Sermon on the Song of Songs,* which treats *ordinata caritas.* Abelard, Bernard of Clairvaux, William of St-Thierry, and Hugh of St. Victor, among others, also discuss the topic. By speaking of a *discretissima dilectio* in God, William, like Richard of St. Victor, rejects Abelard's thesis that the divine Trinity is only love in as much as it loves creatures in a condescension of the superior to a needy inferior. With Richard and William, by contrast, the highest and most ordered *caritas* requires that both parties be of the highest as well as equal worth (Arnold, *Perfecta communicatio,* pp. 107–8).

20. SA I 3.3: 31,16ff.

21. SA I 3.3: 31,24. *In tribus ergo personis potuit esse omnimoda communicatio, scilicet divitiarum omnium communicatio sive totius maiestatis et communicatio dilectionis.*

22. Augustine, *De div. Quaest.* 83, q. 35, n.2 (PL 40.24); *Epist.* 187, c.4, n.21 (PL 33.840); *De moribus Eccles.* I, c.11, n.18 (PL 32.1319); *Confess.,* X, c.23, n.33 (PL 32.793).

tion. And so with just three persons there is the highest, because perfectly communicated, beatitude.[23]

William then posits the necessity of a plurality of persons for the existence and experience of the highest beatitude *(beatitudo)* and pleasure *(iocunditas)* within God. He argues that divine beatitude occurs precisely when the goodness of the Father is communicated not only to the Son, but also to the Holy Spirit. Specifically, beatitude *(cognitio* and *dilectio)* and pleasure *(iocunditas)* emerge when the delights *(deliciae)* of communicated goodness between the Father and Son are shared with the Holy Spirit. This is the highest, mutual charity, which realizes the delights of goodness *(deliciae bonitatis)* and love *(deliciae dilectionis)* between the persons.

In sum, beginning with the assumption of God as *summum bonum*, William derives his view of the trinitarian nature of God. The divine nature is characterized by self-diffusive goodness, which flows into a plurality of persons. But the good effects not only the plurality of persons, but also their identity. The Father is the liberal, generous, fecund, self-diffusive font of goodness, who generates a coequal Son, to whom he fully and perfectly communicates all his goodness. In turn, the Son is the Father's perfect *imago* and *speculum*, the express *verbum*. From these proceeds the Holy Spirit as gift and love. In this way, a perfect communication *(perfecta communicatio)* of goodness and love is realized in the Trinity.

Essential goodness also determines the character of the divine interrelatedness. In the Trinity, supreme beatitude and delight *(iocunditas)* arise: beatitude, because the Father realizes complete self-knowledge and self-perception in the Son; delight, because the pleasures *(deliciae)* of the goodness communicated between the Father and the Son are shared with the Spirit, thus realizing perfect and mutual charity. In the Son, essential goodness becomes intelligible. Through the Spirit, essential goodness is understood and experienced with pleasure and delight. Accordingly, the basic principle, introduced in Chapter 3, emerges in a concrete way within William's doctrine of the Trinity: goodness creates the

---

23. SA I.3.3: 31–32,36ff.

conditions for its own perception, its own intelligibility, participation in which produces pleasure and delight. In trinitarian terms, this principle can be articulated thus: uncreated goodness flows *from* the Father, is manifest and perceived *in* the Son, and is perceived with delectation *through* the Holy Spirit.[24] As will be seen shortly, his conception of the appropriated names and the properties *(notiones)* of the three persons in the economy extends this basic principle. It will also be evident below that this principle is the foundation of his concept of the knowledge of God available to rational creatures.

For now, though, it should be noted that for William the beatitude within the Trinity is the foundation of human beatitude. In his account, William describes the intra-divine life using much the same terminology employed to describe human beatitude. God *in se* enjoys the highest and most pleasurable beatitude through cognition *(cognitio)* and love *(dilectio)* among the persons.

The Trinity ad extra: *The Personal Properties*

While the first three tractates of Book I pertain largely to God *in se*, in Tractates 4–8 William turns to the Trinity in its economic manifestations. These later tractates proceed in a very different manner. Here, William is influenced by late-twelfth- and early-thirteenth-century interest in the grammatical and logical analysis of language as a means to knowledge about reality.[25] His theses, accordingly, concerning the names of God[26] are based upon a linguistic investigation of theological state-

---

24. Arnold is quite right to stress the importance of *perfecta communicatio* within William's trinitarian theology. It should be further stressed, though, that *perfecta communicatio* is central for William precisely because it effects beatitude: namely, delightful apprehension, both within God and for rational creatures.

25. Arnold, *Perfecta communicatio*, pp. 120–21. In the twelfth century grammatical analysis was employed by theologians particularly in the interpretation of Scripture. Increasingly influenced by Aristotelian logic, it emerged finally as *Sprachlogik*, which systematically examined grammatical rules as well as the relationship between conceptuality and reality. Some of William's contemporaries and immediate predecessors, for example, Peter Cantor (d. 1197) and Stephen Langton (d. 1228), were critical of this development.

26. The classification of the divine names represents a substantial component of trinitarian theology at the beginning of the thirteenth century. Its roots lie in the works of the pseudo-Dionysius and the John of Damascus. Further influences come from Gilbert of Poitiers and his school, such as Alan of Lille, Simon of Tournai, and others (Arnold, *Perfecta communicatio*, p. 123).

ments.[27] Although this approach is in many ways foreign to modern readers, its influence on the theology of this period was considerable.[28] For present purposes, the details of this analysis are not as important as his conclusions. Accordingly, it need only be summarized here.[29] Concerning the Father, William reiterates without elaboration what he has said in the prior tractates. Besides unbegottenness *(inascibilitas)*, power, eternity, and unity are also appropriated to the first person.[30]

Concerning the Son, William is more expansive. As above, he calls the

27. William regards the levels of language *(vox)*, concept *(intellectus)*, and concrete reality *(res)* as fundamentally parallel (see SA I 6.6: 104,24ff; SA I 4.1: 37,38ff; SA I 4.2: 41,16f). At the least, they follow similar logical laws. Moreover, he assumes that reality is accessible through logical analysis because the rules of language correspond to the structures of being. Thus, he assumes that the inner-trinitarian relations can be represented linguistically and that verifiable correspondences exist between revealed statements and the divine reality itself. Thus, conclusions concerning the Trinity drawn from linguistic analysis are permitted. At the same time, he does not envision a natural transition from linguistic analysis to divine realities. The transcendence and incomprehensibility of God, as well as human sin, rule out an autonomous access by human persons into the trinitarian mystery. Only by revelation do human persons arrive at speech concerning the immanent Trinity. Grammar, however, must be extended or even altered for theological use. In some cases, new grammatical rules are to be derived. Ultimately, language and logic remain dependent on revealed statements; the former simply clarify the latter (see Arnold, *Perfecta communicatio*, p. 122).

28. In relation to linguistic analysis, William is clearly influenced by Praepositinus of Cremona, though he is less concerned with grammar. Despite a general decrease in these logical-linguistic issues among later scholastics, this approach received a significant impetus from Praepositinus and William and remained important in the trinitarian theology of the later period (Arnold, *Perfecta communicatio*, p. 122).

29. In Tractate 4, William analyzes the essential names of God. In Tractate 5, he considers the adjectival names and verbs spoken of God, distinguishing between essential and relative adjectives. In Tractate 6, he asks whether the notion of "person" can be applied to God. In Tractates 7 and 8, he considers the notions *(notiones)* of God, distinguishing between general and special properties. At the end of Tractate 8, "On the Personal Notions," William comes at last to his teaching on the appropriations in Chapter 8, "On the Notions Applied to Individual Persons by Appropriation." In this chapter, he considers the personal properties of the divine persons which bear directly on his doctrine of the knowledge of God.

30. Power *(potentia)* is appropriated to the Father, following Augustine, in order to contrast the usual association of weakness with elderly fathers (SA I 8.8.1: 157,5f). Eternity *(eternitas)* is appropriated to the Father since the Father lacks not only a principle of beginning but also of being (SA I 8.8.4: 174,60f). Unity *(unitas)* is appropriated to the Father for two reasons. First, just as unity is the beginning of all numbers, so the Father is the beginning of all things. Second, just as unity led *in se* only generates itself, so the Father as if *in se ductus* only generates a Son who is of the same substance as himself (SA I 8.8.4: 175,79ff).

Son the image *(imago)*, mirror *(speculum)*, and Word *(verbum)* in which the Father's goodness is perfectly expressed and perceived. Here, however, he subsumes this triad within the category of wisdom *(sapientia)*. "The Son is the Word and the Image of God the Father and the rational Mirror in which all things are seen; for he perfectly speaks the goodness of God the Father and in him can be perfectly seen the goodness of the Father . . . but vision pertains to wisdom." Yet, the Son displays not only the Father's goodness, but the goodness of all created things as well: "but all things are seen there, since the cause of all things, namely the goodness of God, is expressly seen in the Son, and therefore since in him all things are known, the goodness of God is called knowledge of all things or wisdom."[31] Since both the Father's goodness and that of all created things are visible in him, the Son is called wisdom *(sapientia)*.[32]

William adds two further titles regarding the Son's role in the economy—equality and beauty—which continue the sapiential theme while adding an aesthetic dimension. He argues that equality is to be appropriated to the Son because "equality exists first in the Son since he alone precedes immediately from the Father." Moreover, the Son is adequated to the Father since, "just as the Father gives his highest goodness to the Holy Spirit, so also does the Son." And so, William concludes, the Son "gives equality to the Holy Spirit," and there is equality within the Trinity on the Son's account.[33] The rationale for appropriating beauty to the Son is also twofold. First, the Son is the first-begotten from the Father's light and "the first thing which comes from light is splendor." So, the Son is *the splendor of the Father* (Heb 1:3) and *the brightness of the eternal light* etc. (Wis 7:26); "but splendor and candor pertain to beauty and thus

---

31. SA I 8.8.1: 158,27.

32. William justifies this sapiential designation with additional arguments. Associating wisdom with the Son reverses the typical association of foolishness with sons (SA I 8.8.1: 157,8). Moreover, the ancient philosophers noticed that "without understanding there is not beatitude" and that "in understanding there is maximal beatitude." So they assumed that God was the first and highest intellect. Accordingly, they postulated the existence of an "eternal associate" along with God, whom they called *noys* and *mundus archetipus*, who proceeds immediately from the highest intellect. Through this second being, God enjoys the possession of his own understanding. Thus, since wisdom is properly an intellectual word, this title is given to the Son, along with *noys, ars,* and *mundus archetipus* (SA I 8.8.1: 157,16ff).

33. SA I.8.8.4: 174,62ff.

species or beauty *(species sive pulchritudo)* is appropriated to the Son."[34] Second, punning on the Latin word *species,* which refers both to the form which causes a certain thing to be what it is, and also to that thing's appearance and thus beauty, William argues that "the Son is *Sapientia* and *Speculum* and *Exemplar* of all things and the *Ars* of every living rational thing."[35] Hence, since the *"causa formalis* is also the *Species,"* so "species is appropriated to the Son."[36]

Here, wisdom has two dimensions. Through wisdom God operates, creates, establishes, and holds all things together. Wisdom is the art by which God operates *ad extra* in relation to creation; the "interior word" through which all the created things that "express" uncreated goodness can be designated "exterior words"; the exemplar of creation, according to which God makes all things; the *species* or formal cause of all things. At the same time, wisdom is revelatory, expressive, manifesting. The Father understands himself through his wisdom. Wisdom "perfectly speaks" the Father's goodness, and in it that goodness can be "perfectly seen." Because constituted by wisdom, created things also "speak" and "reveal" that wisdom's essential goodness. Because constituted by wisdom, created things reflect that wisdom's beauty.

In sum, under the category of wisdom, William's reflections on the properties appropriated to the Son reveal an extension of the concepts which characterize the Son within the Trinity *ad intra*. In the economy, that same character informs the Son's relation to created reality, which through him becomes a derivative expression and manifestation of un-

---

34. SA I 8.8.4: 175,84f.

35. Subsumed within the appropriation of beauty to the Son is here the complex of ideas including Exemplar or *mundus archetipus, ars,* and *species.* Thus he argues: "It is to be noted that just as an artist *(artifex)* works through his art or his wisdom, so the Father is said to operate through the Son, since the Son is the eternal and interior *Verbum* by which the Father expressly speaks his goodness, as was said above. Creatures by contrast are exterior words, by which as exterior words the Father speaks his goodness. But all exterior speaking is done through an interior word, and thus the Father speaks exterior words through the interior word, that is, he accomplishes his exterior work through the interior word, and thus the Father operates through the Son" (SA I 8.8.2: 158,3ff). In the Son's economic relation to creation, therefore, the Son is not only the rational mirror in which all things are seen, but also the formal or exemplary cause of created reality, the principle according to which it comes into existence and the source of beauty and equality.

36. SA I 8.8.4: 175,90f.

created goodness. In both contexts, the Son fully receives and perfectly expresses the Father's goodness.

Finally, William comes to the Holy Spirit. As with the Son, his consideration of the Holy Spirit begins in the context of the immanent Trinity. Here, however, William lingers longer in that context. As seen above, the proper names of the Holy Spirit are love and gift. William now adds the "breath" or "wind" *(spiramen)* in which the Holy Spirit is "spirated" essentially from the Father and the Son.[37] As the common spiration of the first two divine persons, the Holy Spirit is also the means by which the Father and the Son have their fruition, "since they love themselves by the Holy Spirit."[38]

Just as the Holy Spirit's role within the Trinity *ad intra* is linked directly to its appropriated titles, so the Spirit's appropriated names are intimately related to its role in the economy of salvation. William allocates no little space in this chapter to the mission of the Holy Spirit and its implications. After distinguishing the Spirit's eternal procession from the Father and the Son from its temporal mission, he argues that the primary appropriated name of the Holy Spirit is goodness or kindness *(bonitas sive benignitas)*.[39] He then poses several clarifying questions

---

37. SA I 8.8.4: 172,16. . . . *quia spiratur essentialiter a Patre et Filio, dicitur etiam Spiritus Sanctus spiramen.*

38. SA I 8.8.4: 175,93. . . . *quia Pater et Filius fruuntur se Spiritu Sancto, quia diligunt se Spiritu Sancto.* Related to this is his interpretation of a statement from Augustine, which William calls "most difficult *(difficillime).*" In the *De doctrina Christiana,* the bishop of Hippo had said: "in the Father is eternity, in the Son equality, in the Holy Spirit the eternity of equality, since [the Holy Spirit] is unity *(connexio),* and all things are eternal on account of the Father, equal on account of the Son, and united *(connexa)* on account of the Holy Spirit" (Augustine, *De doctrina Christ.,* I, c.5, n.5 [PL 34.21]). William interprets this to mean that the Holy Spirit completes and consummates the eternity and equality of the Father and the Son. For "just as the Father gives his highest goodness to the Holy Spirit, so also does the Son." But the communication of the Father's goodness is not complete until the Holy Spirit receives it from the Son. Thus, *ad intra,* the Holy Spirit is the unity *(connexio)* by which divine beatitude is completed and consummated (SA I 8.8.4: 174,50–53).

39. As justification, he offers arguments similar to those given for the Son's appropriations. In normal use, the word "spirit" suggests pride and indignation (as in "spirited"), and so, to ensure that this would not be associated with the Holy Spirit, goodness or kindness is appropriated to the Spirit (SA I 8.8.1: 157,10). Also, just as the Son proceeds from the Father, and the Holy Spirit proceeds from both, so wisdom proceeds from power, and from power and wisdom comes good will, that is the goodness of the soul (SA I 8.8.1: 157,13). Commenting on a Pauline formula from Romans 11:36—*from him and through*

concerning the Spirit's mission. Does the Spirit give itself *(det se)* and send itself *(mittat se)*? Is the Spirit properly given or only said to be given? Is the Spirit a single gift or several? As he proceeds, it becomes clear that William is thinking of mission in a specific sense, namely, as an infusion *(infusio)* of the Holy Spirit into the hearts of believers.

The question whether the Holy Spirit is properly given or only after a manner of speaking leads William into a lengthy discussion on the relationship between the Holy Spirit and grace. This produces several helpful insights into his pneumatology. In the main, he argues that while properly speaking the Holy Spirit is not a kind of "thing" which can be discretely given, it nevertheless can be said to be truly and properly given. For "when the Holy Spirit is given, its grace is also given, which is a kind of thing."[40] In this way, "through grace and in grace the Holy Spirit is both possessed and given."[41] William offers an analogy: "By grace the Holy Spirit is given as the contained in the container *(ut contentum in continente)*." For the Holy Spirit "is contained in grace" and "just as when a jar full of wine is given, the wine is properly given, so when grace is given the Holy Spirit is given in it."[42]

William's intent here is to distinguish grace and the Spirit adequately, without separating them. This intimate relation is important for William in light of the purpose of the presence of the Spirit and grace in the life of the believer: namely, to cause fruition. Hence, William argues that "if grace causes us to have fruition of God, God does the same thing and God is the prime matter of fruition, since [God] is the sweetness of fruition and [God] conserves that grace."[43] And, again "grace is given, therefore, so that it may indwell [the believer], but God or the Holy Spirit is given in as much as the free power of having fruition of God is given."[44] Thus, for William, the teleology of the Spirit's grace-ful presence is

---

and in him are all things—William suggests that the preposition "in" signifies "conservation in being, which pertains to the goodness of God" (SA I 8.8.2: 159,29). Yet all these arguments are subordinate to the primary one: it is the Spirit which makes the perfect communication of divine goodness within the Trinity complete and beatifying.

40. SA I 8.8.2: 163,14ff.
41. SA I 8.8.2: 168,35. . . . *nam per gratiam et in gratia habetur et datur Spiritus Sanctus.*
42. SA I 8.8.2: 168,36ff.   43. SA I 8.8.2: 170,111.
44. SA I 8.8.2: 169,83.

fruition—precisely the same role which the Spirit has in the Trinity *ad intra*.

William is not altogether comfortable with the "wine in a jar" analogy, and he does not pursue it. His preferred metaphor for the infusion of the Holy Spirit is spiritual food *(cibus spiritualis)* or, more precisely, spiritual bread *(panis spiritualis)*. For "grace is given so that it may indwell the soul and cause it to have fruition of God, and the Holy Spirit is properly given as spiritual bread."[45] This is the germ of William's doctrine of the Spirit *ad extra*: the Spirit infused into the hearts of the faithful as spiritual bread in order to cause fruition.

It is this idea of spiritual bread which William takes up in a final inquiry concerning the mission of the Holy Spirit: "Whether the Father and the Son are One Bread in as much as They are Given." The complete form of the question is as follows: "[I]t is asked whether the Father and the Son are one bread in as much as they are given or are multiple breads on the part of the persons." The initial position offered is in fact William's own: "It is proved that they are only one bread, since there is a single goodness and suavity and sweetness which nourishes us; hence, they are only one bread." A rebuttal, however, introduces two counterexamples—one pertaining to the Incarnate Christ, one pertaining to the Trinity—which clarify his position. First, the Incarnate Christ "delights us in as much as he is God, but also in as much as he is man." Second, "the Father not only refreshes us in as much as he is God, but also in as much as he generates a Son equal to himself," and again, "beatitude does not only consist in the apprehension of God as God, but also in apprehension of the Trinity." In light of both examples, there seem to be diverse origins of love and refection and thus "several breads."[46]

William's solution is illuminating. He argues that "the Trinity for its own part is only one bread." With respect to rational creatures, however, "it is a manifold bread, just as the Holy Spirit is single, but with respect to us the Holy Spirit is manifold *(multiplex)*." He then responds to the

---

45. SA I 8.8.2: 168,29. *Ad hoc videtur dicendum quod gratia datur ut insit et ut faciat animam frui Deo, et Spiritus Sanctu proprie datur ut spiritualis cibus, et ita uterque datur suo modo.*

46. SA I 8.8.3.4: 171,2–13.

objections. The humanity of Christ delights rational creatures because of its union with the essentially good divine nature, and the Father generates a Son on account of the goodness of the divine nature. Thus, the refection and nourishment contained in the knowledge of God has a single source: "namely the goodness or suavity of God."[47]

With these clarifications concerning the infused presence of the Holy Spirit, William's reflections on the names appropriated to the Holy Spirit under the overarching concept of goodness can be better appreciated. For he asserts that the Holy Spirit is called breath or wind *(spiramen)*, "not only because he is spirated essentially from the Father and the Son," but also because "he is spirated to us, that is, he is secretly infused for the illumination and sanctification of our hearts." The Holy Spirit is *spiramen*, both in the immanent Trinity by way of procession and in the economy by way of infusion. Not only that, but as an infused presence within the believer the Holy Spirit illumines and sanctifies. William is especially interested in the former term, as an additional appropriation reveals. An objector asks "why teaching is appropriated to the Holy Spirit; whence: *the Holy Spirit will teach you all things* (Jn 14:26)?" Should not this be appropriated to the Son who is wisdom, "since to teach, to illumine properly pertain to wisdom, not to goodness." William replies by reminding his readers that indeed "the works of the Trinity are indivisible," and thus, "if the Holy Spirit illumines and teaches, so does the Father and the Son." But, "because the Holy Spirit is properly love and gift ... the posterior gifts [that is, the gifts of wisdom and understanding] which proceed properly from love are appropriated to him."[48] This passage suggests the intimate relationship between wisdom and goodness, between the Son's identity and function and the Spirit's.

William considers this relationship more explicitly as he turns to the next appropriated title, where he calls the Holy Spirit the "*finger of God*" (Lk 11:20). "For just as with a corporal finger we show corporal things to corporal eyes, so by the finger which is the Holy Spirit spiritual things are shown to spiritual eyes" (1 Cor 12:4).[49] Here, William gives his most

47. SA I 8.8.3.4: 171,15ff.
48. SA I 8.8.4: 172,3ff.
49. SA I.8.8.4: 172,20ff.

explicit indication of the identity and function of the Holy Spirit in the economy, and precisely here its implications for the knowledge of God are most clearly evident. In the economy, the Holy Spirit is the breath and wind infused into the hearts of believers precisely in order to reveal and to manifest the goodness of God which has been fully communicated to and perfectly expressed in the Son. The goodness of God is only truly visible and audible in the Son, through the Holy Spirit's infusion and activity within the believer. As the "finger of God," the Holy Spirit teaches, illumines, and "points out" spiritual things to spiritual eyes. For this reason, William appropriates goodness to the Holy Spirit. Only through the Spirit is the uncreated divine goodness perceptible in the Son. Thus, finally, the Holy Spirit is the manifold, delectable spiritual bread of believers.

In sum, the same trinitarian formula concerning God's own self-knowledge—the Father's goodness perceived in the Son through the Holy Spirit with delight—is apparent also in the activity of the economic Trinity. In created reality the Father's goodness is present and perceptible on account of the sapiential activity of the Son, as mirror, word, exemplar, art, and beauty. That goodness is perceptible with delectation through the Holy Spirit's infusion into the hearts of believers which reveals it, resulting in fruition.

Trinitarian Metaphysics of the Good

Thus William's doctrine of the Trinity, both immanent and economic, contains this basic principle: the uncreated goodness of the Father is apprehended in the Son through the Holy Spirit with delectation. At the same time, it will be remembered that in his treatise on the nature of the good, William employed a threefold division of the good—essential, participatory, and graced goodness—which described not only the ontological status of uncreated and created goodness, but also the manner in which the former is apprehended in the latter. It is now possible to integrate these two.

It has already been observed that when William speaks of the Father's goodness as being communicated fully to the Son, and from both of them to the Holy Spirit, he is speaking of the *bonum in essentia*, described in the treatise on the good. It is also clear that created reality exists and exists as good (has *esse* and *bonum esse*) because it receives *bonum esse* and persists in it through the exemplary and mediating function of the Son as wisdom. Because the Son, who *ad intra* is the perfect expression of the Father's goodness, is also, *ad extra*, the sapiential exemplar, art, and formal cause of creation, created things participate in the Son and can therefore also be called good and can express that goodness. This corresponds to William's category of the *bonum naturae*. Finally, William's discussion of the appropriations and corresponding function of the Holy Spirit indicated an intimate relationship between the Holy Spirit and grace in the life of the believer. Thus, the category of the *bonum gratiae* is to be aligned with the Holy Spirit. As in the treatise on the good, where William indicated the necessity of the *bonum gratiae* for apprehending the *bonum in essentia* within the *bonum naturae*, so also here the apprehension of the Father's goodness within the Son requires the Holy Spirit. Just as the perception of uncreated goodness within created goods occurred with delight through the *bonum gratiae*, so too here with the Spirit.

So, the general principle of the knowledge of God from the treatise on the good is seen to have an explicitly theological foundation within the divine life: *ad intra* knowledge of God is the delectable perception and cognition of the Father's goodness within the Son through the Holy Spirit. Accordingly, it also may be given an explicitly theological formulation: *ad extra* knowledge of God is the delectable perception and cognition of essential goodness within the *bonum naturae*, as it participates in the Son, through *the bonum gratiae*, infused by and with the Holy Spirit.

Conclusion

The central implication of William's trinitarian theology is this: knowledge of God comes through the encounter with God's activity *ad extra*, that is, in the encounter with God's created effects. This means that, for William, the knowledge of God as the good is the end of rational creatures, but this in two ways. Essentially and *in se*, God is one and thus there is a single Object *in which (in quo)* knowledge of God is realized. Effectively, however, God's created effects are manifold, and in this way there is a diversity of objects *by which* (the *finis quo*) knowledge of God occurs, a range of modes *through which* God is encountered, namely, the *delectabilia divina*. Essentially the *summum bonum* is a single good, a single object of knowledge, a single bread, but a multiple end, a manifold bread in effect.

In light of the trinitarian foundation and principle of William's doctrine of the knowledge of God, it is possible to appreciate more fully his doctrine of the spiritual senses, as described both in the treatise on the nature of the good and in the treatise on beatitude. In the former, the objects of the spiritual senses are the manifold created effects (the *bonum naturae*) of uncreated goodness (the *bonum in essentia*), delectably perceived through graced virtues (the *bonum gratiae*). In the latter, William not only spoke of the *divina delectabilia*, but also gave the spiritual senses a general Christological orientation: the singular object of the spiritual senses *in patria* is the divine nature of Christ. Both of these descriptions are more fully intelligible from the perspective of William's trinitarian theology. From that perspective, these objects are the manifold operations and activities of divine wisdom (hence, the Christological orientation of the spiritual senses) who, as exemplar, art, and beauty of creation, makes all created things to be words and images and mirrors of uncreated goodness. This sapiential vision is possible, however, only as wisdom is revealed and made manifest to the spiritual senses through the presence and activity of the Spirit within the believer. Accordingly, though ultimately there is a single object of spiritual apprehension—a single "spiritual bread," namely the Trinity—the means to knowledge of the Trinity are the manifold effects of divine goodness present in the Son, revealed by the Holy Spirit. This is the rationale for William's doctrine of the *delectabilia divina* and a primary assumption in his teaching on the spiritual senses. Knowledge of God through the spiritual senses is the Spirit-facilitated perception of the *delectabilia divina* in the Son, or perhaps better, the delectable apprehension of sapiential goodness in the Son through the Spirit.

CHAPTER 5

CREATION

The Manifestation of the *Delectabilia Divina*

FOR WILLIAM, the possibility of knowledge of God through God's created effects is grounded in his doctrine of exemplarity,[1] which he introduced while describing the personal properties of the Son. William's exemplarism posits an analogy between created and uncreated reality, on the basis of which he justifies predicating of God characteristics found in created reality. To speak, as he did in discussing beatitude, of divine *suavitas, dulcedo, calor, pulchrum,* or *symphonia* as the objects of the spiritual senses is, of course, to take up language and concepts drawn from creation. William's doctrine of exemplarity will be examined here in detail, then, as the crucial link between God *in se* and creation, which allows for the possibility of knowledge of God that the spiritual senses enjoy.

Exemplarity in the Theology of William of Auxerre

William's explicit treatment of exemplarity comes in the form of a relatively short tractate, entitled "On the Exemplar," which introduces

1. As with numerous other topics, the medieval theory of exemplarity finds its roots in the thought of Augustine of Hippo, though the doctrine reaches back to Plato. Traditionally, this doctrine has both an ontological and an epistemological dimension; in the Augustinian tradition the latter is closely related to a doctrine of illumination. In the medieval period the theory's most well-known advocate is Bonaventure, for whom it was the center and key of all metaphysics; see Zachary Hayes, *The Hidden Center: Spirituality and Speculative Christology in St. Bonaventure* (New York: The Franciscan Institute, 1992), p. 12. Though, generally speaking, William does not develop this doctrine as far as Bonaventure, one frequently hears an echo of the Franciscan's teaching in William's theology.

Book II of the *Summa Aurea*. Book II considers the topic of creation generally (angels, prophecy, and sin are also included). William's decision, therefore, to begin the book with a discussion of exemplarity signals its foundational position. As an introductory preface, he notes that prior to speaking of the creation, "something must be said concerning how the world was created and the first question is concerning the exemplar, in whose imitation this sensible world was made."[2] This he does under three headings: first, "what the exemplar is," and whether it is properly fitting to his substance to be the exemplar or idea of the sensible world; second, "whether the Son is the archetypal world"; third, "how sensible things proceed from the eternal exemplar."

A consensus among twelfth-century masters had argued that, strictly speaking, the exemplar of all things is the whole Trinity.[3] In this view, the Son is called exemplar only by appropriation.[4] William argues by contrast that the Son should receive the designation "exemplar" not only by appropriation, but also properly. His position is a direct implication of his trinitarian theology, where the Son's proper designations included *Imago* and *Verbum* of the Father. The Son is properly the *Imago* and *Verbum* of the Father because in the Son the Father can be fully seen and the Son perfectly and completely expresses the Father. But here William extends the thought. He argues that the Son is not merely the Image in which the Father is seen, but the one in whom "all things are seen and shine forth *(relucent)*";[5] "the Son is the *Imago* in which all that is to be seen is seen."[6] Similarly, the Son is called the *Verbum* of the Father, not only because he fully expresses the Father's goodness *(expressissime loquitur Dei bonitatem)*, but also because "by speaking this, [the Word] speaks all things."[7] As the full expression, then, of the Father's fecundity,

---

2. SA II 1: 11,1.

3. Among others, the editor notes Abelard, *Intr. ad Theol.* I n.10; *Theol. christ.* IV (PL 178.992–93, 1282); Hugh of St. Victor, *Didascalicon* VII c.1; *De sacramentis* I p.2 c.6 (PL 176.811, 208); and the *Summa Sententiarum* I 11 (PL 176.58s).

4. SA II 1.1: 12,11ff. "Yet for the same reason that wisdom is appropriated to the Son of God, exemplar or idea of the world *(exemplar sive ydeam mundi)* is appropriated, and for this reason the Son is called exemplar, not properly but by appropriation *(non proprie sed appropriate)*."

5. SA II 1.1: 13,28.   6. SA II 1.1: 13,20.

7. SA II 1.1: 13,34.

the Son also expresses all that the Trinity is in relation to the finite. In communicating most perfectly his goodness to the Son, the Father communicated all that he would create as well. The Son is thus the "proper cause of all things."[8] For William, therefore, the Son's proper designation as Image and Word of the Father entails the notion of exemplarity and the Son, accordingly, is to be designated Exemplar both properly and by appropriation.[9]

William expands upon the concept of exemplarity when he asks whether the Son is identical with the archetypal world *(mundus architipus)*. The question was much discussed by his twelfth-century predecessors, and his treatment is shaped by that discussion.[10] He begins with a definition: the archetypal world is "the divine disposition *(dispositio)* or ordination *(ordinatio)* which was from eternity in the divine mind concerning creatures which were to be made."[11] An etymological analysis emphasizes the point: "*architipus* is said from *archos*, that is, the principal, and *tipus*, that is, the figure, as if to say, the principal figure" *(principalis figura)*.[12]

Is the Son identical with the *mundus architipus*? Yes and no. "Archetypal world" does in fact denote the Son. In this respect, it is a synonym for "exemplar," and like it can be applied to the Son both by appropriation and properly.[13] Yet, "archetypal world" also connotes something created, namely those things which would eventually be created in accordance with their archetypes.[14] But this raises a difficulty. Created things

---

8. SA II 1.1: 13,29. "The proper cause *(proprie causa)* of all things is seen there; for every created thing is known and seen *(cognoscitur et videtur)* in its proper cause."

9. SA II 1.1: 13,33. "The Son of God is not only by appropriation but also properly the image, idea, [and] exemplar of all created things *(ymago, ydea, exemplar omnium rerum)*."

10. SA II 1.2: 14,9f. William reports a threefold opinion on this question current in his day. First, "there are some who say that the archetypal world is identical with God." Second, "others say that the archetypal world and the sensible world are the same essentially, but differ by reason, since it is called the sensible world in as much as it is subject to the senses, but called the archetypal world in as much as it is invisible and in the divine mind." Third, "others say that the archetypal world is neither God nor the sensible world, but those ideas which were eternally in the divine mind, which are neither God nor the sensible world, and this was the opinion of Plato. Hence, they say that the collection of those ideas is the archetypal world."

11. SA II 1.2: 15,46.   12. SA II 1.2: 16,63.

13. SA II 1.2: 15–16,48.

14. SA II 1.2: 16,49ff: "This term '*mundus archetipus*' or '*exemplar*' connotes, in addi-

are manifold, while the divine nature is characterized by the highest simplicity, and yet apparently the designation "exemplar" or "archetypal world" refers to both.[15] William does not offer a completely satisfactory answer to this question and, in fact, appears skeptical as to whether such an answer is possible.[16] He simply asserts that "diversity is not denoted in the exemplar, but in that of which it is the exemplar,"[17] namely, created things.[18]

William's essential position on the question is this: within God, the ideas which constitute the *mundus architipus* are not distinct from one another or from the divine essence; logically, though, the ideas can be distinguished in thought and in signification.[19] The distinction between

---

tion to the Son of God or the divine essence, exemplarity in creatures, and this is from the mode of signifying *(ex modo significandi).*"

15. Gilson asks: "Is there a real plurality of ideas in God? The extreme difficulty which we encounter when we undertake the study of this question is due to a sort of contradiction inherent in it. To resolve it we have in fact to discover a method of reconciling the One and the Many. . . . Without ideas, there is no providence or divine liberty; but with them, divine unity disappears"; Etienne Gilson, *The Philosophy of St. Bonaventure* (Paterson, N.J.: St. Anthony Guild Press, 1965), pp. 135–36.

16. SA II 1.2: 18,104.

17. SA II 1.2: 17,98. "For when diverse ideas *(diverse ydee)* are spoken, diversity *(diversitas)* is not understood in the exemplar *(exemplari)* but in that of which it is an exemplar *(exemplatis)*."

18. Later in Book II, William offers a more elaborate rationale for this assertion: "For granted [something] is known indistinctly *in Verbo,* yet in the same Word it is known distinctly and according to its own idea. For just as the first cause according to itself, and so according to the same, is the cause of a singular thing, in as much as it is singular, and the cause of plural things in as much as they are plural, so the same idea according to itself and so according to the same, is the image or exemplar of the singular, in as much as it is singular, and of plural things in as much as they are plural. And this argument is not valid: the image of man, in as much as it is a man, since it is common to all men, is not the image of a particular man, in as much as it is distinct. Similarly the image of white, in as much as it is white, is not the image of a particular white thing, in as much as it is distinct from other white things. Therefore, by the same reason, the idea, since it is the image of all things, is not the image of a particular entity, in as much as it is distinct. For just as in natural things one nature is confined to one act and is not related to every act, so one image is naturally confined so that it is a sign specially of that of which it is an image. But just as the first cause is not confined to a certain effect, or to man in as much as he is man, or toward a donkey in as much as it is a donkey, or to one in as much as it is one, or to plural things in as much as it is plural, but is related to all those things and according to the same, so the first idea is not confined to a certain sign; but all signs signify [it] according to the same thing in all diverse things" (SA II 6.1: 128,107ff).

19. In this treatise, William speaks of a logical distinction and the multiplicity of the ideas with respect to existing things, while maintaining their simplicity and indistinctness

them is not in what they are, but in what they connote, that is, the real multiplicity of created things, not the divine essence.[20]

Significantly, it is at this point that William introduces the role of the Holy Spirit into his exemplarism. If, in the Son, the ideas are one and indistinct, and yet with respect to creation they are manifold, what is the link between the two? For William, in a certain way of speaking *(tropo loquendi)*, God is "diverse ideas" *(diverse ydee)*, since, as he goes on to suggest, the book of Wisdom says that "the Holy Spirit is manifold *(multiplex)* (7:22) . . . on account of the diverse effects, or on account of the power by which [the Holy Spirit] is able to produce infinite effects outside of itself *(ex se)*; yet *in se* God is most simple and invariable *(simplicissimus est et invariabilis).*"[21] The link between the Son, in whose divine simplicity the exemplary ideas are undifferentiated from each other and from the divine essence, and the real multiplicity and manifold diversity of the creation is the Holy Spirit. Denying, therefore, neither the divine simplicity nor the manifold creation, William envisions a direct, intimate, and immediate relationship between Creator and created through the activity and power of the Holy Spirit. He conceives of all created reality as the manifold, even infinite effects of the Uncreated Spirit.[22]

---

in God; cf. SA II 6.1: 129–30,141ff: "Things are said to be in God in a threefold way, namely, *per causam, per gratiam,* and *per cognitionem. Per causam,* as Paul said in Acts: *in whom we live and move and have our being.* Of which Augustine said: 'not as of his substance, are we thus in him, as he is said to have life in himself.' But since we are something different from God, we are only in God because God operates, whence we live and exist. Now the saints are in God *per gratiam.* . . . And, to the extent that things are said to be in God *per cognitionem,* things were in God from eternity, and in this mode they are said to be one on account of the one idea which represents all things; according to which trope Aristotle said that: 'the soul in a certain way is all things' [*De anima,* III], since the images of all things have to be imprinted on the soul. According to this trope the authority [Anselm] says that 'the creature in God is an uncreated essence, but *in se* it is created' [Anselm, *Monolog.,* c. 34; PL 158.189]. But properly speaking it would be heretical to say this."

20. For a discussion of Bonaventure's similar position on this, see Gilson, *The Philosophy of St. Bonaventure,* pp. 138–39.

21. SA II 1.2: 17,90ff.

22. In contrast to the pseudo-Dionysian tradition, William brooks no possibility of created intermediaries which intervene between God and creation. Thus he seems to develop his exemplarism with a view toward refuting dualist modes of thought. See Gilson, *The Philosophy of St. Bonaventure:* "The universe has been created out of nothing and in time by a unique principle. This statement does not merely state the obvious fact that God is one, or even that we cannot admit with the Manichees one principle for good and

The assertion that the manifold creation consists in the direct, intimate, and immediate effects of the Trinity *ex se*, however, raises a final set of questions concerning the relation between creation and the Creator. These William considers in the third and final section of this tractate.

First, it seems that if creation flows directly and immediately from an invariable and immutable source, then it too should be invariable and immutable. In response, William asserts that the mutability and variability of creation arises from the fact that "all things are from God *(a Deo)*, yet they are not out of God *(de Deo)*, but out of nothing."²³ That is, "they proceed through the mode of will *(per modum voluntatis)* . . . and are not out of the divine essence *(de essentia divina)*."²⁴ Hence, "they are reducible to nothing as a first principle." In contrast, the Son is both from the Father *(a patre)* and of the Father *(de Patre)*,²⁵ and, thus, shares in the Father's immutability and invariability.

The assertion that creation is *a Deo* yet not *de Deo* leads to a second question: what kind of causal relation does in fact obtain between Creator and creation. William avers, "God is the efficient, formal or exemplary, and final cause of things," but "in no way is God the material cause" of things.²⁶ Accordingly, "the *exemplum* does not possess a similitude to its Exemplar in all things; for it has a similitude in form, but not in matter" *(similitudinem in forma, sed non in materia)*.²⁷ Thus, "sensible things are variable because of their matter, since they are from nothing."²⁸ The introduction of matter accounts for the diversity and plurality in created things, in contrast to the simplicity of the divine nature.²⁹

A third and final point pertains to the issue of divine freedom in relation to creation. Here, William brooks no possibility of the necessity of

---

another for evil; its chief significance is that God has produced everything of Himself, immediately, and without intermediary" (p. 178).

23. SA II 1.3: 22–23,22. 24. SA II 1.3: 23,37.
25. SA II 1.3: 23,24. 26. SA II 1.3: 23,46.
27. SA II 1.3: 23,28. 28. SA II 1.3: 23,33.

29. Bonaventure seems to hold a similar view. See Gilson, *The Philosophy of St. Bonaventure:* "The plurality of the things which are expressed by [God] owes its multiplicity in fact to the intervention of matter, and, as all matter is alien to God, what is multiple outside of Him must be one in Him; the multiple ideas of creatures cannot then be distinct realities within the divine mind" (p. 138).

creation. Though the creation flows out from the Creator on account of his essential goodness,[30] God's creative act—which William is fond of comparing to that of an artist[31]—is nonetheless an unconstrained act of will and intellect *(per modum voluntatis et intellectus).*[32]

William's exemplarism can now be summarized thus. Properly and by appropriation, the Son is the Exemplar in whom is the full expression, not only of the divine essence, but also of all that God would create *ad extra*. Within himself and without compromise to the divine simplicity, the Son contains the archetypes, the exemplary ideas *(mundus architipus)*, of all created things. Accordingly, the created order has a direct, immediate relationship to the Creator. While in no way *de Deo*, creation is nonetheless *a Deo*, through a completely free and unconstrained act of will and intellect. In contrast to his immediate predecessors, therefore, William brings exemplary causes back into play in his account of creation.[33]

From the perspective of the possibility of the knowledge of God, William's exemplarism has important implications. The link between the Trinity *ad intra* and its created effects *ad extra* is the Son as Image/Verbum/Exemplar. As the Word is the inner self-expression of God, so the created order is the external expression of that inner Word.

---

30. SA II 1.3: 23,39.

31. This theme will be pursued further in Chapter 8.

32. SA II.1.2: 21,198. A final issue affords William the opportunity to clarify the relationship between goodness and wisdom in relation to divine causality. If "all things flow from God through the mode of liberality, why does it say in the Psalm: *you have made all things in wisdom* (103:24), and it does not say: all things in liberality or goodness?" William responds: "when it says: *you have made all things in wisdom*, this preposition 'in' denotes the exemplary cause; but if it had said: all things in goodness, it would have been completely true, since this preposition 'in' would have denoted the efficient cause."

33. See Marsha L. Colish, "Early Scholastic Angelology," *Recherches de théologie ancienne et médiévale* 62 (1995): pp. 99–100. Colish notes that, following Philo and Augustine, William identifies the exemplars with ideas in the mind of God. In his treatment of exemplarism, a primary concern is to refute the Platonic view of the exemplars as standing above, or as existing independently of God, and also that God had to create the universe in virtue of having the *rationes* of all things in His mind. He also refutes the doctrine of the eternity of the world by drawing a clear distinction between the exemplars of all things in God's mind, eternally, and the reification of the creatures whose forms they become in time through God's free creative act. Moreover, William expressly rejects a chain of being or emanationist model of creation.

"Creatures are an exterior word *(verbum exterius)*, by which the Father speaks his goodness," and such speaking occurs "through an interior word *(verbum interius)*." So, "the Father speaks exterior words through the interior word," that is to say, "the Father operates through the Son,"[34] as "an artist *(artifex)* operates through his art or wisdom."[35] William's exemplarism, then, establishes a direct link not only between created things and the Word, but also between created things and the Trinity *in se*. While the Father's goodness is expressed essentially in the Son, that same goodness is expressed derivatively in the act of creation. In this way, created things are exterior manifestations and expressions of the divine goodness.[36] At the same, William has specified an important role of the Holy Spirit within the creative act, in conjunction with the exemplary function of the Son. The reference to the diverse created effects wrought by the Holy Spirit recalls William's discussion of the Holy Spirit in his trinitarian theology. Especially telling is his reference to Wisdom 7:22, concerning the manifold *(multiplex)* character of the Spirit's work. In his trinitarian theology, this aspect of the Spirit's person and work establishes the principle that knowledge of God is the perception of divine goodness within its diverse created effects.

In short, then, William's doctrine of exemplarism is central to his conception of the possibility of the knowledge of God: exemplarism provides the condition for the possibility of the apprehension of uncreated goodness within its created effects. The manifold effects of the Trinity mediate knowledge of God. Because all things are made according to their pattern in the divine mind, they have a relation to their source and reflect their origin.

---

34. SA I 8.8.2: 158,6ff.
35. SA I 8.8.2: 158,3.
36. Again, Gilson's remarks seem apt in William's case: "The relation of the ideas to the divine substance, considered in its metaphysical origin, is therefore one with the relation of the Son to the Father. In conceiving and engendering from all eternity, in the act by which He thinks Himself, what He can and will manifest externally of His own thought, God has expressed all things in his Son" (*The Philosophy of St. Bonaventure*, p. 134).

Toward a Doctrine of Analogy

At the conclusion of his treatment of exemplarity, William raises a final issue which follows directly from the foregoing, but bears most explicitly on the question of the knowledge of God. How can the absolutely simple divine nature be characterized by and, perhaps more importantly, known through manifold attributes or qualities *(notiones)* such as justice, goodness, liberality, and the like? His solution to the question goes to the heart of how the transcendent God can be an object of spiritual apprehension.

In form, the issue is similar to that raised with respect to the exemplary ideas in the divine mind: how can they be manifold when the divine essence is simple? Regarding content, the issue is more directly related to the question of the knowledge of God, for it concerns the attributes and qualities of the divine nature which can be experienced, perceived, and known. William's solution to the issue, accordingly, is formally similar to his solution to the issue of exemplarity. He begins by affirming the divine simplicity. Speaking most properly, God is not, for example, just through something called justice or liberal through something else called liberality; rather God is good, liberal, and just simply as God.[37] It is possible, nonetheless, to distinguish and name various divine attributes. This, significantly, is done with respect to God's created effects; it pertains not to the divine simplicity, but rather to God in relation to created things. Hence, God is called just or liberal "with respect to particular effects *(ad effectus quosdam)*, not with respect to all."[38] Accordingly, statements such as "God is just" or "God is liberal" posit no essential diversity on God's part, but are linguistic *(in modo significandi)* or conceptual *(per modum intelligendi)* distinctions predicated in relation to creatures.[39] For William, such predication is based upon certain similitudes *(similitudines)* and conformities *(convenientiae)*, a certain proportion or imitation which exists between God and God's effects:[40] "but we make

---

37. SA II 1.3: 29,198.
38. SA II 1.3: 29,203. The case is the same for exemplary causality, cf. SA II 1.3: 30,223.
39. SA II 1 3: 30,211.
40. Drawing on his predecessors, William distinguished three kinds of similarity between God and creation: a similitude of conformity *(similitudo conformitas)*, a similitude

such specification ... through the proportion or imitation *(per proportionem sive imitationem)* which created powers have with respect to God."⁴¹ The possibility that God can be named and thus known by human persons is in part a function of the fact that in some way language appropriate to created things can be applied by analogy to divine things. Certain logical and linguistic expressions are appropriate *(conformes)* both to the divine and the created sphere.⁴² Thus, though he does not here explicitly use the term, he posits some form of analogy between created and Creator.⁴³

What kind of conformity or proportion does William envision? He allows, on the one hand, that the concept of being *("ens")*, for example, can in some sense be applied both to God and to creatures. A proper name *(nomen proprium)* for God is "being not from another" *(ens non ab alio)*. As in William's analysis of the good, a creature entails a twofold *esse*: created *esse* in the creature itself and the divine *esse* as the source *(a quo)* of its created being. The *esse* of a concrete existing thing is derived from that which is *esse per se*. At the same time, however, he rejects any essential similitude between God and creation. The divine sphere is too radically transcendent for the word *"ens"* to be referred univocally to God as the first being *(primum ens)* as well as to created beings.⁴⁴ Yet this

---

of representation *(similitudo representationis)*, and a similitude of imitation in concrete acts *(similitudo imitationis in operibus discrete factis)* (SA II 9.1.2: 231,41). It seems that the *similitudo conformitatis* is what William has in mind here. In general the created world resembles its Creator through a *similitudo representationis*. Human persons, created in the image and likeness of God (Gn 1:26), possess a *similitudo imitationis* in relation to God in discrete acts (SA II 9.1.2: 231,53ff). Elsewhere, he offers a different set of similitudes: a *similitudo nature*, a *similitudo gratie*, and a *similitudo glorie* (SA II 3.2: 50,11 ff.), though he does not elaborate on it.

41. SA II 1.3: 29–30,206.
42. SA I 7.1: 114,113ff.
43. SA I 8.6: 146,159f. This observation and the analysis of analogy which follows are indebted to Johannes Arnold's *Perfecta communicatio*, pp. 54–62.
44. SA I 14.1: 264,96ff. Cf. SA I Prol: 19,23f.: "divine things infinitely exceed natural things"; cf. SA II 9.1.2: 231,51f.: "even if there is a certain relatedness *(convenientia)* between humans and God, yet there difference is maximal"; SA I 5.1: 68,84ff.: "For although the *primum ens* flows out *(influens)* into its effects, yet the name 'ens' does not signify this in relation to *(in habitudine)* that or in that outflowing *(fluxo)*." Even though it is not explicitly mentioned in the *Summa Aurea*, William seems to share the sentiments of the Fourth Lateran Council: "*inter creatorem et creaturam non potest tanta similitudo notari, quin inter eos maior sit dissimilitudo notanda*" (DH 806).

does not relegate theological language to complete equivocation. Rather, without explicitly using the term, William seems to posit an *analogia attributionis*.⁴⁵ An agreement (conformity, proportion) exists solely in the effects of the divine and human attributes, such as goodness, justice, mercy. In relation to their effects, for example, both God and Peter can be called "just" without equivocation,⁴⁶ because divine and created justice both consist in rendering to each his due.⁴⁷ Although God is in the actual and comprehensive sense the cause of all things, God is said to be "just" or "generous" respectively regarding certain effects.⁴⁸ Hence "when it is said: 'God is just,' God as justice is signified, that is, in comparison with such acts as created justice elicits from itself; yet God himself is that

---

45. Cf. Principe, *Hypostatic Union:* "Although William of Auxerre does not state the relationship in just these terms, . . . he seems to teach what would now be called the analogy of attribution" (p. 30). "William belongs to that group of theologians who say that some names are transferred from creatures to God according to a likeness in effects produced by the perfection in question. William, however, expressly denies that *ens* is parallel to *iustus* in this respect; hence it cannot be said that he holds for a doctrine of common predication of 'being' according to similarity of effects. . . . William gives the impression that his position with respect to common predication of being is exclusively that of the 'analogy of attribution,' a term that, of course, he himself does not use" (p. 178).

46. In SA I 4.2: 83,34ff, William lists five types of univocation. According to Principe, in William's thought "univocity" lacks its later technical sense and "is used simply in its etymological sense whereby it refers to calling several realities by the same name or word; thus it includes certain technical types of analogy" (*Hypostatic Union,* p. 178). Arnold notes that for William the univocity of two terms assumes their objective agreement: "every univocation is according to a certain agreement (*omnis univocatio est secundum aliquam convenientiam*)"; SA I 6.2: 82,9 (*Perfecta communicatio,* p. 55, n. 108).

47. SA I 5.3: 72,17ff.: "Truly speaking created justice and uncreated justice agree in no way, neither in genus (*in genere*), nor in species (*in specie*) nor in proper things (*in proprio*) nor in accidents (*in accidente*) and for this reason 'just' is properly said of God and of Peter equivocally (*equivoce*). But since in a certain way (*aliquo modo*) they agree in effect (*conveniunt in effectu*), for this reason in this word 'just' they are called the same thing (*univocantur*). For just as it is of created justice to return to everyone that which is his, so that same thing agrees (*convenit*) with uncreated justice, and thus, since uncreated justice agrees with (*convenit cum*) created justice in its essential effects (*in suo effectu essentiali*) for this reason they are called a single thing (*univocantur*)." SA II 9.1.q.2: 230,19ff.: "Created justice and uncreated justice share this (*communicant in hoc*), that just as by uncreated justice God returns to everyone that which is his, so a human being by created justice returns to everyone that which is his; thus the just person, in as much as he is just, agrees with (*convenit cum*) God; thus in this the human person is similar (*similis est*) to God."

48. SA I 5.1: 68,86. "But when it is said: 'God is just,' this word 'just' signifies the divine essence as a relative quality (*qualitatem habitum*), hence it signifies in relation to an act."

comparison *(comparatio)*.⁴⁹ For God in himself is comparable to all his effects."⁵⁰ That is to say, through himself, God allows himself to be in relationship to all God's effects. Strictly speaking, then, only a conceited agreement exists between the created and the divine.⁵¹ An efficient or formal or final cause within the created sphere can be applied in some way to God because God himself is the efficient, formal, and final cause of all things. For example, if humans can beget, then God the Father can also.⁵² Material statements about creatures by contrast may not be transferred to God, because God is in no way a material cause of creation.⁵³ Hence, creatures have a *similitudo in forma* to God as their archetype.⁵⁴ Elsewhere, William argues that the will of God and the rational human will are *conformes*, since both are directed toward virtue.⁵⁵ In other texts, he appropriates power, wisdom, and goodness to the divine persons on the basis of a *conformitas naturalium* or *in naturalibus*, where the dependent relations of created power, wisdom, and goodness correspond to the intra-divine processions.⁵⁶ In these examples *conformitas* obviously represents no agreement of essence, but a correspondence of structures.

---

49. William understands the term *comparatio* in a narrow sense ("comparison," SA III 5: 74,98ff) as well as in the broader sense ("relation," SA II 8.2.9.2: 215,18ff.).

50. SA II 1.3: 30,208. "Hence, when it is said: 'God is just,' God is signified as justice, that is, in comparison *(in comparatione)* with the kind of acts created justice *(iustitia creata)* elicits from itself; yet God himself is that *comparatio*. For God himself is comparable *(comparabilis)* to all his effects."

51. Arius was "deceived by the fanciful similitude of natural things" (SA I Prol: 18,13f; cf. SA II 10.6.1: 302,110ff) when he attributed to each of the three divine persons its own nature, according to the model of creatures.

52. Regarding the divine generation, William frequently refers to the created analogue. See SA I 8.8.4 (Version a): 299,17ff; cf. ibid. (late version): 173,44ff; SA I 11.7: 219,106ff; SA I 8.5: 139,168ff.

53. SA I 3.4: 35,85ff.

54. SA II 1.3: 23,28ff. "An exemplum does not have a similitude with its exemplar in every way; for it has similitude of form but not of matter, just as the image of Achilles, made out of air, had a similarity with Achilles in form but not in matter."

55. SA I 12.4.3: 233,51ff.

56. SA I 8.8.1: 293,5ff. Cf. SA I 14.2: "Every effect in which the creature imitates God is led back to the Trinity, since in them either the Father, the Son, or the Holy Spirit is imitated. So, God is in creatures, either through power, pertaining to the Father, or through presence or wisdom, pertaining to the Son, or through essence or goodness, pertaining to the Holy Spirit."

In sum: William's doctrine of exemplarism, and the notion of analogy entailed by it, establishes the possibility of predicating various attributes of the divine which are drawn from the realm of creation. Though William's examples in this section include goodness, justice, and the like, it is clear that the kinds of things he describes as apprehended by the spiritual senses are included. To speak of the harmony, beauty, suavity, or sweetness of God is justified on account of the fact that these are created concepts applied to the divine effects experienced in the soul.

Conclusion

As seen in the preceding chapters, William's theological metaphysics and his doctrine of the Trinity ground the possibility of the knowledge of God. The essential goodness of the Trinity, the *summum bonum*, "overflows" *ad extra* into manifold created effects, the *bonum natura*. The metaphysical possibility of something other than God *in se* which reflects and manifests the divine is grounded in the trinitarian goodness. The possibility of created *esse*, which is also *bonum esse* and in which the *bonum essentia* shines forth, is grounded in the primal fecundity of the *summum bonum*. In short, the possibility that there is an object of spiritual apprehension is grounded in the nature of God.

This chapter, however, has shown the next step in William's metaphysics. That created reality in fact imitates and reflects its source, that created goodness is in fact an intelligible and delectable reflection of uncreated goodness is a function of something further: namely, the Son as Exemplar of created reality and the Spirit as the power which brings about manifold created effects. *Ad extra*, the Holy Spirit is the Power by which the created effects of the Trinity are wrought *ex se*. *Ad extra*, the Son is Exemplar, containing within himself the ideas of all created reality. As Exemplar, the Son is the efficient cause of created reality. Moreover, because all things have their archetype within the Word and because the Word is the agent of their becoming and existence, they reflect their Source and can mediate knowledge of the Creator. In this way, the Son as Exemplar establishes a kind of analogy between created and uncreated reality, establishing the possibility that God can be known in the *speculum creaturarum*.

The implications of the foregoing for William's doctrine of spiritual apprehension are not far to seek. Knowledge of God is the apprehension of uncreated trinitarian goodness within its created effects. For William, God's created effects mediate knowledge of the divine attributes, which in turn pertain to the very being of God. William's doctrine of exemplarism and its concomitant (though inchoate) notion of analogy allow him to speak, not only of divine justice, goodness, mercy, impassibility, innascibility, but also of the divine *suavitas, dulcedo, pulchritudo, symphonia*, etc., in short, the objects of spiritual apprehension. These are a subset of the manifold effects of the Holy Spirit *ex se*, through which the Trinity is apprehended.

Symbolic and Mystical Theology

As argued above, William's conception of the good, of Trinity, and of exemplarism constitute the foundation upon which he builds his doctrine of the knowledge of God. With these discussions in place, it is now possible to revisit the centerpiece of that doctrine, his teaching on the spiritual senses. Early on in Book I, after considering the existence and nature of God *in se*, but before launching into his discussion of the economy, William considers a series of questions concerning the possibility of the knowledge of God. In these questions, he explicitly locates the role of the spiritual senses within his general doctrine of the knowledge of God.

"What is the principal name of God?" and "What does the word 'God' signify?"—William poses these two questions as he begins. The first question is spawned by an apparent contradiction between John of Damascus, who asserted that the first and principal name of God is "He Who Is," and Pseudo-Dionysius, who claimed "the good" for this designation. Conceding to the Damascene that "the first and principal name of God *simpliciter* and truly is 'he who is' (Ex 3:15)," he nonetheless upholds the Dionysian teaching. The good "is the first [name] with respect to us *(quoad nos)*, for we must understand God first according to the outflow *(flux)* of his goodness." *Bonum*, then, "is not the first name of

God, but the more principal and more worthy" and so *bonum* is spoken of God "above and beyond being *(ens)*." Why? Because the good "connotes effects in creatures beyond the divine essence, namely *quietem* or *delecationem* or *fruitionem,* by which the rational creature has fruition in God, which is the end *by which (quo)* it rests in God. For God is the end *in which (in quo)* [the rational creature rests]."[57] William's answer to these questions contains much that is by now familiar: his predilection for the category of the good, which encompasses the category of *ens* or *esse;* the diffusion of essential goodness into created goods which participate in it; participation in the "outflow" of divine goodness and participation through rest, delight, and fruition in the highest good; the *summum bonum* as both source and end of created things; the twofold end—the end "by which" *(finis quo)* and the end "in which" *(finis in quo)* there is fruition; and the general principle that the knowledge of God comes through the encounter with God's created effects. Significantly, William is keen to emphasize this implication of this theology of the good for the knowledge of God. The beginning of the knowledge of God is in the encounter with the general outflow of divine goodness, in the "works of God's goodness." In particular, he refers to certain "effects in creatures" namely, rest, delight, and fruition.

A second question—"What the name 'God' signifies"—pursues these issues further. Properly speaking, does "God" signify the divine nature *(natura),* or does it refer to divine activity *(operatio)?* Properly and principally, he concedes, "*Deus*" refers to the divine nature. But, he continues, "as an aid to understanding *(adminiculi ad intelligendum)* God," "*Deus*" refers to the divine acts. Here, he adduces a telling illustration: "just as a demonstrative pronoun is said to signify properly and principally a substance, nevertheless the accidents, which the eyes are able to see, are said to signify not properly, but as an aid to understanding *(cognoscendum)* a substance."[58] Is "*Deus*" thereby used equivocally? No,

---

57. SA I 4.2: 42,34.
58. SA I 4.3: 44,22f. William here offers two other defenses against the charge of equivocation: "The first is that God does not have only one image but many, since he is not like a determinate nature, as Aristotle said concerning the human intellect, which is not of a determinate nature, but is capable of anything whatsoever [*De anima* III.4]. The second

says William, returning to the pronoun illustration. "Just as the pronoun 'him' does not become equivocal by referring to Socrates today and by referring to Socrates tomorrow, even though Socrates is seen under diverse accidents today and tomorrow."[59]

In short, for William, the knowledge of God's substance, of God *in se*, comes through the encounter with God's varied and manifold acts within created reality. This encounter, moreover, is compared to the perception of the accidental attributes or properties of an object of sense perception. Though these objects of perception are not properly the substance, they are an "aid to the understanding of the substance."

Finally, William arrives at the last refinement to his principle that knowledge of God is mediated through creatures—a refinement of no little significance for his doctrine of the knowledge of God and its centerpiece, the spiritual senses. An objection to the assertion that *in se* God is beyond the ken of rational creatures introduced the Dionysian distinction between symbolic and mystical theology.[60] It then argued that while symbolic theology names and knows God through creatures, mystical theology pertains directly to God and thus arrives at knowledge of God *in se*. William refutes the conclusion, but incorporates the distinction between the two kinds of theology into his own position. Symbolic theology names God "by inferior things." For it names God through the fittingness or appropriateness of created things *(per convenientiam rerum)*, such as lion, fire, and the like. By contrast, mystical theology names God "by superior things." For mystical theology "names God through that which it perceives *(sentit)* in secret concerning God, through intellectual vision or contemplation, as when it calls God suave or beloved or the like." William clarifies: both types of theology name God through creatures. Symbolic theology takes up exterior creatures; mystical theology, for its part, names God "through interior and hidden and more worthy effects which the soul receives from the contemplation of God above itself. And the soul imposes such names through the gift of

---

cause is that although there are diverse images of things, all things here are according to the same relationship, namely according to the relation of effect to cause."

59. SA I 4.3: 44,28f.

60. See Pseudo-Dionysius, *Epistola IX* (PG 3.1105d); *De mystica theol.*, c. 3 (PG 3.1034; PL 122.1174).

wisdom, of which it is properly and maximally to know experientially what God is like."[61] Put simply, William here distinguishes between two kinds of creatures: inferior things which are exterior to the soul, and superior, worthier things which are located within the rational creature but which come to it from above. The former is the domain of symbolic theology, in which God is nameable and thus knowable in the mirror of inferior, external creatures. Mystical theology, on the other hand, also has to do with creatures, but with those which William calls the "interior, hidden and more worthy effects" received from God. As the passage indicates, the latter kind of theology is a kind of contemplative or intellectual perception *(sentire)* which comes with the gift of wisdom and results in experiential knowledge of God.

Though William's language here is compact and terse, both the content and vocabulary of his definition of mystical theology make it abundantly clear that he is referring to the kind of knowledge which occurs through the spiritual senses, as described in the treatise on beatitude. In this passage, mystical theology is a kind of perception *(sentire)* which results in experiential apprehension *(cognoscere experimento)* of God. That which is perceived is the sweetness of God and other similar things. Moreover, as in the treatise on beatitude, William is comfortable speaking of this knowledge as intellectual and contemplative at the same time. The reference to the gift of wisdom is also crucial. William's doctrine of the spiritual senses *in via* will be developed explicitly in relation to this particular gift of the Holy Spirit.

This passage is significant not only because it contains a clear reference to and rationale for William's doctrine of the spiritual senses, but also because it is a kind of lapidary summary of William's entire theological project. As noted above, the bulk of William's analysis in this first book pertains to describing and justifying how it is that God can be

---

61. SA I 4.2: 40,117ff. *Mistica vero theologica, que dicitur mistica, id est occulta, nominat Deum per id quod in occulto de Deo sentit per intellectualem visionem sive cnotemplationem, ut cum vocat Deum suavem, dilectum, et huiusmodi. Utrobique tamen per creaturas nominatur; sed in simbolica per exteriores creaturas, in mistica vero per interiores et occultos et digniores effectus quos anima a Dei contemplatione supra se recepit, et talia nomina imponit anima per donum sapientie, cuius maxime et proprie est cognoscere experimento qualis sit Deus.*

named and thus known. Accordingly, the consistent reference to the act of naming God in these definitions of symbolic and mystical theology suggest that these two forms of theology encompass all forms of knowledge of God. It is also clear in this passage that, for William, mystical theology represents the climax, the goal of all other forms of naming God, and as argued in this chapter, William's entire theology moves toward this climax—the delectable and beatific perception of spiritual realities. Thus, what has been labeled "spiritual apprehension" of God is the goal of William's theology. It is that, ultimately, which he labors to justify throughout Book I, and it is that with which the *Summa Aurea* concludes in Book IV, in the treatise on beatitude.

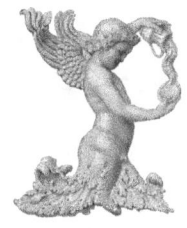# PART III
THE VIRTUES OF SPIRITUAL APPREHENSION

CHAPTER 6

FAITH
Knowledge of God in a Visual Mode

AS WE HAVE SEEN, for William beatitude is the apprehension in the next life of the Trinity, its manifold *delectabilia*.¹ More precisely, *fruitio* consists in the acts of *cognitio* and *dilectio,* and these three are the endowments of the beatified soul. *Cognitio* and *dilectio* are the perfected acts of the rational and concupiscible powers,² acts which are enabled by the virtues of faith and charity, respectively. Into this framework, William introduced his doctrine of the spiritual senses, relating their activity directly to the virtue of faith.³ In a particularly lyrical passage that bears repeating, he proposes diverse, faith-enabled acts of spiritual perception:

> By faith we see *(videmus)* spiritually. By faith we hear *(audimus)* what Jesus says. For *faith comes by hearing* (Rom 10:17). By faith we perceive scents *(odoramus)* spiritually. For by faith we cognize *(cognoscere)* that the Son of God was made man for us, that he wept for us and was tormented for us, that he sorrowed, that he suffered. And when we recall the benefits of this kind, we perceive *(odoramus)* the good odor of Christ *(bonum odorem Christi)* as an aromatic perfume flowing from him. . . . When by faith we meditate upon these things which we know, as if by chewing *(masticando),* we taste *(gustamus)* the sweetness of God *(dulcedinem Dei),* and this is by faith. By faith we touch *(tangimus)* the suavity of God *(suavitatem Dei).*⁴

---

1. See Chapter 2 above. SA IV 18.3.3.2.2: "We will delight in the beauty *(pulchritudo)* and symphony *(simphonia)* and aroma *(odor)* and sweetness *(dulcedo)* and attractiveness *(suavitas)* of God. But in God these are none other than delectable things *(delectabilia).*"
2. SA IV 18.3.3.1: 499,99ff.
3. SA IV 18.3.3.2.3: 590,18ff. "There is only one spiritual sense, the intellect, and only one virtue which perfects the spiritual sense, namely faith."
4. SA IV 18.3.3.2.3: 510,60ff.

In some way, faith facilitates the beatific activities of the spiritual senses. William thus gives priority to faith in the experience of fruition: "by the spiritual senses alone and by faith alone we have fruition of God formally and properly." Yet, he does not neglect the role of charity. Though, properly speaking, "charity does not delight in God nor does it have fruition of God except by faith," yet "charity moves faith to the act of having fruition of God." In this sense, charity too experiences delight—but always through faith: "charity always has delight, since it is never without faith."[5] Faith and charity, therefore, figure centrally in William's account of beatitude. At the same time, he does not of course relegate faith and charity to the next life; rather, they begin to function in these ways in the present.[6] In William's theology, their activity thus bridges the two states of life. An analysis of these virtues is necessary for a fuller appreciation of his doctrine of the spiritual senses; the following will focus on the nature of faith and charity in the present life *(in via)*.

William's account of these virtues *in via* relates them to two forms of spiritual sensation: *visus* and *tactus*. For him, the Trinity is delectable in two primary modes: to the *intellectus* or rational power in a visual modality *(per modum visus);* and to the *affectus* or concupiscible power in a tactile modality *(per modum tactus)*. It will be argued, moreover, that in relation to faith and charity, *visus* and *tactus* stand by way of synecdoche for whole spiritual *sensorium*. Faith will be analyzed in this chapter; charity is the topic of the following chapter.

The Graces of Christ the Head and Spiritual Sensation

William's primary discussion of the virtues constitutes nearly the whole of Book III of the *Summa Aurea*, beginning with Tractate 10. Before examining his views on faith and charity, it will be helpful to locate this discussion within two larger trajectories in that book. First, like Peter Lombard in his *Sentences,* William links the virtues with Christology,

---

5. SA IV 18.3.3.2.2: 507,72ff.

6. SA IV 18.3.3.2.1: 503,22ff. "For just as the grace of God is the perfection of nature, so the glory [of God] will be the perfection of grace.... that is, begin to see God through faith so that afterwards you may see God by sight. For this ... beginning is had [now], the perfection of which will be had in the future."

which he treats in the first nine tractates. The person and work of Christ are the foundation and starting point for the remainder of Book III, as the salvation made possible in Christ is appropriated and completed by the possession and activity of the virtues.⁷ This link to Christology provides a starting point for an analysis of faith and charity and a payoff regarding William's teaching on the spiritual senses.

A question is raised: how, and according to which nature, is Christ the Head of the Church?⁸ William's answer relates Christ's headship directly to the possibility of spiritual sensation in the members of the ecclesial body. Christ, he argues, is the Head according to both natures. With respect to divinity, Christ is Head "since he vivifies and gives sense *(sensificat)* to [the body] spiritually."⁹ With respect to humanity, Christ is the Head in a metaphorical sense, "since just as the head vivifies and gives sense to the whole body, so from Christ, as from a head, flow the spiritual senses and movements *(sensus et motus spirituales)* into the Church as into a body."¹⁰ In this way, William establishes the possibility of spiritual perception on the foundation of Christology and ecclesiology,¹¹ as in his treatment of beatitude.¹²

---

7. SA III 10: 112,2. "Having spoken of the liberation of the human race, namely, Christ, something must be said concerning those things through which Christ liberates, namely, concerning the virtues."

8. SA III 4.2: "On the Dignity According to which Christ is the Head of the Church."

9. SA III 4.2: 63,9ff.

10. SA III 4.2: 63,15ff. According to Rahner, William's remarks here are part of a larger early scholastic discussion which has its proximate source in a controversial remark of Peter Lombard's, but whose remote source is Augustine. Relying on Augustine's *Letter 187* (c.13, n.40), the Lombard asserted that just as all five bodily senses reside in the head, but only the sense of touch resides in the other members, so in Christ the Head all the senses reside, while only the sense of touch exists in the saints (*III Sent.* d.13, c.1: "Ita vero habitat, ut ait Augustinus Ad Dardanum, *quod omni gratia plenus est; non ita habitat in Sanctis. Ut et in nostro corpore inest sensus singulis membris, sed non quantum in capite; ibi enim est visus est et auditus et olfactus et gustus et tactus, in ceteris autem solus est tactus:*" ita et in Christo habitat omnis plenitudo divinitatis, quia ille est caput, in quo sunt omnes sensus. In Sanctis vero quasi solus tactus est, quibus datus est spiritus ad mensuram, cum de illius plenitudine acceperunt [Jn 1:16]). This remark sparked a debate on the question among later commentators since it appears to contradict an assertion of Origen's transmitted by the *Glossa ordinaria* (Rahner, "The Doctrine of the 'Spiritual Senses,'" pp. 104–34).

11. Like the endowments *(dotes)* of the blessed, the *sensus gratiae* are first the possession of the ecclesial community of believers, and only secondarily are they the possession of individual believers.

12. See Chapter 2 above. Christ's headship is analogous to his role as Spouse in the

The second trajectory pertains to the larger process of the reception, possession, and activity of the virtues. Here, too, William proceeds with an eye toward spiritual perception. He depicts progress in the cardinal virtues as a purging and preparation of the soul's capacity for spiritual sensation.[13] The fear of the Lord, to begin, expels sin, and so "cleanses the palate of the heart *(palat[i]um cordis),*" after which "the sweetness of God *(dulcedo Dei)* is sensed *(sentitur)*";[14] "little by little the eye of the mind *(oculis mentis)* is purged, so that God may be clearly seen and perfectly loved."[15] The theological virtues for their part are infused directly by God and relate the soul directly to God. They are distinguished from the other virtues in that through them the soul experiences a more immediate perception of, and delight in, God.[16] In fact, William seems to envision progress in the virtues as moving along a continuum of increasing capacity for spiritual sensation. "He who only possesses the cardinal virtues *(virtutes politicas)* does not taste the sweetness of God." Through the purgatorial virtues *(virtutes purgatorias),* however, one "senses *(sentit)* [the sweetness of God] somewhat." But the completely purged soul, possessing the theological virtues, "perfectly senses the sweetness of God."[17] William typically describes the transition from cardinal to theological virtues as a transition from exteriority to interiority: one is "recalled to interior things, where there are greater pleasures *(delicias).*"[18] Both of these trajectories reflect William's interest in spiritual perception and anticipate his fuller teaching on the spiritual senses.

---

context of beatitude. In his human nature, Christ is Head and Spouse of the church in a unique way which goes beyond the more general relationship to the Trinity, which both angels and humans enjoy. William relates this vivifying role of Christ as Head to the Holy Spirit as well. The church is called the body of Christ because "just as members of one man are vivified by one soul which has its seat in the head, so all the faithful are vivified by one soul, that is, by the Holy Spirit, who principally has its seat in the head which is Christ" (SA III 4.5: 67,5ff).

13. SA III 10.1.3: 121,54ff.
14. SA III 38.4: 726,33.
15. SA III 14.5: 264,40. Cf. SA III 16.5: 329,89. Increasingly, the soul "senses *(sentit)* the sweetness of God."
16. SA III 11.2: 181,182. "For it is not possible for there to be formed a medium between God and the delight by which we properly delight in God, since nothing is closer to God than such delight by which we delight in him."
17. SA III 30.3: 597,84ff.
18. SA III 30.3: 597,96.

Progress in virtue prepares the members of Christ's body for the "spiritually sensuous" beatific vision in the next life.[19]

The Theological Virtues: The Twofold End of Faith and Charity

In order to appreciate William's teaching on respective sense modalities of faith and charity, it will be necessary to lay out his fundamental conception of the theological virtues. In a generally Aristotelian sense,[20] William sees the virtues as habits *(habitus)*.[21] In this view, each *habitus* has its own proper act *(motus)*, of which it is the cause—"from a virtue an act is elicited as from its cause."[22] This act, moreover, has an associated delight or passion which is unique to it and which arises from its encounter with its proper object. William cites Aristotle's *Nicomachean Ethics* with approval: "each virtue has its own good and its own delightful things *(delectabilia)*."[23] Precisely speaking, this delight is neither the virtue itself nor its act, but a kind of "second movement."[24] Still, the

---

19. SA III 11.2: 177,58. "For it belongs first to the human person that he reason; second, that through reason he acquire the virtues; and third that through the virtues he acquire beatitude."

20. See Lottin, *Psychologie et morale,* vol. 3, pp. 103–15. For a discussion of twelfth-century views of *habitus,* see Cary Nederman, "Nature, Ethics, and the Doctrine of *Habitus:* Aristotelian Moral Psychology in the Twelfth Century," *Traditio* 45 (1989): pp. 87–110, but also Marcia Colish, "*Habitus* Revisited: A Reply to Cary Nederman," *Traditio* 48 (1993): pp. 77–92.

21. SA III 14.1: 254,50. "As the first light *(prima lux)* only illumines the intellect for believing through the medium of a habit, which is faith, so the first charity *(prima caritas)* only inflames the affection through the medium of a habit, which is created charity."

22. SA III 10.4.5.3: 164,35. "Thus a virtue gives to its act its that-it-is and its that-it-is-good; therefore it gives to it its goodness. Every virtue is *simpliciter* better than its act, since nothing is better than the virtue by which man is made like to God. For the virtue gives to its *motus* the goodness that it possesses. Hence, the act of virtue has its goodness accidentally, but the virtue has its goodness substantially."

23. SA III 11.2: 178,106f. "The philosopher says that 'in every potency or in every power of the soul there is its proper delight.' For each power delights in the obtaining of its end; thus, how much more does every virtue have its own delight."

24. SA III 39.5.2: 757,192. "The delight, by which the soul delights in God, even though it is annexed to the act, yet it is only from the sweetness of God, and it is not *from* the act, but *with* the act, through what it receives from its virtue, namely that for God's sake it is moved into God. Hence, since that delight is the end of the virtue properly, for this reason it is better than the virtue, and that virtue causes delight in God through that which it does in the act. But the act, through what it receives from its virtue only (since that act is posited with that delectation, as annexed to it), is better than the virtue, not on account of itself, but because of the annexation of the delight, which is annexed through its virtue."

presence of delight is determinative of the virtue and its act; the absence of delight reveals the absence of the virtue.[25] Finally, it is through a virtue's act, strictly speaking, and not the virtue itself, that persons experience fruition of God.[26]

Beyond these generalities, William's conception of faith and charity[27] is governed by his conviction that they are defined individually and distinguished respectively according to their diverse, proper ends *(finis)*. This notion of end, though, is twofold. There is an end toward which a virtue tends and in which it rests *(finis in quo)*. Here, end has the sense of a proper object. There is also an end by which *(finis quo)* a virtue moves toward and rests in its proper object. In this sense, end is a proper operation or act *(motus)*.[28] This prompts William to observe that the end *in which* faith and charity rest is ultimately a single reality, namely God; there are, however, diverse ends *by which* they rest in God, "since there are diverse delights by which ... we delight in God."[29]

Regarding these diverse ends *by which* faith and charity rest *(finis quo)*, William sees the substantial or proper act of faith as delighting "in

---

25. SA III 11.3.1: 187,89ff. "Delight and sadness, in as much as they are pure passions, are not virtues nor the acts of virtues; but they are determinative of virtues and their operations. Similarly, sorrow and joy, in as much as they are a second act, are determinative of those virtues, for ... if someone abstains and rejoices in that fact, he is chaste, since he rejoices in his abstinence and it pleases him, and this determination is a sign that he has true bodily chastity. But if he is sad in abstaining, it is a sign that he does not have true chastity."

26. SA III 10.4.5.3: 165,62ff. "We say that this is twofold: 'by the act of the virtues we have fruition of God and not by the virtue,' since if this ablative 'by the virtue' denotes the formal cause, in the same way that the ablative 'by the acts of the virtues,' it is true. But if it denotes the efficient cause, it is false, since both by the virtue and by the act of the virtue we have fruition of God, but in one way and in another. By the virtue we have fruition of God effectively, but by the act of the virtue we have fruition formally."

27. William's primary interest lies in the rational and concupiscible powers and their associated virtues, faith and charity. These two powers, their acts and the virtues which perfect them, have a permanent place in the soul's experience of beatitude, while hope and the irascible power are not so perfected. Thus, he is most concerned with two aspects of the soul, the *intellectus* and the *affectus* and the virtues of faith and charity. Cf. SA III 13.5: 251,86: "We say that there are two things in the soul: *intellectus* and *affectus*. By the intellect we delight in the first truth *(in prima veritate)* immediately; but by the *affectus* in the first goodness *(in prima bonitate)*. For the intellective power is properly directed toward the true; the concupiscible power is properly directed toward the good."

28. SA III 11.2: 181,174.

29. SA III 11.2: 181,175ff.

the highest delectable through the mode of estimation and cognition *(per modum estimationis sive cognitionis)*"; while for its part charity delights "through the mode of union *(per modum coniunctionis)*, since 'delight is the union of the lover with the beloved.'"[30] Reflecting his abiding tendency to pattern knowledge of God on physical sensation, William justifies this account by appealing to the forms of delight found in physical sense perception. As with sensible delights *(delectabili sensibili)*, he argues, there are only three ways of delighting in the highest delectable *(summo delectabili)*. "For when someone desires a sensible delectable, if he estimates that he is able to have it easily, and if he hopes that he will have it, and when he is united to it either through acquisition or possession, he delights in that which he had earlier desired."[31] Faith's substantial act, then, is cognition/estimation; charity's is union.

As just noted, the ultimate end *in which* faith and charity rest is God. But William is not content to leave the matter there. Regarding the proper objects of faith and charity *(finis in quo)*, he begins with a dilemma. On the one hand, all the virtues must have the *summum bonum* as their common, singular end. It might seem, then, that they are not substantially distinguished from each other. Some of William's twelfth-century predecessors had in fact affirmed this position,[32] but he rejects it. For him, "the species of [the virtues] are to be distinguished according to their principal (and nearer) ends, not according to their final ends."[33] But what then are the principal objects according to which faith and charity might be distinguished? For William and his contemporaries, this dilemma pertains in particular to the virtue of faith. How and in what sense is faith a virtue? The dilemma arises in part from the Aristotelian distinction between intellectual speculation, an act of the speculative intellect oriented toward the true *(verum)*, and moral virtue, an act of the practical intellect oriented toward the good *(bonum)*.[34] If faith

30. SA III 11.3.5: 194,51. "Delight is the joining of the lover with the beloved *(coniunctio diligentis cum dilecto)*."
31. SA III 11.3.5: 194,42.
32. See Lottin, *Psychologie et morale*, vol. 3, pp. 100–101, 144.
33. SA III 11.2: 176,44.
34. SA III 12.2: 200,4f.: "The philosophers say that the end of speculation *(speculationis finis)* is truth *(veritas)* or the true *(verum)*; the end of virtue *(virtutis finis)* is the good

is a virtue, it seems that it must reside in the practical intellect and be oriented toward the good. But what then of any speculative truth-content in faith, which would be oriented toward the true? On the other hand, is it truly possible to give speculative knowledge the status of a virtue? For his part, William refuses the dilemma, arguing that faith is a "speculative virtue," pertaining both to the good and the true. But how?

William agrees with Aristotle that a virtue must be oriented toward the good *(summum bonum)*, not merely as its final end, but as its substantial, principal, or material end. The *bonum* must belong to the essence of faith; the good must not be related to it only accidentally, otherwise faith would not be a virtue in the same sense as charity. If charity alone is substantially directed toward the good, alone having the good as its proper end—while faith is only accidentally related to it, only related to the good as its final end—then faith would only be a virtue accidentally, not substantially. For faith truly to be a virtue, it must have the *bonum* as its substantial end, and the *bonum* must be its substantial end in another, specifically different way than it is for charity.

Toward this end, William argues that, although in one sense the end *in which* the virtues delight is the good as a singular object,[35] yet as such an end the *summum bonum* must be spoken of in two ways: "with respect to himself God is a single end in essence *(unicus finis)*, but in effect God is a manifold end *(multiplex finis in effectu)*"[36] in which *(finis in quo)* the virtues delight and rest, "just as the Holy Spirit in the book of Wisdom is called *multiplex*, on account of the many effects which he has in us."[37] "In a certain way," William surmises, "there are diverse ends of those delights."[38] More precisely, he posits three such ends, correspon-

---

(bonum);" SA III 12.2: 200,8f.: "The intellect is twofold, speculative and practical; in the speculative intellect are knowledge *(scientie)* and the speculation of the truth *(speculationis veritatis);* in the practical intellect is virtue *(virtus)* and good work *(bona operatio).*"

35. SA III 11.2: 180,163. "If [the end in which] is understood of the good essentially, then the good will be the mediate and final end of the virtues, but not on account of the identity of this end are all virtues of their most special species."

36. SA III 11.2: 181,189.

37. SA III 11.2: 180,168. See Chapters 4–5 above for a discussion of the Holy Spirit's manifold, created effects.

38. SA III 11.2: 181,193.

ding to the three theological virtues:³⁹ "for faith delights in the first truth *(prima veritate)* immediately; hope [delights] in the first generosity *(prima largitate)*; charity delights in the first goodness *(prima bonitate).*"⁴⁰ With respect to faith and charity in particular, this assumption concerning the manifold manifestations of the *summum bonum* enables William to appropriate Aristotle's assertion in the *De anima* that the good and the true are identical, yet distinguishable. This ontological identity allows the *summum bonum* to be the end for faith in a substantially different way than it is for charity. For faith, the *summum bonum* is the *bonum ut verum*, the good as true.⁴¹ It delights faith as an illuminating light *(lux illuminans)*, as the *prima lux et sapientia* for the intellect.⁴² For charity, the *summum bonum* is the *bonum ut bonum*, the good as good, as pleasuring and delicious sweetness, as the *prima bonitas et suavitas*.⁴³ Faith's proper object, then, is the *bonum* as the first truth *(prima veritas)*, while charity's is the *bonum* as the first goodness or suavity *(prima suavitas)*. In effect, for William, *veritas* and *suavitas* are the primary, cre-

39. SA III 11.3.5: 194,54.: "God, who is the multiplex end of the theological virtues, in a sense, is only a threefold end." Cf. SA III 11.3.5: 195,63ff.: "But all things which are said concerning God have to be reduced to these three. Wisdom and light are reduced to that which is called the first truth. Through that which is called the highest reward and power they are reduced to that which is called the highest *largus;* the highest concord, the highest mercy is reduced to that which is called the highest good or suavity. And thus there are only these three theological virtues."
40. SA III 36.1.1: 684,31. Cf. SA III 14.6: 265,35: "Faith delights in the first light *(prima luce)* and this is a different delight from the delight by which charity delights in the first goodness *(prima bonitate);* therefore, just as charity has its delectable, so faith has its own delectable, since every virtue has its own proper good and its own proper delectable *(delectabilia).*" Here, then, William resorts to the distinction between the *bonum in essentia* and the *bonum* in its manifold, created effects to justify his assertion of three *fines in quo* of the theological virtues (see Chapter 3 above).
41. William's views here are developed in opposition to those of the circle around Stephen Langton and Godfrey of Poitiers. It is inspired in part by pseudo-Dionysius. G. Englhardt, *Die Entwicklung der dogmatischen Glabuenspsychologie in der mittelalterlichen Scholastik vom Abelardstreit (um 1140) bis zu Philipp dem Kanzler (gest. 1236)*, Beiträge zur Geschichte der Philosophie und Theologie des Mittelalters, vol. 30 (Münster: Aschendorff, 1933), p. 266.
42. SA III 36.1.1: 684,37. "The operation of the intellect tends toward some end, in the attainment of which it delights and rests, and this end is the first truth, for if the intellect is delighted by this, that 'the diagonal is incommensurate with the side' [Aristotle, *Topics* I.15], how much more will it be delighted by the first truth."
43. SA III 13.5: 251,86f.

ated modes of the *summum bonum* and the principal objects of these virtues.

Integrating both types of end—the *finis quo* and *finis in quo*—William sums up the basic nature of faith and charity: faith tends immediately toward the first truth through its act of cognition, while charity tends immediately toward the first suavity through its act of desire.[44] In light of this view of faith and charity, William arrives at a quite literal interpretation of Augustine's statement that "every virtue is love":[45] for love *(amor)*, he argues, can be understood broadly so as to pertain to every virtue, "as it is not only of the concupiscible power to love and desire the first things, but also of the rational power since 'all men by nature desire to know,' as Aristotle said (*Metaphysics* I.1), and that is reason's desire."[46] Both faith and charity are oriented toward their immediate and substantial ends with a kind of love *(amor)*.[47] Faith is the love of the first truth; charity is the love of the good.[48]

---

44. SA III 36.1.1: 687,103. "There are three motive powers, the irascible, the concupiscible, and the rational, and they have three general ends: the truth, the highest or most glorious, or most honored, and the good or the delectable. The rational power tends toward truth generally, by whatever truth it is true; the irascible power tends toward the highest or the most glorious, by whatever height it is high; the concupiscible power tends toward the delectable by whatever delectability it is delectable. Tending toward these same ends are the three theological virtues, which are situated in the three aforesaid powers; faith is oriented toward the truth and to the cognition of the truth, but hope is oriented toward the heights, charity towards delectation."

45. Englhardt notes that William's interpretation of the statement *omnis virtus est amor* and its application especially to faith introduces a rather non-Aristotelian element into the otherwise very Aristotelian approach to the nature of faith. Subsequent scholastics did not follow his thesis that faith and love are virtues in a univocal sense; the statement was taken up later in a more metaphorical sense, as later scholastics became increasingly familiar with the Aristotelian theory of virtue (Englhardt, *Glaubenspsychologie*, pp. 272–76).

46. SA III 36.1.1: 685,44.

47. SA III 11.2: 179,124ff. "Love is understood sometimes narrowly, sometimes broadly. Taken strictly it is the same as friendship *(amicitia)*; and in this sense it is in the concupiscible power, and in this sense only charity is the love of God. But sometimes the desire of whatever good is called love, and in this sense every virtue is love essentially *(per essentiam)*, since every virtue loves its good, namely, its act. . . . And, in this sense, Augustine said that 'every virtue is love.'" Cf. SA III 38.2: 722,57; SA III 39.1: 729,52.

48. SA III 10.4.3: 152,72: "The love of the cognition of the first truth is of faith; but the love of the highest good, in as much as it is good, is charity." SA III 11.2: 179,138: "Faith is the love of the first truth. Charity is the love of the first suavity."

The Virtue of Faith

Throughout his *ex professo* treatment of faith,[49] William everywhere builds upon these fundamental assumptions. As a virtue, faith is substantially and materially related to the good; but as an act of the speculative intellect, it is directed toward the good *as true.*[50] But how precisely does he conceive of faith's relation to the *bonum* as *verum?* He does so by leaning heavily upon the notion of *aestimatio,* a technical term that draws on two twelfth-century intellectual traditions. This notion enables him to conceive of faith as both an intellectual cognition or speculation *(in speculativo intellectu)* of the true and as an appraisal or judgment of the true as the good. "Faith consists in speculation of the first truth and in estimation of the good: for as long as by faith the intellect speculates the first truth, it estimates it to be the highest delectable and the highest good for itself and is moved toward that in order to delight and rest in it."[51] In short, faith is a speculative estimation of the good as true.[52] William offers what will turn out to be a telling analogy: "Just as a sheep

---

49. SA III 12: *"De Fide."* Englhardt suggests that the tractate on faith marks an important stage in the development of the scholastic treatment of the topic. He notes further that William's understanding of faith, especially his psychology of faith, was once thought to be largely inspired by Hugh of St. Victor. In reality, however, the issues and problems he considers and the solutions he provides have their source in the thought and writings of Peter of Corbeil, Praepositinus, Stephen Langton, and Godfrey of Poitiers (Englhardt, *Glaubenspsychologie,* p. 211).

50. Englhardt argues that with William the tradition which understood faith as contemplative knowing directed toward the highest truth proves stronger than the Aristotelian influences. For William, nodding uneasily at both Aristotelian virtue theory and Neoplatonic metaphysics, virtue does not consist merely in the avoidance of evil and the pursuit of the good, but also in *cognitione et suavitate* (Englhardt, *Glaubenspsychologie,* pp. 271–72). See O. Lottin, "Les dons du Saint-Esprit chez les théologiens depuis Pierre Lombard jusque'à S. Thomas d'Aquin," *Recherches de théologie ancienne et médiévale* 1 (1929): pp. 41–61.

51. SA III 12.2: 200,20ff.

52. William understands "good" here, not in the sense of good acts associated with the practical or political virtues, but with the uncreated, essential goodness of the Trinity: "the end of faith is the eternal good, not in the first place the good in acts, such as the political virtues. Yet that faith does move toward the good in acts through the middle political virtues which it moves. For faith vivifies both the interior and the exterior man, as the Apostle said: *but the just shall live by faith.* Thus when the philosophers said that virtue is located in the practical intellect, they understand this only of the political virtues which consist in acts; of faith they did not understand it" (SA III 12.2: 201,38ff).

flees a wolf through estimation *(per estimationem)*, so by estimation faith is moved into the first truth."[53] A proper appreciation of William's view of faith requires an analysis of this concept as it emerged in the twelfth-century intellectual milieu.

Excursus on Aestimatio

The Latin verb *aestimare* has classical pedigree. Its primitive sense is that of an evaluation of material or moral value.[54] By extension, it also came to mean "to believe, to think, to judge," and both senses (with the variants *existimare* and *extimare*) passed into medieval usage.[55] Two distinct medieval traditions of this term antedate the thirteenth century.[56] On the basis of its extended meaning, the term acquired a technical sense in the course of the twelfth century among Christian authors, for whom it meant an uncertain knowledge, inferior to other more certain forms. Peter Abelard's definition of faith found in his *Theologica scholarium,* uses *existimatio* as a synonym for *substantia* found in the Hebrews' definition of faith: "the conviction of things not seen, that is, things not available to the corporeal senses."[57] In context, Abelard appears to contrast faith's knowledge and lesser degree of certainty with scientific knowledge in the Aristotelian sense and the absolute certainty of logical demonstration. This was an innovative and controversial use of the term, which evoked a storm of protest.[58] Bernard of Clairvaux and

---

53. SA III 12.2: 200,25f.

54. Pierre Michaud-Quantin, *Études sur le vocabulaire philosophique du Moyen Age* (Rome: Ateneo, 1970), pp. 9–10. It is an evaluation that is neither self-evident nor fixed, made by someone whose personal qualifications make such judgments authoritative. One might, for example, estimate the price of goods, the weight of an object, the merit of an act.

55. Michaud-Quantin, *Études,* p. 13.

56. For much of what follows, I am indebted to Marcia Colish's excellent study on Peter Lombard, *Peter Lombard,* Brill's Studies in Intellectual History, vol. 41 (Leiden: Brill, 1994), pp. 494–95.

57. Peter Abelard, *Theologica "scholarium"* 1.2, 1.11–15, ed. Constant J. Mews, *CCCM* 13: 318, 322–25: *Fides est . . . existimatio rerum non apparentium, hoc est sensibus corpories non subiacentium,* cited in Colish, *Peter Lombard,* pp. 494–95.

58. The verb *existimare* is used in the Vulgate translation of the New Testament to describe epistemic states generically, regardless of their content. Cf. Rom 2:3; Rom 6:11; Rom 8:18; Rom 14:14; 1 Cor 7:26; 1 Cor 7:36; 1 Cor 8:2; 1 Cor 10:12; 2 Cor 10:2; 2 Cor 11:5; Phil 3:8; 2 Thes 3:15; Jas 1:2. It can be rendered in English in most of these contexts as "to consider," "to deem," "to esteem," "to expect," "to suppose," "to regard."

William of St. Thierry understood Abelard to mean "opinion," uncertain knowledge, and saw it as a purely subjective judgment. In response, Abelard's disciples sought both to clarify what he meant and to show that his intent was Pauline and had patristic support. They suggested that Paul's *argumentum non apparentium* in Hebrews 11:1 is basically the same cognitive state as the one to which the apostle refers in Romans with the use of *existimare*, and that Abelard intended to emphasize the relative degree of faith's certitude in the absence of empirical evidence. A moderating voice in this debate was found in Hugh of St. Victor. He agreed with Abelard that this was an issue requiring clarification, and supported the orthodoxy of *existimatio* against Abelard's critics.[59] For his part, Hugh (like his Cistercian counterparts) often associated estimation with opinion,[60] and saw it as an intermediate position, between affirmation and negation, in the examination of two ideas. Yet he too attempted to grant it a relatively high degree of certitude, which emerges in his own definition of faith: "a certitude concerning things that are absent, above opinion and below knowledge."[61] Finally, Roland Bandinelli (later Pope Alexander III) made a final effort to salvage Abelard's definition by adding the adjective *certa*, allowing him to distance *aestimatio certa* from mere opinion.

A quite different meaning of the term *aestimatio* made its appearance in the second half of the twelfth century with the introduction of Latin translations of Aristotle and his Arabic commentators. With these, the idea of an inferior knowledge is maintained, but on a different plane, and enriched by other notions.[62] The Latin root *aestim* renders the Arabic root *wahm* used by the Arab commentators[63] on Aristotle to describe an act *(aestimatio)* or faculty *(vis aestimativa)* whereby an animal, with-

---

59. Colish, *Peter Lombard*, pp. 494–95.
60. Hugh of St. Victor, *De sacramentis* I, 10, 2 (PL 176.330–31), cited in Colish, *Peter Lombard*, pp. 494–95.
61. *Fides est certitudo rerum absentium supra opinionem et infra scientiam constituta* (PL 176.330–31), cited in Colish, *Peter Lombard*, pp. 494–95.
62. See Harry A. Wolfson, "The Internal Senses in Latin, Arabic, and Hebrew Philosophical Texts," *Harvard Theological Review* 28 (1935): pp. 250–314. See also Michaud-Quantin, *Etudes*, pp. 19–21.
63. Wolfson mentions Alfarabi and Avicenna as authors who incorporated this act/faculty into their accounts of the internal senses ("The Internal Senses," pp. 254–55).

out previous experience, perceives the insensible forms (*intentio*—that concerning the sensible thing which is not sensed by the external senses) connected with the impression of sensible objects, such as the sheep's perception of hostility at the sight of a wolf or its perception of friendliness at the sight of its young.[64] In this act, the animal perceives *(cognoscit)*, judges *(judicat)*, but above all apprehends *(apprehendere* is the classic term for this knowledge) non-sensible *intentiones*, determines their practical value, and dictates the appropriate response (attraction or aversion).[65] An important aspect of this act/faculty is its certitude. The instinctive and natural *aestimativa* was considered incapable of error. Moreover, this faculty in animals was thought to correspond to human intelligence *(dianoia, logistike, bouleutike)* and to be analogous to human sagacity *(synesis)*, art *(techne)*, prudence *(phronesis)*, forethought *(pronoia)*, or wisdom *(sophia)*. While this faculty exists primarily in animals, it also came to be attributed to humans and was seen in human judgments not affected directly by reason.[66] As a translation of the Arabic *wahm*, then, this medieval usage of the Latin term *aestimatio* retains the sense of a knowledge inferior to that obtained by reason, and of a knowledge which evaluates an object for the advantages and disadvantages which the object will procure. *Aestimatio*, moreover, relates to something that affects the estimator: what advantage or disadvantage will be gained, what goodwill be acquired.[67]

These twelfth-century developments regarding the notion of *aestima-*

---

64. See ibid., pp. 256–57. The verb *aestimare* and the adjective *aestimativa* are found in the translations of the *Book of Definitions* of Isaac Israeli as descriptions and characteristic of the animal in contrast to human behavior.

65. Wolfson, "The Internal Senses," p. 268. Aristotle does not mention this faculty, and Wolfson argues that this faculty arose from a perceived defect in Aristotle's account of the actual motion of pursuit and avoidance in man and animals.

66. Ibid., pp. 270–74. Whether animal or human, estimation involves an act of abstraction. In its judgment, estimation transcends the level of abstraction found in the imagination, for its object is only accidentally material. Neither goodness nor malice, for example, are in themselves material. Yet estimation apprehends these "in" material things. Accordingly, its judgment is not definitional (as are the wholly immaterial concepts employed by the intellect), but imaginable, conjoined with singularity and sensible form. Estimation's judgment is of two kinds: one is that which is not *per se* sensible, like friendliness or malice; the other is something not now sensed, but *per se* sensible, such as the sweetness of honey which is seen but is not now sensed, though properly it is a sensible quality.

67. Michaud-Quantin, *Études*, p. 24.

tio, finally, must be located within the larger context of discussion of the Aristotelian notion of the "internal senses" of the soul, a term coined to refer collectively to those post-sensationary faculties (in contrast to the five physical senses) which Aristotle discussed in *De anima* and in *De memoria et reminiscentia*.[68] When the term "internal senses" first appears in the Latin philosophical texts,[69] it is used as synonymous with a single post-sensationary faculty of the soul. In Augustine, for example, the *interior sensus* or *interior vis* functions in the same way as Aristotle's "common sense."[70] In the early thirteenth century,[71] under the influence of the Arabic commentators, scholastic thinkers began to incorporate this Aristotelian psychology more extensively into their theories of human knowing, and this particularly with respect to *aestimatio*. Increasingly, the concept of animal *aestimatio* was integrated into construals of human sense perception and psychology.[72] In fact, William's use of the vocabulary transmitted by the Arabic translations is one of the first wit-

---

68. Wolfson, "The Internal Senses," pp. 250–66. These internal senses are also sometimes referred to as "spiritual," "separable," or "cerebral" and are so called because they reside within the brain and operate without bodily organs.

69. Wolfson finds no reference prior to Augustine. He does mention Cicero's *tactus interior*, but argues that it has an entirely different meaning. He also asserts that Galen does not actually use the term, though Arabic philosophers who reproduced his classification use it ("The Internal Senses," p. 252, n. 12).

70. The observation is Wolfson's: For Augustine, cf. *Confessions* I, 20; VII, 17; *De libero arbitrio* II, 3–5. Similarly, Gregory the Great's *"sensus cerebri,"* which presides within *(qui intrinsecus praesidet)*, also functions like Aristotle's "common sense" (*Moralia* XI, 6 [PL 75.957B]). In Eriugena, this power is identified with the Greek term *dianoia*, which in his view stands below *ratio (logos)* and *intellectus (nous)* but above the five external senses and imagination (*De divisione naturae*, II, 23 [PL 122.577D]). All texts cited in Wolfson, "The Internal Senses," p. 269.

71. See Wolfson, "The Internal Senses," p. 265. Perhaps even earlier: Isaac of Stella speaks of the following list of soul powers: *sensus, imaginatio, ratio, intellectus,* and *intelligentia*. This is perhaps a conflation of Boethius with the addition of intellect from Augustine. The *De spiritu et anima*, probably by Alcher of Clairvaux, draws on all possible sources. It contains the list from Isaac noted above and speaks of interior and exterior senses.

72. Cf. Wolfson, "The Internal Senses," p. 263. Through the Latin translations from the Arabic in the twelfth and thirteenth centuries, the Avicennian and Averroian classifications of the internal senses became known to the scholastics. John of Spain translated from Avicenna's *Al-Shifâ'* the section dealing with the soul, which is generally referred to as *VI de naturalis* or as *De Anima*. It is likely John of Spain also translated al-Gazali's *Maḳâṣid al-Falâsifah*, the third part of which, dealing with physics and containing the discussion on the soul, is referred to as *Physica*. Later, Gerard of Cremona translated Avicen-

nesses to the construction in humans of a sensible psychology copied from that of animals.⁷³

Aestimatio *in William of Auxerre's View of Faith*

Turning to William's use of the term *aestimatio* in his discussion of faith, it is evident that he is indebted to these two traditions.⁷⁴ In general, his use of this term is reminiscent of his twelfth-century predecessors in the tradition inaugurated by Abelard.⁷⁵ At the same time, his frequent use of sheep-wolf examples reveals an apparent Arabic-Aristotelian inspiration.⁷⁶

Most basically, for William, *aestimatio* is a judgment *(arbitrium)*.⁷⁷ He will use *aestimare* and *arbitrari* as synonyms. For example,⁷⁸ "contempt for worldly love is said to *estimare* or *arbitrari* such love as vile and noxious to the soul; and this judgment *(arbitratio)* is of faith." Moreover, *aestimatio* judges non-sensible realities *(intentiones)*; specifically, it judges the value or worth of these non-sensible, spiritual realities. So, "contempt for the world is . . . an *estimatio* of the world as vile in com-

---

na's Canon. John of Rochelle is the first scholastic thinker to systemize Arabic *aestimatio* within a complete system of human sense perception and psychology.

73. Michaud-Quantin, *Études*, p. 24.

74. The frequent recurrence of this term in numerous texts scattered throughout Book III, in addition to the text cited above (see SA III 35.1; III 36.1.1; III 38.2; III 39.5.4; III 40.1; III 42.2.1.2) make it abundantly clear that *aestimatio* describes the fundamental act of faith. So significant is *aestimatio* to the act of faith that William even describes the first sin in Eden as at root an improper estimation or judgment of the good. While other authors had posited pride, omission, or doubt as the root of the first sin, William opts for infidelity, which is the result of improper estimation. "The apprehended good moves. Since it happens in estimation that the good moves the appetite, as is clear through the contrary. For a sheep does not flee the wolf unless it estimates the wolf to be noxious to itself; therefore before the woman wished to be like God she estimated that she was able to be as God. But such estimation was infidelity; thus her first sin was infidelity" (SA II 9.3.1: 254,15ff).

75. Michaud-Quantin, *Études*, pp. 22–23.

76. O. Lottin, "La théorie du libre arbitre au treizième siècle," *Revue thomiste* 32 (1927): pp. 359ff.

77. SA II 10.3: 281,92ff.

78. Michaud-Quantin suggests that William prefers the verb *aestimare* over the substantive *aestimatio* and that this reflects the fact that the pejorative sense of the latter did not extend to the former. He offers this text as an example in which William uses both *arbitrari* and *aestimare* side by side in the verb form, but only *arbitratio* in the noun form (*Études*, p. 23). In actual fact, though, William appears to have no qualms about using the substantive *aestimatio* and does so frequently (see the texts cited below).

parison with spiritual goods." As in the Arabic usage, a key feature of faith's *aestimatio* is its certitude: "faith is the certain estimator *(certa estimatrix)* of all things."⁷⁹ Yet, though it draws on both traditions, William's use of this term is unique.⁸⁰ In this respect, he has the distinction of being the first and last scholastic thinker to give to *aestimatio* a special meaning in relation to faith.⁸¹

How precisely does *aestimatio* function in faith? In contrast to the Aristotelian tradition, William locates *aestimatio* in the intellectual (not the animal) part of the soul and views it as a rational judgment of the speculative intellect. For "to apprehend *(apprehendere)* something is to cognize *(cognoscere)* it, and to cognize is the same as to judge *(iuidicare);* hence, since the intellect alone is held to comprehend *(comprehendere)* and to cognize insensible things, it is only of the intellect to judge of insensible things."⁸² Yet, his usage also contrasts with the twelfth-century theologians in that he grants to faith's *aestimatio* the highest degree of certitude and confidence, placing the knowledge of faith not only above opinion (as did Hugh of St. Victor), but above even Aristotelian *scientia* and syllogistic demonstration (in contrast to Hugh).⁸³ A final and

---

79. SA III 35.1: 668,61f.

80. Englhardt observes that William's understanding of the nature of faith *(Glaubenspsychologie)* is a synthesis of various elements: the psychology of Praepositinus, some well-known sections of the *Nicomachean Ethics,* Augustinian and pseudo-Dionysian philosophies, the contrast between Peter of Corbeil's Pauline Commentaries and the direction of Stephen Langton (*Glaubenspsychologie*, p. 279).

81. Michaud-Quantin, *Études*, pp. 17–18. When, in his *De bono,* William of Auvergne uses the term *aestimatio* several decades later in the same context, he clearly has in mind the older, and for him pejorative, notion associated with William of St. Thierry and Bernard on the equivalence of *aestimatio* and *opinio*. It is similar to the knowledge of something only obscurely seen; the vision of the truth which it gives is analogous to that of night animals which cannot bear the light of day. Humans make their estimations in the blindness of darkness. William of Auvergne uses the word *credulitas* as a synonym. He also defines it as *opinabilis apprehensio*. It is not only deprived of certitude, but is radically imperfect and susceptible to error.

82. SA II 10.6.1: 300,70ff.

83. SA III 12.2: 201,47ff. "We say that faith is not only above opinion, but also above science, even above demonstrative science. For the intellect illumined by faith believes in the first truth more than in a syllogistic demonstration. Hence, when it is said [by Hugh of St. Victor]: 'faith is midway between opinion and science,' this is understood concerning the opinion of unformed faith and concerning the manifest science by which we will see God in the future *facie ad faciem*."

unique aspect of William's view of *aestimatio* is that it is generative of rational rather than animal desire. Just as "a sheep would not flee a wolf, unless it estimated the wolf to be noxious to itself, so no brute animal naturally desires something unless it first estimates it to be amicable to itself." So, just as in animals, "estimation generates attraction *(appetitum)* and aversion *(fugam)*," so in rational creatures, "the estimation of reason generates rational desire and rational aversion."[84] As will be seen, this causal link between estimation and desire will prove determinative in William's view of faith.[85] In sum, then, modeled on certain Aristotelian conceptions of sense perception, *aestimatio* is a rational, perception-like judgment of the speculative intellect concerning spiritual, non-sensible realities; it possesses the highest degree of certitude and generates rational desire for its object.

The bonum ut verum: *Faith's Object and Its Twofold Act*

This view of faith as entailing an *aestimatio* allows William to resolve the problem, introduced above, of how to maintain faith's cognitive relation to the true, as well as posit a genuine relation to the good as a virtue. As a rational act, faith is a speculative cognition of the true: "faith consists in speculation of the first truth."[86] As an *aestimatio*, though, faith is also a judgment of the good: "faith possesses a judgment by which it determines that God is our highest good, [and] the end and source of unmediated delight."[87] Hence, faith "does not consist purely in speculation, neither is its end only the true, but also the good. For as long as by faith the intellect speculates on the first truth, it estimates it to be the highest delectable and the highest good for itself and is moved toward it in order to delight and rest in it."[88] Thus, though William tends to speak of faith's object as the *bonum ut verum*, the good as the true (and so positing its

---

84. SA III 8.2: 721,121ff.
85. Englhardt notes that the "psychological bearer of *aestimatio* and the affective acts following from it, the *desiderium, tendere, amare, delectari,* and *quiescere*, is the speculative intellect" (*Glaubenspsychologie*, p. 280).
86. SA III 12.2: 200,22.
87. SA III 36.1.1: 690,215. Cf. SA III 38.2: 721,127: "The estimation of the good is of faith."
88. SA III 12.2: 200,20ff.

virtuous nature as directly related to the good), he will also shift the perspective and speak of faith's object as the *verum ut bonum:* the true, known in intellectual cognition, which faith's *aestimatio* judges to be the good as well, and, more precisely, as the delectable good, the proper human end: "[faith itself] is the cognition and estimation of the end."[89]

In effect, William posits two inseparable, yet distinguishable moments within faith. Behind this distinction lies the above-noted assumption, Aristotelian in origin, concerning the ontological identity of goodness and truth. William's conception of faith corresponds to this identity. Enlisting the Stagarite's authority, he avers that "the true and the good are the same; but it is called *verum* as the end of the intellect or speculation, the *bonum* as the end of desire and action. Whence, Aristotle, in the *De anima:* 'the good and the true are the same; but it is called the truth in as much as it is without act, the good in as much as it is with act.'"[90] Aristotle's distinction prompts William to argue that in as much as faith is oriented toward the true *qua* true, through cognition or speculation, it relates to its end without movement. The logic behind this "motionless act" is the assumption that "to believe or to assent is not properly an act, since an act is properly toward possessing or acquiring something." As for Aristotle's notion of cognition, so for William's view of faith, a speculative act is without movement: "The first truth is the end of faith, toward which it tends, in which it has to rest *(quiescere);* but rest in that is only the end *by which* it rests and delights in that end; and thus it does not have to be moved into that rest properly."[91] Paradoxically, then, faith's cognition of the true is not actually an act: "though faith, properly speaking, does not have an act . . . nevertheless it possesses the act which conjoins the soul to God without motion."[92] Faith's first act, its end *by which (finis quo)* it rests, then, is cognition or speculation of the first truth. Thus: "the desire for the first truth *(prima veritas)* by efficient or perfect cognizing, which is of faith, is the first act of the rational soul, by which the intellect through faith desires the first truth, either cognition or vision of it, so that it may rest in it."[93]

---

89. SA III 36.1.1: 690,219.
90. SA III 10.4.3: 153,86. Cf. Aristotle, *De Anima* III 428a 22–23; III 431b 10–11.
91. SA III 39.1: 732,154.   92. SA II 8.2.9.5: 224,35ff.
93. SA III 39.1: 731,124. William continues the thought: "But that this kind of love of

It is subsequent to and from this first act that faith's *aestimatio* of the true as identical with and so constitutive of its good emerges. Faith judges the true to be its desired end,[94] which judgment generates the desire to possess and move toward rest in it.[95] "Faith must rest in the first truth; but everything which must rest in something it can acquire is moved toward that; so faith by its nature is only moved to the first truth by desire or appetite *(desiderium sive appetitum).*"[96] Faith's second moment, then, is *aestimatio*'s perception of the *verum* as its *summum bonum* and the concomitant movement toward this end born of desire or appetite. This second moment appears to correspond to the so-called "second movement" of any virtue, noted above, namely, the attendant experience of delight arising from the encounter between a virtue's primary act and its proper end. Here, the estimative moment is this moment of delight.

In faith, William concludes, "there is a twofold movement *(duplex motus)* toward the first truth." The first is a quasi-movement "toward cognizing *(ad cognoscendum)* the first truth." That is, the soul is moved to that act *by which (quo)* it rests in God. In the second, though, there is "a true movement toward possession *(ad habendum),*"[97] toward the object in which *(in quo)* it desires to rest. William explicitly concedes that the term *motus* is used equivocally here:[98] "these two acts are not univocal, since the act toward possession follows the cognition of the thing to be possessed."[99] The first is not properly an act at all, while the second is. "The true in as much as it is true is without movement *(sine motu)*, the good, in as much as it is the good, is with movement *(cum motu).*"[100]

God is in the intellect is clear through that which Augustine said: 'to love God with the whole heart is to love God in the intellect without error, to love God with the whole soul is to love God in the will without contradiction or contrariety;' but the love of God by which we love God in the intellect, so that by seeing we may rest in God, is of faith, and 'the first act toward God,' as Dionysius said."

94. SA III 38.2: 723,177. 95. SA III 38.2: 724,216.
96. SA III 38.2: 723,171. 97. SA III 39.1: 731, 118.
98. SA III 39.1: 731,110ff. "It is true that by the act of faith the soul is moved to the first truth, so that it may rest in it; but this proposition is not generally true: 'if something is moved to something, etc.' This is true for univocal acts, all of which are toward possession, . . . but it does not hold for the act toward cognizing but for the act toward resting in or possession."
99. SA III 39.1: 731,117. 100. SA III 38.2: 723,180.

Faith, then, has its own substantial relation to the good, has its own desire for, possession of, rest in its proper end—"the good is still the material and end of faith . . . but with respect to the true":[101]

> For *within itself,* faith possesses an estimation . . . and so it possesses joy and delight of *itself.* . . . For faith *in se* is the cognition and estimation of its end and is moved by the act of love toward its end by that cognition and estimation; and so it possesses *in itself* the reason *(ratio)* of its act, for it is the first master *(prima magistra)* of the virtues.[102]

In this way, William gives faith an essential integrity as a virtue, having not only a proper act, a specific desire for its end, and concomitant delight, but also a proper object or end in which it is to rest.[103] This desire for possession of and rest in the good, born here, as it were, with faith, will come to maturity in the theological virtue which grows out of it, namely, charity.[104]

In sum, by incorporating an Arabic-Aristotelian *aestimatio* into his conception of faith, William puts forward a unique view of this virtue.[105] Faith is a cognitive act of the speculative intellect, which apprehends the *prima veritas* precisely as the *summum bonum* through an *aestimatio,* an affective judgment. Faith can be characterized as a speculative discernment *(discernere),* a contemplative consideration *(consideratio),* "a savorous judgment,"[106] desire-generating and affection-satisfying, of the

---

101. SA III 38.2: 723,177. Cf. SA III 14.6: 266,36: "Thus, faith is inclined toward its own good *per se* and according to itself; so in its very self is the virtue perfected. . . . faith tends toward its own proper good, namely toward the first illuminating."
102. SA III 36.1.1: 690,210ff.
103. SA III 38.2: 722,157ff.
104. SA III 38.2: 723,177. "The good is first the substance of faith before it is the substance of charity." The virtue of charity will be explored in the following chapter.
105. Englhardt's comparison of William's conception of faith with Hugh of St. Victor's is instructive. Hugh sharply separated the function of the intellect and that of the will, comparing the relation of intellect to will to that of matter to form: he assigns the decisive role to the will in the whole faith-act. Hugh thus contrasts with Abelard, who stressed the intellectual moment in believing. For his part, William everywhere unites the Hugonian poles, stressing the speculative nature of faith's knowledge. To that extent the superficial viewer could find a similarity between William and Abelard. But William's intention does not deny the participation of the affection or reduce its significance for faith. Faith's speculative aspect, which he construes as virtuous, differentiates it from the other virtues. But he seeks in faith's speculation the affection's ardor, which Hugh had pulled too far apart (Englhardt, *Glaubenspsychologie,* p. 279).
106. William J. Conlan coined this useful phrase for William's view of faith in his

good as true.[107] Because of its *aestimatio* (and here the germ of William's doctrine of the spiritual senses emerges), faith is a kind of intellectual perception or perceptual judgment, which carries over from its original context in animal sense perception an association with sensation. For Aristotle, intellectual knowing is analogous to sense perception; William too finds this view fruitful. Faith's cognition of the true is somehow like the sense perception of its own good, of its end to be desired, possessed, united with, rested in.[108] Speculation has an affective dimension. With *aestimatio*, the intellect transcends a purely speculative, ethically neutral posture and experiences a virtuous and delectable union with its end. Faith is thus both a virtue and a science and might best be called a "speculative virtue."[109]

Faith's Substantial Mode of Delight: per modum visus

When William comes at various points in the *Summa Aurea* to sum up this act of faith, he characterizes it as a form of spiritual vision *(visus)*: "The first good, that is, the first delectable *(primum delectabile)* which is God, in as much as God is an illuminating light, is delectable to the intellect through the mode of sight *(per modum visus)* or through the mode of cognition *(modum cognitionis)*; and such delectable love . . . is of the substance of faith."[110] Examples of this orientation toward vision are easily multiplied: "faith is a certain vision or knowledge of eternal things";[111] "vision is properly of reason (the power perfected by faith)";[112] "faith is a vision of the truth";[113] "therefore to delight in the vision of God is . . . of faith, whose it is to see God in the present."[114] In the

---

article "The Definition of Faith According to a Question of Ms. Assisi 138: Study and Edition of Text," in *Essays in Honour of Anton Charles Pegis*, ed. J. R. O'Donnell (Toronto: Pontifical Institute of Medieval Studies, 1974), p. 26.

107. SA III 11.3.5: 194, 61.

108. In effect, William assimilates the Aristotelian notion of prudence (discernment of good or evil, what is to be pursued or avoided) within the sphere of speculative theology. See Edgar de Bruyne, *Études d'esthétique médiévale*, 3 vols. (Bruges, 1946), vol. 3, p. 75.

109. Englhardt suggests that William's lasting merit lies in the fact that he offered for the first time a complete and coherent system of faith-psychology (*Glaubenspsychologie*, pp. 279).

110. SA III 10.4.3: 151–52,52ff.   111. SA III 12 7.3: 223,14.
112. SA III 36.1.1: 687,126.   113. SA III 12.3: 206,131 (alt).
114. SA III 36.1.1: 686,84.

medieval Neoplatonic tradition stemming from Augustine and Dionysius, William uses the term beauty *(pulchritudo),* apparently referring precisely to the good as true, to describe the object of this vision: "the vision of the highest beauty suffices for the love of it, just as the estimation of the horrible and noxious suffices in a sheep so that it flees the wolf."[115] As is his wont, he offers an explanatory analogy from physical beauty: "Just as there is delight in the vision of sensuous beauty; so there is delight in the vision of intelligible beauty."[116] Again, "corporal sight is delighted by corporal beauty; thus, how much more is spiritual sight *(visus spiritualis),* namely the intellect, delighted by the highest spiritual beauty *(summa pulchritudine spirituali),* except by faith; hence, faith is essentially delighted by the first truth or the first beauty *(prima pulchritudine).*"[117] Thus, faith is "the habit of loving . . . the first beauty,"[118] or "the apprehension of the beauty of the first truth,"[119] and faith finds fruition when it sees the First Beauty unveiled before it as its highest delectable.[120]

Faith's Delight and the Spiritual Senses

William thus sums up the nature of faith as having a primary visual modality, as spiritual vision or sight *(visus).* Certainly, in one sense, *visus* functions here as a metaphor—to be sure, it is the primary metaphor in medieval illuminationist epistemologies generally, of which William's is an instance. Yet, for him, *visus* is more than metaphorical. As seen above, faith entails a kind of intellectual perception of the *bonum ut verum,* analogous to an animal's perception *(aestimatio)* of its kin, and as just noted it is spiritual *visus* that sees divine beauty. Moreover, as noted in Chapter 2, William's discussion of beatitude assumed an actual, distinct spiritual sense of sight. At key points, then, regarding both this present life and the next, he refers explicitly to the spiritual sense of sight in relation to faith.

115. SA III 42.2.1.2: 806,25.
116. SA III 36.1.1: 685,40.
117. SA III 38.2: 718,36ff.
118. SA III 38.2: 719,40.
119. SA III 42.1.3: 802,94; cf. SA III.38.2: 722,159: "Faith is the love *(amor)* of the first truth *(prime veritatis)* or of the first beauty *(prime pulcritudinis).*"
120. SA II 8.2.9.5: 224,39. "After faith and charity are deep within [it] . . . the faithful soul sees the first beauty openly."

Yet in the quotation with which this chapter began, William links faith with the activity of all the spiritual senses. How then is faith's primary visual modality to be related to that description of faith's relation to the whole *sensorium*? What exactly does he mean by the spiritual sense of sight? Does he wish to associate spiritual sight exclusively with the virtue of faith and the rational power of the soul? By implication, is each spiritual sense to be coupled with a distinct theological virtue? That is, as William puts it: "if the suavity *(suavitas)* of God delights the spiritual touch and for this delight there is a certain virtue," then, there ought to be a distinct virtue for "the sweetness *(dulcedo)* of God" delighting "spiritual taste *(gustus spiritualis)*" and for "the melody *(melodia)* of God" delighting "spiritual hearing *(auditus spiritualis)*" and so forth, such that "there ought to be five theological virtues according to the five delights of the five spiritual senses *(quinque sensum spiritualium)*."[121]

An answer to this question must begin by recalling from his discussion of the spiritual senses in the context of beatitude that, for William, there is fundamentally only a singular spiritual sense, namely, the intellect or rational power of the soul:[122] "Even though logically *(secundum rationem)* there are five spiritual senses, yet essentially *(in essentia)* there is only one sense, namely the intellect." Accordingly, here as there, William denies the need for a specific, one-to-one alignment between the various theological virtues and the spiritual senses: "it is not necessary that there be five virtues perfecting the five spiritual senses, rather one suffices, namely faith." For, "there is only one spiritual sense, the intellect, and only one virtue which perfects the spiritual sense, namely faith."[123]

Also germane, from the same discussion of beatitude, are William's remarks on the essential singularity of faith, despite its diverse objects of

---

121. SA III 36.1.1: 686,95ff.
122. See above Chapter 2 and the quotation with which this chapter began. Cf. also SA III 36.1.1: 685,43: "the intellect has its delight in its end and perfection; but the perfection of the intellect is faith; therefore by faith the intellect delights in God, and so by faith we have fruition of God."
123. SA IV 18.3.3.2.3: 509,18ff. Cf. SA IV 18.3.3.2.4: 514,70f. As noted in Chapter 2, William refers to this singular spiritual sense as the "the *sensus communis*," a designation of Aristotelian psychology for one of the inner senses.

belief. This singularity obtains due to faith's singular formal object. "Though there are diverse things to be believed *(credentia)* and diverse believable things *(credulitates)*, yet faith is singular, since the formal object *(ratio)* of believing is the same." William sees a parallel between faith's singularity and that of the spiritual sense: "even though there are diverse acts of the spiritual senses, there is, nevertheless, one virtue and one habit, since there is one formal object of perceiving *(ratio percipiendi)*, namely, through faith."[124] And so, "the spiritual sense is one, even though it has many objects." Materially, there are diverse sense objects, diverse acts of spiritual sensation, and diverse forms of spiritual delight. Yet, formally there remains a singular spiritual sense, the intellect, and a single perfecting virtue, faith.

In William's view of beatitude, then, the intellect through faith apprehends and delights in the Trinity in a "spiritually sensuous" manner through its singular spiritual sense. Yet, because of the manifold nature of the *delectabilia divina*—the real diversity of the Holy Spirit's effects within the soul—this encounter involves a real diversity of spiritual perceptions. So, to accommodate both a singular intellect and its manifold spiritual sense delights of beatitude, he shifts from spiritual sense in the singular (i.e., the rational intellect) to plural spiritual sense acts (spiritual sight, sound, smell, taste, and touch) in his description of the soul's experience of fruition. Perfected and enabled by faith, the intellect apprehends the Trinity through a "spiritually sensuous" encounter of all the spiritual senses with all the *delectabilia divina*.[125]

William, therefore, does not wish to identify or exclusively associate

---

124. SA IV 18.3.3.2.4: 515,95f. *Sicut enim dictum est in questione de fide, licet sint diversa credentia et diverse credulitas, tamen una est fides, quia eadem est ratio credendi. Similiter, licet sint diverse operationes sensus spiritualis, unica tamen est virtus, et unicus habitus, quia unica est ratio percipiendi, scilicet per fidem.* Cf. SA IV 18.3.3.2.3: 511,88ff: "For faith is one, even though it has many objects, such as hell, eternal life, and many other things. And this is the case since there is one formal object *(ratio)* of all things to be believed. Similarly, since there is one formal object *(ratio)* of sensible delighting in spiritual things, the spiritual sense *(sensus spiritualis)* is one, even though it has many objects."

125. In light of this fundamental understanding of spiritual perception, it must be observed that for William the spiritual senses are not, properly speaking, resident capacities of the soul; still less are they permanent faculties; rather they are faith-enabled acts of spiritual perception on the part of the singular intellect or spiritual sense.

the virtue of faith with spiritual sight. Here, it must be noted that the distinction between the singular intellect and its diverse spiritual perceptions corresponds to the above-noted distinction between a virtue's substantial act (first act, cognition in the case of faith) and its concomitant delight (second act, estimation's delight and rest in the case of faith). This distinction between speculation and delectation creates a certain space for all the spiritual senses, not just spiritual sight. The substantial act (primary *motus*) of the singular intellect is speculative cognition of *veritas*, but its experience of manifold delight in the *verum ut bonum* (secondary *motus*) occurs through diverse spiritual perceptions. Hence, the acts of spiritual senses are the occasion and means of faith's delight: delight occurs through, and is concomitant with, spiritual sense perception. Most precisely, the intellect is oriented toward speculation of *veritas*, not toward the delight that is concomitant with speculation through the spiritual senses: "To delight in the vision of God is of faith; but faith does not tend properly toward delighting, but toward vision, which is accompanied by delight."[126] Again, "faith is not properly oriented toward delight, but is properly oriented toward the cognition of the first truth, which is concomitant with delight."[127] Strictly speaking, faith's movement is toward apprehending the first truth with the result that delight occurs there. The end *in which* faith delights is properly *veritas*, not the accompanying *delectatio*.

Why, then, does William characterize faith as a form of spiritual *visus*, as *per modum visus*? The answer is best seen in light of the above-noted distinction between a virtue's proper object (*finis in quo*) and its proper act (*finis quo*). As seen, the end *by which* faith rests is cognition. This is faith's substantial act and William described it paradoxically as a "motionless act." Properly speaking, it is this act of cognition which he construes as having the modality of spiritual *visus*. Faith is best described as *visus* because it perceives the beauty of the *prima veritas* in some sense without motion, perhaps in the same way that physical sight seems to see immediately without being moved, without any change in the "distance" between viewer and object.

126. SA III 36.1.1: 688,136.
127. SA III 36.1.1: 687,117.

In effect, then, William has appropriated spiritual *visus* to the act of faith. Yet, *visus* is understood here by way of synecdoche: it stands for, and sums up, all other acts of spiritual perception. As William described it in his treatment of beatitude,

> By seeing God we will hear spiritually, since by seeing we will have cognition *(cognitio)*; and this is to hear by seeing *(audire videndo)*. We will assemble the goods given to us by God and this will be to perceive the odor *(odorari)* of God by seeing *(odorari videndo)*. We will know the internal *rationes* of God; and this will be to taste *(gustare)* spiritually. Likewise, by seeing God we will be inflamed by his love . . . and this will be to touch *(tangere)* him. . . . so will that vision have in itself every delectable thing.[128]

In a synaesthetic manner, the single act of faith's vision contains the experience of every *delectamentum* associated with the other spiritual senses. Following on the act of faith, primarily construed as spiritual *visus*, is its concomitant delight which pertains to all the spiritual senses. Given the intimate connection between faith's speculation and concomitant delight through the spiritual senses, he "reads" back into faith's substantial act the sense modality of spiritual *visus* which, in light of its particular characteristics in the realm of physical sense perception, is especially apt for describing faith's primary act.

Conclusion

A remarkable feature of William's conception of the virtues generally, and of the theological virtues in particular, is its consistent orientation toward spiritual perception through the spiritual senses. The graces of Christ the Head flow into the ecclesial body as senses of grace *(sensus gratie)*, as spiritual senses and movements *(sensus et motus spirituales)*. Progress in the virtues prepares the soul's capacity for spiritual perception or sensation: it cleanses the "palate of the heart" *(palat[i]um cordis)* so that the soul increasingly "senses *(sentit)* the sweetness of God."

In particular, the virtue of faith relates the soul directly and immediately to God as the perfecting *habitus* of the soul's rational power. Faith has its substantial twofold act *(motus)* of *cognitio* and *aestimatio*, and as-

---

128. SA IV 18.3.3.2.4: 513–14,56ff.

sociated delight, which arises uniquely from its encounter with its proper object, the first truth *(prima veritas)* or, rather, the *bonum ut verum*. This gives faith's speculative *scientia* an essentially virtuous affectivity. All of this, William sums up in the construal of faith as spiritual *visus* of divine beauty, encompassing the good as true. Precisely at this juncture, in order to describe fully faith's experience, he resorts to his doctrine of the spiritual senses. Faith's delight in the *bonum ut verum* comes from its manifold perception of it. This fundamental notion of faith as perception undergirds his expansion of faith's primary visual modality into diverse modes of spiritual perception and their associated delights.

CHAPTER 7

CHARITY
Love of God in a Tactile Mode

FOR WILLIAM, as noted at the outset of the preceding chapter, beatitude entails a role for *dilectio,* for the *affectus* or concupiscible power and its perfecting virtue, charity: "beatitude occurs in the concupiscible power through *affectio* or perfect *dilectio.*" At the same time, faith is primary, both in this life and the next, because charity depends upon faith: "charity does not delight in God nor does it have fruition of God except by faith." This dependence, however, does not relegate charity's role to insignificance. Rather, William will argue that ultimately charity consummates faith's fruition, for charity's act culminates in contact, leading to union between God and the soul. By charity, the soul delights "through the mode of union *(per modum conjunctionis)* because 'delight is the union of the lover with the beloved.'"[1] This assumption prompts William to appropriate a distinct sense modality to this virtue. While the predominant sense modality for the act of faith is *visus,* for charity it is *tactus.* Charity is a form of spiritual touch, and to it God is delectable "in a tactile modality *(per modum tactus).*"[2] William's conception of charity is thus directly related to his doctrine of the spiritual senses.

While faith and charity have essential differences and unique functions, they do not operate in isolation from each other. William posits an interconnectedness between them that implies that they act in concert

1. SA III 11.3.5: 194,52f.
2. SA III 10.4.3: 152,56f.

with one another. They are acts of one and the same soul in its relationship to God. He describes this relationship thus: "the rational power has been given for the purpose of apprehending *(ad cognoscendum)* the highest good and the highest truth," while "the concupiscible power has been given for this, that it is moved into the highest good *(ad summum bonum).*"[3] Charity, then, can be defined generally as a desire-born movement for the delight experienced through faith. Charity moves faith to the act of delighting and having fruition, since, as William is fond of saying, "wherever love is, the eyes follow."[4] Ultimately, these two virtues, and the activities of the soul which they enable, provide the basic framework for the activity of the spiritual senses.

The Initial Relationship between Faith and Charity

An analysis of William's teaching on charity begins with this virtue's dependence on the virtue of faith. The priority William gives to faith rests upon two assumptions. First, in his view of the soul, "the rational power is to command the concupiscible and irascible powers,"[5] and, accordingly, the virtue that perfects reason (i.e., faith) ought to govern the virtues which perfect the other two powers.[6] So, "just as reason must first discern and command, before the concupiscible power desires . . . so the act of formed faith must precede the act of charity."[7] Second, from an epistemic standpoint, it is axiomatic for William that cognition of an end must precede desire for it.[8] Since nothing is loved before it is known,

---

3. SA IV 18.3.3.1: 499,90ff.

4. SA IV 18.3.3.1: 502,166. "For love *(dilectio)* tends toward this, that it might delight in loving through vision *(per visionem)*. Hence, 'where love is, the eyes follow.'"

5. SA III 38.2: 718,21. "For reason is the spiritual king of the kingdom of the soul, hence on that verse in Ecclesiastes: *woe to that land whose king is a child*, the Gloss says: 'the king, that is, reason'; if, as king, reason has to govern the virtues and the other powers, then the virtue which is located in reason has to rule all the other virtues."

6. SA III 38.2: 721,118. "For it is a common, natural conception of the soul that reason ought to govern the concupiscible and irascible powers."

7. SA III 38.2: 718,25.

8. SA III 38.2: 718,17: "'To know the end in the right way is prior to being moved to that end in the right way'; but faith is the true cognition of the end; but charity is moved to that end; thus faith is naturally prior to charity." SA III 39.1: 730,60: "But that faith is substantially prior to charity is proved through this: that the cognition of the end is naturally prior to the act of the virtue naturally oriented toward that end; thus the cognition of the first goodness is prior to the desire for it; and so faith is prior to charity naturally."

the *primum bonum* is first the *bonum intellectus* before it is the *bonum affectus*.⁹

Faith not only precedes charity, but also generates it. As described in the previous chapter, there is a twofold movement toward the *bonum ut verum*. First, faith "moves" toward cognition of the *prima veritas* by a paradoxical "motionless act"; second, it truly moves to the *verum* when by *aestimatio* faith perceives it as *bonum* and as *pulchritudo*—that is, as delectable and desirable¹⁰—and moves to delight and rest in it. Thus, within faith itself, *aestimatio* generates a desire for the good. It is precisely this appetite for the good which becomes charity, desiring the good as good. The good is first the object of faith before it is the object of charity.¹¹ Yet, once faith has apprehended the beauty of the first truth, it necessarily generates love in the affection, and the soul desires God by charity.¹² Again, since the good is not revealed as *veritas*, without also simultaneously being revealed as *suavitas*, the movement of charity *(motus caritatis)* develops immediately.¹³ In short, faith's estimation generates the desire that is charity.¹⁴

9. SA III 40.1: 765,122. "We say that faith is the necessary cause of all the virtues, and faith necessarily generates all the virtues, especially since all the virtues tend to the end of faith, since the cognition of the highest good necessarily generates the love of God, and so of the others."

10. SA III 38.2: 721,133ff. "Formed faith precedes all the other virtues, especially for this reason, that the cognition of the end naturally precedes the act ordained toward that end. . . . And that this is so is taken from a simile with brute animals, since the sheep would not flee the wolf, unless it estimated the wolf to be noxious to itself, for if it estimated the wolf to be a dog, it would not flee, in the same way no brute animal desires something naturally unless it first estimates it to be friendly to itself; therefore, since it is the case in brutes that their estimation generates attraction *(appetitum)* and aversion *(fugum)*, it is similar in rational animals, that the estimation of reason generates rational desire and rational aversion; but it is agreed that the estimation of the good is of faith; hence, faith precedes charity, the charity of which is to desire the good."

11. SA III 38.2: 723,177.

12. SA III 42.2.1.2: 806,25. "So faith immediately generates charity, for the vision of the highest beauty suffices for the love of it, just as the estimation of the horrible and noxious suffices in a sheep so that it flees the wolf." Cf. SA III 42.1.3: 802,93: "That we concede saying that charity is in faith as an effect in a cause, for as was shown above, [faith] is the cause of charity, for since faith is the cognition of the beauty of the first truth, of necessity it generates love in the affection and thus charity, ergo faith is the cause of charity."

13. SA III 38.2: 724,216.

14. SA III 38.2: 723,200. "The estimation, by which someone judges God to be the highest good or highest delectable through faith, is generative of the desire for that good. This is clear through a simile with brute animals. For when a dog estimates a bone to be delec-

The good must first belong to the estimation before [it belongs to] to desire, for how would it desire this kind of good unless first it were estimated and judged to be true and good, since in that case it would be moved toward an end, which was not predetermined to be the end; but estimation or judgment or predetermination of the good or the end is the work of faith.[15]

Faith produces charity because it creates a new apprehension of divine things, which in turn generates a new appetite or love for those things.[16] William concludes, then, that since "faith is the sufficient, first and principal cause of charity,"[17] charity is the effect of faith and faith's most perfect work. Hence, even as he grants that the theological virtues are inextricably linked, that all are infused simultaneously, and that whoever has one has all,[18] he yet gives faith a logical or natural priority and causality.[19] By way of summary, he offers a trinitarian analogy:

---

table or amicable for itself, it is moved immediately to it, and that animal estimation immediately generates animal desire; therefore, similarly, the estimation of faith by which someone estimates God to be his highest good immediately generates the desire for that highest good; therefore, that act [of faith] immediately generates the act of charity."

15. SA III 38.2: 723,181. Cf. SA III 40.1: 762,27: "A sheep, seeing a wolf, estimating it to be unfriendly and dangerous to itself, immediately flees; but just as judging something to be horrible for oneself causes aversion, so the estimation of something delectable causes appetite; but with the estimation of the horrible aversion comes necessarily; so with the estimation of the delectable, appetite for it comes necessarily; thus estimating God to be delectable for oneself, it necessarily desires God for itself; but that which is done by nature with difficulty is done easily by virtue; thus, when someone by faith estimates God to be delectable for himself, he desires God for himself; but this appetite is nothing but charity; thus he has charity, and consequently all the other virtues."

16. SA III 10.1.3: 120,22. "But when man is in the old state he cannot be moved by the act of love into God, rather he is first moved by the act of cognition; thus for the same reason, the new man in justification cannot be moved by the act of love into God; rather he is first moved by the act of cognition in his new mode, namely the motion of faith; and in justification the act of faith must be first."

17. SA III 36.1.1: 687,129: "Since love is an immediate effect of faith, Augustine said . . . that 'charity is in faith.'" SA III 14.7: 268,31: "The understanding of faith is the cause effecting the love of God." SA III 38.2: 719,50: "Commenting on the verse in Galatians: *in Christ neither circumcision nor uncircumcision avails for anything, but faith that works through charity,* Augustine [*In I Joan.,* tr. 10, n.2 (PL 35.2055) via the Lombard's *Gloss]* said: 'the work of faith is love or delight'; thus, faith is the efficient cause of charity; hence, it is naturally prior to charity."

18. SA III 14.1: 255,84. "The intellect is the beginning of all the virtues materially; and from it all the virtues proceed not effectively, but materially; but they proceed effectively from God. . . . Charity proceeds from faith and hope as from its original cause; yet all the virtues are infused simultaneously and are simultaneous through the nature of the connection, not through the nature of the causality."

19. SA III 38.1:715,64. "We say that all the virtues are naturally simultaneous. For faith is

Just as the Son proceeds from the Father, and the Holy Spirit from both, so hope is generated by faith, and charity [is generated] from faith and hope. And, just as the Father spirates the Holy Spirit—since he gives to the Son to spirate the Holy Spirit—so faith immediately generates charity, for the vision of the highest beauty suffices for the love of it.[20]

As the Father generates the Son and the Spirit proceeds from both, so faith generates hope, and from faith and hope comes charity; yet ultimately charity also proceeds immediately from faith, in the same way that the vision of the highest beauty immediately produces love and desire for it.

In light of faith's primacy over charity, William rejects a common assumption of his contemporaries: that faith receives its essential formation from charity and that charity is the mother of all the virtues.[21] Rather, he credits God directly with the essential formation of both faith and charity,[22] rather than love or grace.[23] With him, then, faith acquires a new status among scholastic theologians,[24] and in a radical way—by giv-

---

the necessary cause of hope and charity, but charity is the necessary cause of all the other virtues. But this argument is not valid: 'all the virtues are naturally simultaneous, ergo none is naturally prior to any other,' for faith, in as much as it is the cause of hope and charity, is naturally prior to them, but in as much as it is their necessary cause, which being established, they are established, it is simultaneous with them, and so from the same nature it is prior to and simultaneous with them, but in one way and another."

20. SA III 42.2.1.2: 806,19ff.

21. See Lottin, *Psychologie et morale*, vol. 3, pp. 197ff. William, in effect, does not admit without restriction the axiom received in the schools on the subject of charity as the mother of the virtues; he even denies this view the title of an "authority," judging that the axiom stems from a false conception of the Lombard regarding the Holy Spirit. Cf. SA III 14.6: 266,47f. "That authority which called charity the mother of all the virtues was not the authority of the saints, but the authority of the Lombard who said that charity is nothing other than the Holy Spirit; and thus we are not required to consent to such an authority. Yet charity can be called the mother of all virtues on account of its act. For there is not any virtue which charity does not move to its act, sometimes it even moves faith. Whence the Apostle: *charity believes all things*."

22. SA III 14.6: 266,54. "In the absence of charity all the virtues are unformed; yet the advent of charity does not perfect them; but God who gives faith perfects them; and to the extent to which God perfects faith, God generates charity in persons."

23. SA II 8.2.9.5: 224,34: "It should be said that God alone essentially perfects faith and charity at the same time." SA III.38.2: 719,45: "Faith is essentially love, even though it is not that which is charity; and [faith's] love is gratuitous, since it tends only toward God; thus, [faith's] love is meritorious; thus, it is perfect; thus, it is not perfected by charity; thus, it has neither its essence nor its perfection from charity."

24. Englhardt, *Glaubenspsychologie*, p. 220. Prior to William, the scholastics understood the supernatural formation of faith to occur only by the addition of love. He is the

ing faith its own substantial integrity and priority in the salvific process—he thereby avoids an ultimate absorbing of faith into charity.²⁵

The Substantial Nature of Charity

When William comes to define the substantial nature of charity, he proceeds in a manner parallel to his treatment of faith. He describes charity in relation to the power of the soul which it perfects, in relation to its proper act, object, and mode of delectation by which it relates to God. As faith perfects the rational power of the soul, so charity is a *habi-*

---

first theologian, who, as a principal condition of true faith, sees the fact that one believes God for God's own sake and above all as the most substantial circumstance of *fides formata*. This occurs without the addition of charity. Cf. SA III 14.6: 265,29ff: "Believing is prior to loving; . . . to believe the first truth for its own sake and above all else is prior to loving the first goodness for its own sake and above all else; so the act of formed faith is prior to the act of formed charity; therefore, formed faith is prior to formed charity; thus, charity does not inform faith." Cf. SA III 14.6: 266,37: "Faith thus is inclined toward its own proper good through itself and according to itself; thus in itself it is perfected; thus it is not perfected or formed by charity. . . . Charity in no way inclines faith toward its proper good, nor toward any other good; that is agreed; so charity does not perfect faith in as much as it is a virtue; therefore, charity does not inform faith." Cf. SA III 14.1: 254,47: "Just as the first cause, that is God, is capable of inflaming the affection to love, so is the first light capable of illuminating the intellect for believing; so, just as the first light does not illumine the intellect for believing except through the medium of a habit, which is faith, so the first cause does not inflame the affection except through the medium of a habit, which is created charity."

25. Englhardt, *Glaubenspsychologie*, p. 220. The circle around Stephen Langton, with which William is familiar, had credited charity alone with everything. Throughout the early scholastic period, thinkers had increasingly emphasized the role of love. Love induces the other virtues to the final end; love is the driving strength of the soul, the *pondus animae*. No merit or virtue is possible without it. With the Pauline commentary of Peter of Corbeil, Godfrey of Poitiers, and their disciples, William posits the thesis that each soul power has its own inherent, unique love, with which it moves toward its own end (see the chapter on faith above). He thus takes the Augustinian statement *omnis virtus est amor* in a completely literal, nonmetaphorical sense. There are different types of *amor*, and each soul power has its own. William's theory of the relation between faith and love is thus not original in its basic lines. But in his reasoning William goes deeper. His distinctiveness is that out of the controversy between the *Corboliensis* and the *Cantuariensis* over the formation of the virtues, in which he sides with the former, he approaches the problem of whether faith is a virtue from a newly introduced Aristotelian perspective, and follows this view in its psychological implications. He thus inaugurates among thirteenth-century scholastics an interest in empirical faith-psychology, which persists to the end of the century. Among the early scholastics, William thus represents a contrast, not only to Stephen Langton and his circle, but also to the theory developed by Richard Fishacre (Englhardt, *Glaubenspsychologie*, pp. 264–69; 250–57).

tus which perfects the concupiscible power. As faith's substantial act *(finis quo)* by which it relates immediately to God is cognition, so charity's substantial act *(finis quo)* by which it relates the soul to God is *dilectio*, which is best rendered as "desire." But what precisely does charity desire? This raises the question of charity's object, the end in which it rests *(finis in quo)*. Although, as noted in the prior chapter, the *summum bonum* is the substantial end of all the virtues, these still relate to the good in some qualified fashion.[26] Even faith apprehends the good as true. By contrast, William posits an immediate and direct relationship between charity and the *summum bonum:*

> for the good, which is the mediate end of the other virtues, is the immediate end of charity; faith tends immediately toward the true, but desires the truth, because it is good; . . . charity, however, desires the good, because it is the good.[27]

Charity's substantial end and object, therefore, is the good *qua* good:[28] "Charity rests the heart in the highest good";[29] "inasmuch as God is good, God *in se* attracts the affection";[30] "to delight in the good, in as much as it is good, is of charity alone."[31] Accordingly, William refers to charity's object as the "first goodness" *(prima bonitas)*[32] or the "highest good" *(summum bonum)*. As a synonym he also speaks of the first or highest pleasure *(prima suavitas)*.[33] Charity is the good as pleasure *(suavitas)*. For "by charity the soul delights in the first sweetness immediately and properly,"[34] "since in the *affectus* charity is drawn immediately by . . . the suavity of God."[35] William also depicts charity's encounter with the good *qua* good as the experience of divine sweetness *(dulcedo)*—"charity . . . joins the human mind to the sweetness (*dulcedi-*

---

26. SA III 11.2: 179,140. Cf. SA III 10.4.5.2: 162,70.
27. SA III 36.1.1: 685,53ff.
28. SA III 10.4.3: 152,72. "The love of the highest good, in as much as it is good, is charity."
29. SA III 14.1: 255,99.
30. SA III 14.4: 259,50.
31. SA III 35.2.4: 672,25.
32. SA III 36.1.1: 684,32.
33. SA III 11.3.5: 195,67.
34. SA III 11.2: 179,140.
35. SA III 10.4.5.2: 162,72. Cf. also SA III 11.2: 179,124ff; SA III 39.1: 729,57; SA III 11.3.5: 194,58–62.

ni) of the Holy Spirit"[36]—as well as the experience of "overflowing delight" *(jucunditatis).*[37]

Finally, with respect to charity's mode of delight, the heart of William's reflections on charity emerges. In a general way, charity can be described as a desire for delight in the good. Citing Aristotle's dictum "concupiscence is the desire for delight,"[38] he defines charity as a desire *(dilectio)* for delight or fruition: "by charity we have fruition, maximally, and properly and *per se*"; hence, "fruition is better defined by the love of charity."[39] Elsewhere he argues that "the concupiscible power tends toward the delectable by whatever delectability it is delectable," and accordingly it can be said that essentially "charity tends towards delight."[40] But this is not quite sufficient. Rather, William prefers to define charity more precisely as a desire for a particular kind or mode of delight in the good, namely, as spiritual touch. The *summum bonum* "is delectable in as much as God is delighting and delicious pleasingness *(suavis delectans sive delicians)* to the *affectus* . . . through the mode of touch *(per modum tactus).*"[41] Hence, just as he described faith's mode of delight as spiritual vision *(visus),* so he links charity's delight with spiritual touch *(tactus).* Charity is the desire for immediate delight in the good *qua* good through the mode of touch.

Charity's Desire for Faith's Delight

A full appreciation of charity as *tactus* requires that this initial description of the relationship between faith and charity now be extended

---

36. SA III 14.3: 258,27. Cf. SA III 14.4: 261,116ff: "'This person loves God for God's sake' can denote the motive or efficient cause, so that it means: God or the sweetness of God is the motivating cause why this person loves God, just as the benefits which some one confers upon him are the cause why he loves that one. It can denote the final cause, so that it denotes God himself to be the final end of that love in its meaning, just as the bee loves honey on account of its sweetness." William will also speak of the "spiritual joy *(letitia spiritualis),*" which is in the love of God. Cf. SA III 15: 269,2ff: "Whence in the Canticle of Canticles the spouse says: *the king has brought me into his storerooms; he ordered charity in me.* The king, that is Christ, brought me into his storerooms, that is, into the church, in which is drunk the spiritual wine of joy, through which all temporal things which are not to be loved are made vile *(vilescunt)."* Cf. SA III 14.1: 255,78: "In the act by which one loves something sweet, sweetness is loved by that love which is concupiscence."

37. SA III 14.1: 254,70.
38. SA III 36.1.1: 686,74.
39. SA III 36.1.1: 685,53–57.
40. SA III 36.1.1: 687,107ff.
41. SA III 10.4.3: 152,56f.

Charity ❧ 147

and completed. William's assumption that charity is generated substantially from faith creates a permanent relationship between these two virtues, which he describes rather tersely:

> The desire for the delectable or the good, in as much as it is delectable or good, is the act of perfect charity and possesses of itself delight on account of the determination of the end, but the determination of the end is by faith, for charity desires the good . . . on account of the good, and this is so because charity judges *(estimare)* it to be good, and this judgment *(estimatio)* is of faith; hence . . . charity has delight from faith, yet [it possesses] delight *per se* substantially, for that determination, which faith provides, is of charity substantially.[42]

As depicted here, charity perpetually depends on faith for its essential nature as a virtue. In a sense, the whole structure of faith's relation to the good is "transferred" to charity. In this relationship, charity receives, in effect, three things from faith: the good as its proper object;[43] its desire for the good; and its initial delight in the good.[44] Charity receives its object—the good as good—from faith's act of estimation, which sets the good before it precisely as its proper and substantial end. Moreover, faith's ensuing desire for and delight in the good become the proper act and delight of charity too. So much is this the case that in places William will attribute faith's act of *aestimatio* to charity. Yet, this in no way undermines charity's integrity as a virtue, nor makes its delight less proper to it.

The structure of this relationship is clarified helpfully when it is noted that it corresponds to a fundamental distinction in William's thought: the distinction between desire and delight, discussed in Chapter 2. This distinction, it is important to note, is derived from his understanding of physical sense perception. William distinguishes between the desire for a physically delectable thing and the experience of possessing and delighting in it.[45] Noting that "only with the physical senses do we delight in

---

42. SA III 36.1.1: 689,197ff.
43. SA III 38.2: 723,186. "The good is first of the substance of faith before it is of the substance of charity."
44. SA III 36.1.1: 690,205. "We say that faith gives the pleasure *(delicias)* of charity."
45. SA III 10.4.3: 152,83. "That this solution is true can be seen in corporal desire, since the desire for delight in sensibly delectable things is in the concupiscible power; but the delight which is the end of that desire is in the senses."

physically delectable things *(in delectabili corporali)*," he observes that "the desire for physically delectable things does not possess delectation, but moves the corporal senses to the act of delighting."[46] So, generalizing, there must be two distinct powers of the soul each with an associated act, "one power of desiring and another of delighting."[47] Examples relating to culinary and sexual appetite are adduced: "we are delighted not by desiring food, but in eating it";[48] "the desire by which someone desires to delight in a woman is moved by concupiscible things, but that delight is not in the concupiscible power but in . . . [the sense of] touch *(in tactu).*"[49] For William, then, properly speaking, delight occurs not in the desire for, but only in the act of, sense perception.

As William conceives of it, the relationship between faith and charity is similar. So "in the case of one who desires the truth so that he may be delighted by it, the desire is in the concupiscible power, but the delight is [in the spiritual sense of] taste *(in gustu).*"[50] Spiritual taste stands here for spiritual perception in general. Spiritual delight occurs in faith's apprehension through all the spiritual senses. Charity desires the delight which occurs in and through faith's apprehension:[51] "the desire for spiritually delectable things does not experience delight, but moves the spiritual senses to the act of delighting spiritually."[52] Delight is fundamentally an adjunct of faith's apprehension, an experience proper to the rational power of the soul. Desire is fundamentally an impulse, a movement, an appetite for delectation, and is an act of the soul's concupiscible power.[53] In the end, charity is a desire for, and a movement toward, a

---

46. SA IV 18.3.3.2.2: 506,35ff.
48. SA IV 18.3.3.2.2: 506,36.
50. SA III 36.1.1: 686,79.

47. SA III 36.1.1: 686,71.
49. SA III 36.1.1: 686,76.

51. SA III 36.1.1: 688,138. "The following argument is not valid: 'charity desires to see God,' by the fallacy of accidents, since the desire for every good or delectable is of charity, but its desire, which is the good or the delectable, is of diverse virtues, hence the desire for seeing God, in as much as it sees God, is of faith and not of charity."

52. SA IV 18.3.3.2.2: 506,37.

53. William makes the same point in his treatment of beatitude: SA IV 18.3.3.2.2: 507,72. "By the spiritual senses alone and by faith alone we have fruition of God formally and properly. Hence, charity does not delight in God nor does it have fruition of God except by faith, and in the future it will not have fruition of God except by vision. But it is true that in a way charity moves faith to the act of having fruition of God. Hence, charity always has delight, since it is never without faith and hope. Hence, it always moves

delight which it receives from "outside" itself through faith's apprehension. William, accordingly, contrasts faith's vision with charity's desire in relation to spiritual delight:

> delight pertains both to vision and to love, but to vision in one way, to love in another: to vision as that in which *(in qua)* there is delight, to love as that by which *(a qua)* delight is grasped and augmented. For love tends toward this, namely, that through vision it may delight in loving. Hence: "wherever love is, the eyes follow."[54]

Vision—here a synonym for faith's apprehension—is that *in which (in qua)* there is delight, while love is that *by which (a qua)* delight occurs, in as much as charity pursues it. In short, charity desires, hungers for, pursues, effects, maintains, and augments that delight which occurs in faith's apprehension. "Charity has sweetness and delight; but not from itself, rather from its adjunct, namely cognition."[55]

Yet, in a crucial way—and here at last the tactile dimension emerges—William affirms that the delight concomitant with faith's apprehension is more proper to charity than to faith, and, in fact, comes to fruition with charity. The desire for possession of the good, "conceived" as it were with faith, comes to maturity, arrives finally at its fulfillment in the virtue of charity. Through charity, the soul comes to touch the Good. Here, it must be recalled that *in se* faith tends properly not toward delight, but toward the cognition of *veritas,* which is accompanied by delight through the spiritual senses.[56] Strictly speaking, faith's primary act is apprehension of the first truth, with the subsequent and in some sense secondary result that delight occurs there. As noted, William's dominant category for faith is vision *(visus)*. Charity's act, in contrast, is specifically and primarily toward that delight which occurs in its immediate en-

---

[faith/vision] to the act of delighting and having fruition, since 'where love is, there are the eyes.'"
54. SA IV 18.3.3.1: 502,164.
55. SA IV 18.3.3.2.2: 508,92.
56. SA III 36.1.1: 687,117: "Faith is not properly oriented toward delight, but is properly oriented toward cognition of the first truth, which cognition is concomitant with delight." SA III 36.1.1: 688,135: "To delight in the vision of God is of faith; but faith does not tend properly toward delighting, but toward seeing, which vision of God is accompanied by delight."

counter with the good, even though that delight comes from faith's act of apprehension:[57]

> The movement toward possession follows the cognition of that which is to be possessed; thus, there is a twofold movement of the soul toward that truth or a twofold love for the first truth: one by which *(qua)* the soul moves *toward cognizing the truth*, so that it may delight in it, so that this word *"ad"* denotes the end *by which* it rests, not *in which (in quo)* it rests; the other by which it is moved into that, that is, *to possessing the truth*, so that the first movement is toward delight; and afterwards it is the movement of charity.[58]

Faith's first "movement," its proper act (its end by which it rests, its *finis quo*), is cognition or apprehension. More precisely, though, what is described is not properly a movement; rather it is charity that properly moves toward this resting in the good:

> The first truth is the end of faith, toward which it tends, in which it has to rest; but the rest in that is only the end *by which* it ceases to move and delights in that [that is, cognition]; and thus it does not have to be moved into that rest properly; but that other virtue [must be moved], namely charity, which is in the concupiscible power, which desires delight, so that it tends toward it, of which it is the *investigatrix;* and so it is clear that even though that rest in a certain way is the end of faith, yet it is not the material of it nor the end of it; and thus the desire for that rest is not of faith but of charity.[59]

Charity tends properly and immediately toward the delight found in the possession of, union with, and rest in the *summum bonum*. Charity's task is to be the *investigatrix,* the seeker and pursuer of delight. Charity's desire is the efficient cause, moving faith to the act of delighting, and

---

57. SA III 36.1.1: 687,112. "When charity desires to delight in the vision of God, it commands faith to be moved toward seeing God."

58. SA III 39.1: 731,117. *Quoniam ad habendum motus sequitur cognitionem rei habende; est ergo duplex motus anime in illam veritatem sive duplex dilectio prime veritatis: una qua movetur ad cognoscendum ipsam, ut delectetur in ipsa, ita quod hec dictio "ad" notet finem quo quiescitur, non in quo quiescitur, alia qua movetur in ipsam, id est ad habendum ipsam, ut motus sit primo in ipsam delectationem; et sicut est motus caritatis.*

59. SA III 39.1: 732, 154ff. *Prima veritas est finis fidei, ad quem tendit, in quo quiescere habet; sed quies in illa est tantum finis, quo sistit et delectatur in illa; et ideo non habet moveri in illam quietem proprie; sed alia virtus, scilicet caritas, que est in vi concupiscibili, cuius est appetere delectationem, ut ad quam tendit, cuius est investigatrix; et ideo patet quod, licet illa quies quodam modo sit finis fidei, tamen non est eius materia neque eius finis; et ideo desiderium illius quietis non est fidei sed pocius caritatis.*

conserving and augmenting it. "Charity moves toward that conjunction, and makes it and holds it in existence."[60] Hence, charity brings about the soul's final rest in its divine end. Precisely for this reason, William construes charity as a form of *tactus*. Charity desires "to delight in the suavity of God, which delights the [sense of] touch *(tactum)* spiritually."[61] For, "as the highest good moves faith and hope through the mode of estimation, so it moves charity through the mode of touch *(per modum tactus)* toward God's suavity."[62] In short, charity culminates in contact with, in touching, the Beloved.

Here, it must be noted that as with faith's *visus*, William understands charity's *tactus* by way of synecdoche: it represents all the spiritual senses, but is singled out in order to emphasize and clarify a particular dimension of the soul's encounter with God. The assignment of *tactus* to charity is appropriate from William's perspective, because in his account of physical delight, touch is the most intense form of sense perception and causes the greatest delight: "the delight, which charity desires, is similar to sensible delight, which is through the [physical sense of] touch, which is the greatest among the sensible delights."[63] Accordingly, in a veritable summary of his teaching on faith, charity, and the spiritual senses, William specifies:

the delight which is according to spiritual *tactus* is [not] charity, but it is the end of the act of charity. So also, the delight which is in spiritual *gustus* or *odoratus* is not charity, but the end of the act of charity; spiritual *visus* is to be understood similarly. Hence ... the desire for cognizing God is the *intellectus* of faith; but the desire for delighting in God either in the mode of *visus* or *odoratus* or *gustus* or *tactus* is of charity. For this is the desire for the good as good, that is, the delectable as delectable.[64]

Charity then is the desire for the delight arising from the "spiritually sensuous" apprehension of the good, which occurs in the intellect through faith. As with faith, William is not attempting to allocate rigidly a particular spiritual sense to charity; rather, his reference to touch is meant to evoke broadly its substantial nature and act. Hence:

60. SA IV 18.3.3.2.2: 507,72ff.
62. SA III 10.4.5.2: 162,76.
64. SA III 10.4.3: 152,73ff.

61. SA III 36.1.1: 686,92.
63. SA III 36.1.1: 686,94.

Charity tends towards delight, not only the delight which is in spiritual touch *(in tactu spirituali)*, but toward the delight of every spiritual sense *(sensus spiritualis)*, since, when charity desires to delight in the vision of God, it commands faith to move toward the vision of God.⁶⁵

Faith cognizes, estimates, apprehends—in short, faith is *visus*. Charity desires, pursues, possesses, conjoins, rests in—in short charity is *tactus*. Between vision and touch, the remaining spiritual senses enter in to complete the spiritually sensuous encounter.

Charity's Consummation of Faith

Finally, William views charity, rather than faith, as the consummation of the soul's experience of delight and fruition. This consummation depends on charity's *tactus* in two ways. First, as the *telos* of its essential act, charity's *tactus* culminates in union.⁶⁶ For as "charity moves through the mode of touch *(per modum tactus)* to God's suavity," so it "in a greater way unites itself to God."⁶⁷ For this very reason, charity's love can be described as conjunction or union: "Charity unites and conjoins to God, for love *(amor)* is the conjunction of the lover with the beloved, *for he who adheres to the Lord* through charity *is made one spirit with him*."⁶⁸ But perhaps more importantly, on account of its tactile modality William credits charity with a more intense delight, a greater pleasure than faith:⁶⁹ "just as there is greater delight *in tactu* than in the other senses, so there is greater delight in charity"⁷⁰ and "there is greater pleasure *(jocunditas)* in charity than in faith, just as there is more pleasure in touch than in vision."⁷¹ Although faith has fruition in God, yet charity

---

65. SA III 36.1.1: 687,111. This remark, concerning charity's imperative toward faith, confirms the "location" of the delight that charity pursues: it is the adjunct of faith's apprehension.

66. SA III 11.3.5: 194,53. "By charity through the mode of union, since 'delight is the union of the lover with the beloved.'"

67. SA III 10.4.5.2: 162,69ff.

68. SA III 42.1.2: 795,42.

69. SA III 36.1.1: 689,180: "Every virtue has its own proper delight substantially . . . but there is greater delight in charity than in faith." SA III 10.4.5.2: 162,69: "in a greater way [charity] causes [us] to delight in God." SA III 41.2: 785,75: "charity . . . is more intense and more pleasing *(jocundior)*."

70. SA III 10.4.3: 152,59.

71. SA III 14.6: 266,66.

has fruition, "maximally, properly and *per se*,"⁷² despite the fact that charity receives its delight from faith:

> faith gives the pleasure *(delicias)* of charity, nevertheless charity has greater pleasure than faith, since charity possesses not only pleasure from faith, but also from its proper matter, which exceeds that of faith.⁷³

This is so precisely because charity's *tactus* entails a more immediate, direct encounter with the good: "charity has greater delight . . . since it is immediately at . . . the font of delight" *(fonti delectationis)*.⁷⁴ For these reasons, William attributes the consummation of the soul's fruition in God to charity.

To capture this final relationship between faith and charity in the experience of fruition, William employs a comparison with eating, to which he often turns, especially and appropriately in the context of his Eucharistic theology. He is fond of comparing, respectively, charity's desire for God with physical hunger for food and faith's apprehension of God with the physical act of savorous eating. As always, it is first and foremost faith which perceives and apprehends the good, faith which eats with savorous and spiritually sensuous delight through the spiritual senses. Yet William is quick to point out that the delight found in eating is proportioned to the degree of love's unsatiated hunger: *the one who eats me will yet hunger* (Eccl 24:29). The greater the intensity of charity's desire, the greater faith's delight:⁷⁵

---

72. SA III 36.1.1: 685,53.
73. SA III 36.1.1: 690,205. Cf. SA III 36.1.1: 688,163ff. "Augustine said: 'the delights of charity are drawn from an alien heart and the delights of wisdom [are drawn] from its own heart' [see Lombard *Sent.* d.1, c.3 (I, 57); *Summa Sententiarum* I c.10 (PL 176.57)]. Therefore, charity possesses its delight *(delicias)* from an alien heart, namely from faith, for in this is the love of God most delicious to someone, that he believes himself to be loved by God."
74. SA III 36.1.1: 689,172.
75. SA III 38.2: 722,137: "Even though the act of faith is *in se* delectable, yet it is more delectable from the consort of the act of charity, for since the act of charity (*rectius,* faith), with which someone believes that he will have fruition of the highest good in eternity, is delectable *in se*, yet it is more delectable from the desire of charity, by which man desires to have fruition of that highest good. For the more delectable faith and hope are, the greater the desire for the thing; thus since charity perfects faith in the delectation of its act, it is rightly called its form."

Those who eat through vision, will hunger through charity. For they will have hunger, that is, the desire of charity, so that they may eat delectably; and so it is clear that love augments delight, which will be in vision.[76]

As one who eats without hunger eats without savor, so there is no savorous apprehension for faith unless the hunger of charity provides it. Accordingly, even though faith's apprehension "is the most worthy and acceptable *(dignissimum et acceptissimum)* gift," is "beatitude and *eternal life* (Jn 17:3)," contains "every delight *(omnes delicie),*" since "to eat with desire is to eat delectably," yet "charity is the *most excellent (excellentissumum) gift* (1 Cor 13:3) in as much as it consummates . . . fruition in God."[77] In sum, just as union consummates the desire born of vision, so charity's touch consummates the delight born of faith's apprehension and its hunger ultimately enables faith's savorous delight.[78]

Conclusion: Faith, Charity, and the Spiritual Senses

Fundamentally, William conceives of both faith and charity as forms of spiritual sense. Faith is an apprehension, best described as *visus*. It is primary: from its *aestimatio*, desire for delight in the good and movement toward the same are generated; in a word, faith produces charity. But charity's dependence on faith does not marginalize its role in the soul's knowledge of God. Though the experience of delight occurs first in the intellect, occurs in its apprehension of the *bonum* as *veritas*, occurs through the singular spiritual sense in its various acts of spiritual sensation, yet faith's experience "passes over" into charity. Here, though, the soul relates to the *summum bonum* under a different formal aspect, namely, that of the good *qua* good or as *suavitas*: charity's end is the *summum bonum* in as much as it is good. Accordingly, charity is associated with desire, with hunger, and with the movements and acts which flow from these. It is the efficient cause of delight, desiring, pursuing, effecting, maintaining, augmenting, and ultimately consummating the soul's fruition.

In light of charity's orientation toward the good as *suavitas*, William

---

76. SA IV 18.3.3.1: 502,167f.
78. SA III 38.2: 721,134f.

77. SA II 4.1: 89,86ff.

transposes the soul's encounter with the *bonum* and its experience of delight into a different sense modality, namely, that of spiritual touch *(tactus)*: charity desires delight of the *bonum* through the mode of touch *(per modum tactus)*, culminating in union *(conjunctus)*. This is charity's substantial nature. In light, moreover, of charity's *tactus*, its experience of delight is greater than faith's. Charity delights in the end set before it by faith with a greater intensity than faith alone. For, as William argued, "as there is greater delight *in tactu* than in the other senses," so there is greater delight in charity than in faith.[79] Precisely as *tactus*, charity consummates faith.

Ultimately, love and knowledge, charity and faith are intimately related and mutually informing in the soul's experience of fruition. They act in concert with one another: faith apprehending, delighting, savoring; charity desiring, pursuing, hungering—yet charity is only sated by faith's repast, while faith only savors in proportion to charity's desire. Charity, as hunger, arises from faith's prior savorous perception, yet faith's savor is only realized, ultimately only consummated, by charity's hunger. The structure of this relationship is governed by William's conviction that knowledge of God is best described as spiritual sense perception, and sense perception is a function of intellect and cognition, not of will and affection. Accordingly, the spiritual senses are to be associated with the *intellectus*, the rational power, and the virtue of faith. At the same time, the weight of biblical and patristic emphasis on the role of charity pushes William, not only to give charity the final word in his account of fruition, but also to see charity as the cause of faith's act,[80] in the same way that the desire to see a beautiful object moves one to look at it,[81] or

79. SA III 10.4.3: 152,59f.
80. SA III 38.2: 722,144: "Because charity often moves faith to its act and then perfects its act, like a governor *(sicut rector)*, with respect to its end; for whenever charity moves faith, like someone who, from the desire for enjoying *(ex desiderio fruendi)*, desires too little to see it *(ipsum)*, natural love *(naturalis amor)* causes it to believe that which it loves, as the Apostle said: Charity believes all things." Cf. SA II 8.2.9.5: 224,35ff: "But after faith and charity are deep within the soul, charity itself through the act of desire, which is its proper act, elevates faith and does not cease, until faith has arrived at that which it intends and rests in its end, which then it chooses alone, since the faithful soul sees the first beauty openly."
81. SA III 38.2: 722,149. "Charity is called the head of the virtues for this reason, that the maximal sweetness moves and draws all, for the desire of the thing loved moves toward

because the intensity of charity's sweetness entices faith to its act.[82] (Only in this sense does William grant charity the title "head" or "mother" of the virtues.)[83] In the end, a certain circularity characterizes William's account of these virtues. Faith is primary, and generates charity; yet faith is only fully actualized by the presence of charity.[84]

In the last analysis, the sense metaphors for faith and charity, *visus* and *tactus*, seem well suited for their respective roles in William's analysis of the soul's apprehension of God. While faith initiates the divine-human encounter, there remains a "distance" between perceiver and perceived analogous to that implied in visual sensation. Charity's role—to desire and pursue the object known by faith to the point of unitive consummation—is viewed appropriately as a more direct touching of, and more intimate union with, God. William's account of faith and charity does not yet reveal the full scope of his doctrine of the spiritual senses, but it does unveil the basic spiritual-aesthetic orientation at the heart of his understanding of the knowledge of God.[85]

Finally, in light of William's conception of faith and charity, a fuller appreciation of his reflections on beatitude is now possible. In that discussion, he was keen to differentiate the experience of the two primary powers of the soul, the rational and the concupiscible, according to two

---

seeing that which is loved, toward causing that to be willed; hence faith is the head as origin and as commander of the regime, but charity is the head by the power of moving and drawing through its excessive sweetness. Whence it is that Scripture sometimes attributes all goods to faith, sometimes to charity, for the same reason, the Gloss said that 'charity has primacy among the virtues.'"

82. SA III 39.1: 731,99. "Charity is the perfection or the fulfillment of the law, and because its sweetness moves and draws all the virtues to their end, namely faith and hope, as Paul said: *charity believes all things, hopes all things, endures all things*; and since all the *motus* of the virtues are perfected and meritorious, for this reason that they are referred to the proper end of charity, namely to the highest good, and since charity by its sweetness augments the delectation which is in the other virtues, and that which is in faith, for the soul is more greatly delighted when by cognizing God it loves God."

83. SA III 38.2: 722,149. "Charity is called the form of the virtues, since it informs all the subsequent virtues, by giving them their essence and perfection; but faith can be called formed [by charity] for three reasons."

84. M.-D. Chenu, "L'amour dans la foi," *Bulletin thomiste* (Notes et communications) 9 (1932): pp. 97–99. Unfairly, Chenu seems to characterize William's approach to the relative roles of faith and charity as excessively opposed to affectivity.

85. Englhardt speaks of a "certain fundamental aesthetic tendency in William's psychology of faith" (*Glaubenspsychologie*, p. 269).

self-expressive manifestations of the Trinity that are by now familiar: "There will be two delights [*in patria*] by which we will immediately delight in God, namely, by seeing his beauty *(pulchritudinem)* and by loving his goodness *(bonitas)*."[86] Correspondingly, "there are two ways [by which we are assimilated to God] . . . either through beauty or goodness . . . beauty is of faith; goodness is of charity."[87] Faith, perfecting the rational power of the soul, finds delight in the divine beauty, while charity, perfecting the concupiscible power, delights in the divine goodness. Thus, in beatitude, "the *intellectus* as much as the *affectus* will rest."[88] The following text from Book III finely recapitulates his entire teaching on this matter:

Beatitude consists not only in the vision of God, but also in the love [of God], since Augustine said that "eternal life is to see what you love and to love what you see." Since the whole reward is attributed to vision or apprehension, for this reason apprehension is generative of love. And, properly and primarily fruition is in that vision, since Augustine said in *De immortalitate animae*, that to *intelligere* or to *videre* God is the same as to *audire* God, and to *audire* God is the same thing as to *olfacere* God, and *gustare* is the same thing as to *tangere*, which is properly to have fruition of God.[89]

Here, the singular beatitude consists of knowledge and love in intimate relation: to love what you know and to know what you love. As always, William grants primacy to the apprehension of the *intellectus;* from it charity is generated in the *affectus*. But here, once again, he subsumes under the single *visio Dei*, in a synaesthetic fashion, all the other spiritual senses in a way which also charts the progression, from apprehension

---

86. SA III 39.5.2: 753,59ff.
87. SA III 29.3: 578,178. *Duobis enim modis intellgitur, quia assimilamur Deo vel in pulcritudine vel in bonitate; velle autem assimilari Deo in pulcritudine fidei est, in bonitate autem caritatis est.*
88. SA III 39.5.2: 753,68.
89. SA III 41.2: 786,108ff. *Dicimus quod beatitudo non consist solum in visione Dei, sed etiam in amore, sicut dicit Augustinus quod "vita eterna est videre quod amas, et amare quod vides," quia totum premium attribuitur visioni vel cognitioni, ideo quia cognitio est generativa amoris et quia proprie et primo fruitio est in ipsa visione, quoniam Augustinus dicit, in libro De immortalitate anime, quod intelligere sive videre Deum idem est quod audire ipsum, et audire idem est quod olfacere, et gustare quod tangere quod est proprie frui Deo.* (The latter passage credited to Augustine is not found by the editors; the sense is in *Epist.* 147, c.2, n.7 [PL 33.599; CSEL 44.281]).

to union. Starting with *videre*, the soul moves to *audire*, to *olfacere*, to *gustare*, and finally, to *tangere*, which, as William notes in the end, is the consummation and full experience of fruition. Thus, faith and charity, through the spiritual senses, collaborate to arrive at the fulness of spiritually sensuous knowledge of God: to touch as well as to see God.

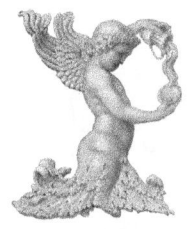

PART IV
THE FORMS OF SPIRITUAL APPREHENSION

CHAPTER 8

SYMBOLIC THEOLOGY
Exterior Perception of God's Effects

CREATION FINDS ITS ULTIMATE PURPOSE as a partial, finite expression of infinite plenitude and as a fragmentary manifestation of the fullness of divine glory: this is a conviction that William shares with later scholastic thinkers.[1] In various places throughout his *Summa Aurea*, most notably in his treatment of the six days of creation,[2] he elaborates this intuition into a profound vision of creation's capacity, not only to reflect the self-communicating goodness of the Trinity, but in so doing to be a source of knowledge of the Creator. In this regard, as with other topics, William initiates a scholastic tradition of profound reflection.

William assumes that *in se* and *ex se* God cannot be known by rational creatures, on account of the weakness of their spiritual sight and the smallness of their intellect. And yet, in spite of these limitations, he affirms that God can be known "in and from created things" *(in creaturis et ex creaturis)*, as "in a mirror" *(sicut in speculo)*. Though *in se* God cannot be seen in this life—*since no one has ever seen God* (Jn 1:18)—yet through faith the human intellect can be illumined in order to see God

---

1. Gilson, *The Philosophy of St. Bonaventure*, p. 181. "What profit then to the divine glory is the fact of creation? Simply to communicate itself, to manifest itself, to extend beyond itself something of the infinite goodness which constitutes it in multiplying around itself fragmentary images of the perfection on which it rests. This glory therefore which God enjoys from all eternity radiates around itself partial gleams which reflect without increasing it; in doing so it shows itself, and it is this very manifestation of the divine perfection which constitutes the immediate end of creation."
2. SA II, Tractate 8.

"in the mirror of creatures" *(in speculo creaturarum)*.³ All knowledge of God, therefore, is mediated by God's effects. They are a mirror in which the divine goodness can be perceived.

In this regard, as noted at the conclusion of Chapter 5, William distinguishes between two kinds of created effects, external and internal, and two corresponding forms of theology: symbolic and mystical (a distinction he borrows from Pseudo-Dionysius, but to which he gives a very different meaning). Mystical theology pertains to created effects, but to those which are perceived within the interiority of the rational creature. By contrast, symbolic theology "names God from inferior things," applying the "meaning or sense" *(sententia)* of visible realities to the Trinity as is "fitting" *(convenientia)*, when, for example, Scripture calls God a lion, fire, and such like.⁴ Symbolic theology considers the Trinity as perceived in the *speculum* of its external, created effects. For William, therefore, symbolic theology can be defined as the apprehension of uncreated goodness (the *summum bonum*) within its visible effects (the *bonum per participationem*). While this knowledge of God does not involve the spiritual senses, it is nevertheless a perception of trinitarian effects and thus a prelude to its mystical counterpart.

An Aesthetic Orientation

William's interest in the visible manifestation of divine glory reflects what might be termed an aesthetic orientation in his theology.⁵ He takes

---

3. SA I 4.1: 38,73ff. "But to us [God] is nameable in one way, unnameable in another way: unnameable *in se* and *ex se*, but nameable in creatures and from creatures, since we understand in no other way except in creatures as in a mirror *(in speculo)* and through creatures *(per creaturas)*. . . . Properly speaking, then, God is unnameable because, since he who is the true light illumines our intellects, he illumines our intellects not in order that we may see God *in se*, which would be properly to see, for *no one has ever seen God* (Jn 1:18) on account of two reasons: 'on account of the weakness of our sight which due to its infirmity has eyes for seeing the true sun like the eyes of an owl for seeing the material sun' [*Metaphysica* II.1], and because of the smallness of our intellect which is not sufficient for comprehending God's infinite magnitude. And so, in the present time God does not illumine our intellect so that we may see God *in se*, but only in the mirror of creatures *(speculo creaturarum).*"

4. SA I 4.2: 40,117f.

5. See Edgar de Bruyne, *Études d'esthétique médiévale*, 3 vols. (Bruges, 1946); Umberto Eco, *Art and Beauty in the Middle Ages*, trans. Hugh Bredin (New Haven, Conn.: Yale University Press, 1986); Henri Pouillon, "Le premier traité des propriétés transcendentals, La

the lead among scholastic thinkers in treating the concept of beauty *(pulchritudo)* as an explicit theological category.[6] This is evident in, but not limited to, his conception of symbolic theology. Broadly considered, William's aesthetic is typically medieval—a melange of biblical, patristic, and classical inheritances.[7] Nonetheless, his approach is uniquely his own.

To begin, William's aesthetic is primarily a theological concern. It is not pursued independently for its own sake, but is rather conceived indirectly as he pursues other theological questions. Accordingly, it has a pronounced religious character, typical of thirteenth-century aesthetics: the beauty of things is a function of the Creator's beauty.[8] In a related vein, William's overarching interest is intelligible beauty.[9] Sensible beauty is a reflection of—and sometimes even a contrast with—its intelligible counterpart. He seeks to discern in the visible, concrete object a reflection of, and participation in, the eternal beauty and metaphysical splendor of God. His, thus, is a pancalistic vision of creation:[10] every part of creation, as well as the cosmos as a whole, is an expression of divine beauty.[11] Moreover, William's conception of the beautiful is developed in close relation to his views on the metaphysical good. As will be seen below, he posits an intimate relationship between the beautiful and the good.

A particularly important aspect of William's interest in the visible appearance of invisible beauty is the moral sphere. For him, there is a

---

'Summa de bono' du Chancellier Phillipe," *Revue néoscolastique de philosophie* 42 (1939): pp. 40–77; Władysław Tatarkiewicz, *Geschichte der Äesthetik*, vol. 2, *Die Äesthetik des Mittelalters* (Basel/Stuttgart: Schwabe & Company, 1980), pp. 243–50.

6. De Bruyne, *Études*, pp. 4–5; cf. Pouillon, "Le premier traité," pp. 40–45.

7. Eco, *Art and Beauty*, pp. 2–5.

8. See de Bruyne, *Études*, pp. 6–7.

9. Eco, *Art and Beauty*, p. 5. The inspiration of this is Platonic, but actually the Christianized Neoplatonism of Pseudo-Dionysius, especially his *On the Divine Names*. There, "the universe is an inexhaustible irradiation of beauty, a grandiose expression of the ubiquity of the First Beauty, a dazzling cascade of splendors."

10. "The medieval aesthetic tends to integrate all levels of aesthetic experience into a grand system" (Eco, *Art and Beauty*, pp. 6–7).

11. "From the philosophical point of view, it is the metaphysical character of the aesthetic which is primary: the whole is considered as a function of being and its first principles" (Eco, *Art and Beauty*, pp. 8–9).

beauty *(honestum)* of the soul that is manifest in its external, visible acts, which themselves have a certain beauty. This accounts for his frequent association of beauty *(pulchrum, decorum)* and utility or goodness *(aptum, honestum)*.

Another dimension of William's aesthetic that emerges in symbolic theology is its subjective element. He stresses the centrality of the experience of pleasure—*delectatio*—on the part of the theological perceiver. In fact, as has become evident, the category of *delectatio* is a leitmotif in his theology. One context in which this subjective element will emerge prominently is that of mystical theology, where the apprehension of the *divina delectabilia* through the spiritual senses produces delight.[12] But William also stresses this subjective experience of delight in the context of symbolic theology, where physical sense perception and corresponding knowledge are also to be accompanied by pleasure. While in both contexts he stresses the proper reference and ultimate source of this aesthetic perception—namely, the Trinity—he nonetheless allows for the fact that the immediate object of theological apprehension is created things: *I have delighted myself in your works, O Lord* (Ps 91:5) is the motto of symbolic theology.

Finally, it must be noted that the derivative character of created beauty does not undermine its objective reality. Rather, for William, visible beauty is an objective property, actually inhering in things. Precisely in this regard, he makes perhaps his most important contribution to scholastic aesthetic theory.[13] While various concepts were enlisted in the medieval period to give expression to the objective presence of created beauty, that most often employed (and that to which William will devote considered attention) was the sapiential triad of measure, number, and weight *(mensura, numerus, pondus)*—from Wisdom 11:20, *Lord, you have ordered all things in measure, number, and weight*—or other similar triads derived from it.[14] The tradition of an aesthetic built around this Sa-

---

12. Discussed at length in Chapters 6, 7, and 9.
13. See de Bruyne, *Études*, pp. 4–5.
14. Other triads include: *modus, forma*, and *ordo* (dimension, form, and order) or *substantia, species, virtus* (substance, nature, and power), or *quod constat, quod congruit, quod discernit* (that which determines, that which proportions, that which distinguishes). These triads have a dual purpose: to define not only the beautiful, but also the good.

lomonic triad begins with Augustine, is sustained throughout the early medieval period, and then flourishes with the scholastics,[15] who were especially intrigued by the bishop's remarks on beauty. Here, William initiates a scholastic tradition of reflection on this triad and its relation to created beauty by explicitly asserting that the presence of the triad constitutes the beauty of created things.[16] Consequently, although he does not develop a comprehensive theory of the beautiful from the Salomonic triad, William may be considered the inaugurator of a medieval "sapiential" aesthetic,[17] which emerges in the early thirteenth century.[18] Fittingly, then, the phrase "symbolic sapience" is here enlisted to refer to the object of symbolic theology: the visible self-manifestation of divine wisdom, revealed in the beauty of created things, and characterized chiefly by measure, number, and weight.[19]

15. De Bruyne notes that the dualist movements of the Cathars and the Albigensians are important though indirect causes of the advancement of aesthetics in the thirteenth century. It was not only on the political plain that the war against the Albigensians was waged; the theologians and the philosophers of Paris attacked these movements and they were forced to demonstrate the nonexistence of evil. It is above all William of Auxerre, Philip the Chancellor, and William of Auvergne who were the champions of Christian optimism (*Études*, p. 3).

16. These assertions will be explored further below: "these three are the beauty of a thing" (SA II 13.1) and "its beauty and its goodness are the same substantially" (SA II 9.4). See de Bruyne, *Études*: "But these are the aesthetic principles to which Augustine consecrated a long development! If Philip the Chancellor, preoccupied above all with the parallelism of the one, the true, and the good, passes over beauty in silence, the other authors are struck by Augustine's remarks on beauty. It is first and chiefly William of Auxerre, who in his *Summa Aurea* announces the capital proposition: *haec tria (scilicet species, numerus, ordo) est rei pulchritudo, penes quae dicit Augustinus consistere bonitatem rei* (SA II 13.1). It follows that '*idem est in substantia ejus bontias et ejus pulchritudo*' (SA II 9.4). Thus William of Auxerre inaugurates the aesthetic which we are calling 'sapiential': we will find it with John of Rochelle, Alexander of Hales, Albert the Great, among others under the profound influence of Philip the Chancellor" (pp. 3–5).

17. As is the case with so many synchronic treatments of various scholastic topics, William's contribution to this issue is often presented in isolation from the rest of his thought and thus appears "dropped from nowhere." It is hoped that this chapter will give a more coherent and integrated account of this aesthetic orientation in William's theology.

18. De Bruyne mentions William of Auvergne, Philip the Chancellor, and, especially, John of Rochelle, Alexander of Hales (and in the *Summa Halesiana*), and Albert the Great. See Tatarkiewicz (*Geschichte der Ästhetik*, pp. 243–50), who notes that, building upon a Cistercian and Victorine foundation, the first generation of scholastic theologians (including William of Auxerre, Alexander of Hales, and William of Auvergne) initiated the scholastic discussion of beauty, and typically did so using the sapiential categories of measure, number, and weight.

19. William stands in a long and venerable Christian tradition of reflection on

The Beauty of the Trinity

A proper starting point for an analysis of William's view of symbolic theology is found in his doctrine of the Trinity. His aesthetic orientation—his theological interest in the concept of beauty *(pulchritudo)*—first emerges there. William's justifications for a triad of divine persons involve various aesthetic notions, including beauty, harmony, fittingness, symmetry, and interrelatedness,[20] typical of twelfth- and thirteenth-century aesthetic canons.[21] He sees the inner-divine life to be characterized by an interrelatedness *(germanitas)*, a perfect communication *(perfecta communicatio)* among the persons, which entails these characteristics. Within the divine life, there is an immediate procession, that of the Son, and a procession which is both immediate and mediate, that of the Holy Spirit from the Father and the Son. This arrangement, according to William, is the most ordered *(ordinatissima)*, most beautiful *(pulcerrima)*, and most fitting *(convenientissima)*. In it the Son is related as much to the Father as to the Spirit. In receiving, the Son is related to the Father; in giving, to the Spirit. If a fourth person were introduced, the perfect interrelatedness *(germanitas)* of the Trinity would be destroyed.[22] In a general sense, then, William sees the divine nature as characterized by beauty, ordination, and fittingness.

William's doctrine of appropriations within the trinitarian life further reflects this sapiential aesthetic. For William, the Son is the interior and eternal Word *(Verbum)* of the Father.[23] As *Verbum* He "perfectly

---

Wisdom 11:21, extending as far back as Irenaeus of Lyon, Origen of Alexandria, and Augustine of Hippo, and continuing into the Middle Ages in such authors as Cassiodorus, Isidore of Seville, Bede, Rabanus Maurus, and Boethius. See Peri von Israel, "*Omnia Mensura et Numero et Pondere Disposuisti*: Die Auslegung von Weish 11,20 in der Lateinischen Patristik," in *Miscellanea Mediaevalia: Veröffentlichungen des Thomas-Instituts der Universität zu Köln*, vol. 16/1, *Mensura, Mass, Zahl, Zahlensymbolik im Mittelalter* (Berlin: de Gruyter, 1983), pp. 1–22.

20. See above, Chapter 4.

21. Arnold, *Perfecta communicatio*, pp. 111–14: Arnold notes the important mathematical dimension (apparent in the triad: measure, number, proportion) of the twelfth- and early thirteenth-century aesthetic sensibility shared by William and his contemporaries. This promoted a certain aesthetic approach to the doctrine of the Trinity. Already in the first half of the twelfth century, Thierry of Chartres sought arithmetic and geometrical proofs for the Trinity, as did Alan of Lille.

22. SA I 3.4: 33–34,52ff.   23. See Chapter 4.

speaks" the Father's goodness, and in Him that goodness can be "perfectly seen." As such, the Son is the Father's perfect and full expression, the Image and Mirror of the Father's goodness. At this juncture, William associates the notion of beauty *(pulchritudo)* with the Second Person.[24] The rationale for this appropriation is twofold. The first pertains to the Trinity *ad intra:*

> the Father is the first light or first intelligence or natural memory, from which ... the Son proceeds ... ; but the first thing which comes from light is splendor and the Son is *the splendor of the Father* (Heb 1:3), as it says in Hebrews, and in the book of Wisdom it says: *the brightness (candor) of the eternal light* etc. (Wis 7:26); but splendor and candor pertain to beauty and for this reason species *(species)* or beauty *(pulchritudo)* is appropriated to the Son.[25]

As the Son is the radiance *(splendor)* and brightness *(candor)* of the Father's light, so he is the divine beauty. Here, the category of expressiveness emerges. Precisely as the Father's expression, as *Verbum,* as His perfect self-manifestation, the Son is the *candor* and *splendor*—the beauty —of the Father.

In the second rationale, William shifts vocabulary, punning on the Latin word *species*—referring both to the form which causes a certain thing to be what it is and to that thing's appearance and thus beauty. He also shifts the focus of the appropriation to the context of the Son's relation to creation *ad extra:*

> The second reason is that the Son is *Sapientia* and *Speculum* and *Exemplar* of all things and the *Ars* of every living rational thing *(omnium rationum viventium);* hence as the formal cause he is also the species, for this reason also species is appropriated to the Son.[26]

Here, the appropriation of *species* to the Son is derived from the Son's function in relation to the act of creation and, by extension, to created things—the function of formal causality. The visible appearance and beauty, the form or species of created reality, is a function of its relation to the divine beauty. In this regard, William appears to build upon the

---

24. Prior to William, Peter Lombard made a similar appropriation: "the most perfect beauty is the Son, that is the Truth of the Father, which never in any way departs from him ... And which is the model of all things" (I *Sent.* d 3 [163a]).
25. SA I 8.8.4: 175,84f.   26. SA I 8.8.4: 175,90f.

appropriation of beauty within the inter-trinitarian relations, finding in the inner-divine appropriation of *pulchritudo* to the Son a basis for the Son's role as *species, ad extra*.

As these justifications for the appropriation of beauty to the Son reveal, moreover, the notion of divine exemplification *(exemplar)* is crucial for William's theological aesthetic.[27] The Son's role in linking the Trinity *ad intra* and its created effects *ad extra* pertains to Him as *Verbum*/Exemplar. The divine creative act is wrought through the Son, who contains within himself the forms and patterns of all that can and would be created. William's favorite designation for the Word as Exemplar is Wisdom and it is precisely this which created reality reflects. Of greater significance, William associates divine wisdom *(sapientia)* with divine artistry *(ars)* in the act of creation:

Just as an artist *(artifex)* works through his art or his wisdom, so the Father is said to operate through the Son, since the Son is the eternal and interior *Verbum* by which the Father expressly speaks his goodness. . . . Creatures by contrast are an exterior word *(verbum exterius)*, by which as exterior words the Father speaks his goodness. But all exterior speaking is done through an interior word, and thus the Father speaks exterior words through the interior word, that is, he accomplishes his exterior work through the interior word, and thus the Father operates through the Son.[28]

As the full expression *(Verbum)*, therefore, of all that the Father is, the Son is the Exemplar of all that could be and would be created *ad extra*. As Exemplar, the Son is the Art *(Ars)* by which the Father-Artist *(Artifex)* acts in creation.[29] Precisely in the *Artifex-Ars* relationship, divine wisdom *(sapientia)* emerges:

Speaking of the first creation, Moses said . . . *In the beginning,* that is in the Son or in Wisdom; just as an artist *(artifex)* makes something through his wisdom,

---

27. See Chapter 5 for a discussion of William's doctrine of exemplarity.
28. SA I 8.8.2: 158,3ff.
29. Cf. SA II 1.1: 21,187: "For human artists *(in artifice creato)* three things are required in order that he might make something, but for the first artist *(in primo artifice)*, namely, for God, these are not required." Cf. SA II 1.3: 26,115. SA I 8.8.2: 158,3ff: "Just as an artist *(artifex)* works *(operatur)* through his art or wisdom *(per artem sive per sapientiam suam)*, so the Father is said to work through the Son *(per Filium)*, since the Son is the eternal and internal *(eternum et internum)* Word, by which the Father expressly *(expresse)* speaks his goodness."

so God through his eternal Wisdom created the world. Hence: *you O Lord, have made all things in your wisdom* (Ps 103:24). And in John's Gospel: *all things were made through him* (1:3).[30]

In short, the Son as Wisdom is the Son in relation to the Father's artistic act of creation.[31]

Though the Son is central in his sapiential theology, William does not neglect the Holy Spirit. Within the divine life, he appropriates the notion of goodness *(bonitas)* to the Spirit, and this title also pertains to the role of the Spirit in relation to creation. The divine goodness is the "motivation" for creation and is also shared or "communicated" to created reality. For William, moreover, the role of the Spirit in the divine self-expression in creation continues this sapiential motif. In his view, the Spirit mediates between the divine simplicity *ad intra*, and its manifold, even infinite, diversity of created effects *ad extra*. William's scriptural authority for the multiplicity of the Spirt's effect is the same sapiential book which specifies the triad of measure, number, and weight:

> God is diverse ideas under diverse modes of speaking, of which it is said in the book of Wisdom, that the Holy Spirit is manifold *(multiplex)* (7:22), and in John's Gospel: *all that is mine is yours;* for this is said on account of diverse effects, or on account of the power by which [the Holy Spirit] is able to produce infinite effects outside of itself *(ex se);* yet *in se* God is most simple and invariable.[32]

---

30. SA II 8.1: 166,7ff.

31. William, like later scholastics, uses the opening verses of Genesis to refute various errors of pagan philosophers and heretics, specifically those of Aristotle, Plato, and various dualists. Cf. SA II 8.1: 167,16ff. "Through this which was said: *In the beginning,* that is the beginning of time, the opinion of Aristotle is excluded, who said that the world was eternal; whose opinion was disproved above. . . . Through this which was said: *he created,* the opinion of the Platonists is excluded, who said there were three eternal principles: the *artifex,* matter, and the ideas. . . . And this omnipotence of God working *per se* Moses showed when he said: *God created,* that is, he produced in being from nothing, thus excluding the opinion of the Platonists and the Epicureans, who posited two principles of being: *athomos* and *inane,* from which the world was said to be made, not created. Also, through this which was said: *God created the heavens* etc., the opinion of the Manicheans is excluded, who posited two principles of things, namely a good God, the beginning of incorporeal things, the God of light and of the New Testament, and another evil god, whom they called the god of darkness and the god of the Old Testament. . . ."

32. SA II 1.2: 17,90ff.

The link between the Son, in whose divine simplicity the exemplary ideas are undifferentiated from each other and from the divine essence, and the real, manifold diversity of the creation is the Holy Spirit. Denying, therefore, neither the divine simplicity nor the manifold creation, William envisions a direct, intimate, and immediate relationship between Creator and created through the activity and power of the Holy Spirit. He conceives of all created reality as the manifold, even infinite effects of the Uncreated Spirit.[33]

For William, then, the notion of sapiential expression suggests itself as an overarching description of the divine life and its relation to creation. Within the Trinity, the Father expresses himself perfectly in the Son, who is his Wisdom, and this expression is consummated by the mutual gift of the Holy Spirit. But this divine self-expression is not confined to the divine life. Rather, its uncreated and essential goodness "overflows" *ad extra* and is refracted in manifold, created, and participatory effects. This "overflow" is a trinitarian act. The presence of uncreated goodness within its created effects occurs "in" the Son, who as "Wisdom" is not only the Image, Mirror, and Expression of the Father's goodness, but also the Beauty, Exemplar, and Art by which created things come into and persist in good and beautiful being. Through the Son, the Father's goodness and beauty are expressed *ad extra*.[34] At the same time, the Spirit—"the universal gift in which all gifts are given"[35]—is the principle of diversity and multiplicity in created things, through whom the divine goodness expresses itself in myriad effects.

William's notion of symbolic theology everywhere builds upon these trinitarian assumptions. In a basic sense, creation is an expression, a manifestation of the Trinity which is immanently self-expressive, self-diffusive. Wrought artfully by the divine wisdom—spoken into existence by the Word, given concrete and diverse expression by the Spirit—created things are so many exterior "words," partial, incomplete expressions of the divine candor and splendor which bespeak the beauty of their

---

33. William brooks no possibility of created intermediaries which intervene between God and creation. In many ways, he develops his exemplarism with a view toward refuting the dualism of the Cathars and others.
34. SA III 1: 27,53ff.
35. SA II 1.1: 13,20.

Source. In short, the divine wisdom has expressed itself in creation. Quoting Augustine's *Confessions*, William reminds "all things exclaim: 'God made us.'"[36]

The Metaphysics of Sapience

The dynamic toward self-expression, which characterizes the Trinity both *ad intra* and *ad extra*, is intimately linked with William's convictions concerning divine goodness. Precisely because the Trinity is the *summum bonum*, it expresses itself and that which is expressed and communicated is the divine goodness. William develops his theological conception of beauty in close conjunction with this metaphysics of the good.

On the basis of creation's origin,[37] William argues that all created things are good through their participation in the *summum bonum*. But how, exactly, does he conceive of created goodness? Incorporating Aristotelian categories within a Neoplatonic framework, William envisions the following threefold division of the created good:

> the good is understood in a threefold way, as Aristotle said: namely the "moral good" *(honestum)*, regarding which the Lord said: *you shall be holy as I am holy;* the "delectable good" *(delectabile)*, of which it is said: "that is good whose apprehension is delight," or "the good is that which all things desire," or "the good is that which is desired by all." Also, the good is called "bestowing good" *(conferens)*; and of this Dionysius said: "the good is self-diffusive."[38]

These three forms of the good—the "bestowing good" *(conferens)*, the "delectable good" *(delectabile)*, and the "moral good" *(honestum)*—provide the fundamental framework in which William conceives of creation's goodness. While the moral good will be taken up below, it is primarily the bestowing and the delectable good that provide the categories in which William articulates creation's metaphysical goodness. He relates these two forms of the good to efficient and final causality, respectively:

---

36. SA II 1.2: 15,28; 15,39.
37. SA II 8.1: 174,195ff. Throughout William's description of creation, there is an ongoing polemic against various dualist strains of thought.
38. SA II 8.2.9.3: 221,31f.

As the good is delectable, it can be reduced to the final cause; as it is bestowing [it can be reduced] to the efficient cause; and the final and the efficient cause are the same, on account of the fact that the *summum bonum* said so of himself: *I am the alpha and the omega, the first and the last* (Rev 22:13).[39]

The *summum bonum*, then, is "the alpha and the omega," simultaneously the bestowing efficient cause of all things, that which is self-communicative, and the delectable final cause of all things, that which all things desire.

Corresponding to these two forms of the good, William posits a twofold goodness in creation, conceived of as two dynamic, complementary orders *(ordine)*, a "twofold ordination in things." The first ordination corresponds with the bestowing good. It is that good which "everything that has been infused by the first fount *(primo fonte)* struggles and attempts to diffuse to others, and to the extent that creatures are more noble and superior, the more they are infused, as they are superior creatures, in that they are closer to the font of being *(fonti essendi)*."[40] In this "downwardly" cascading order of the good, the self-diffusive dynamic of the *summum bonum* permeates all that flows from it, so that each created thing attempts to diffuse to that which is "below" it, the good which it has received from "above" it. The second order of created goodness corresponds to the delectable good and moves "upward" toward the highest good. This order is "toward the first good itself in which all things desire to rest, and by this appetite all things are moved so that they might rest in it. . . . For all things tend toward this that they might participate in the divine being in their own way."[41] In this second order, created things are good because they desire, move, and tend toward rest in the highest good. This twofold ordination, in short, constitutes the goodness of created reality: on the one hand, goodness diffuses itself "downwardly" into created effects; on the other, created things desire to move back and tend "upwardly" toward rest in the *summum bonum*. These orders, moreover, are clearly dynamic and complementary. Uncreated good bestows participatory goodness upon created things, which in turn establishes in them an orientation of desire for rest in

39. SA II 8.2.9.3: 221,38f.
40. SA II 8.2.9.4: 222,14f.
41. SA II 8.2.9.4: 222,11f.

their delectable, divine source commensurate with their being and capacity.

Measure, Number, and Weight

In a sense, for William, creation is "suspended" within these two dynamic ordinations established by the *summum bonum*. At this point, in order to describe the goodness of the creation thus constituted, William employs the Salomonic triad of measure, number, and weight *(mensura, numerus, pondus)*, derived, as noted above, from the sapiential text: *you, Lord, have disposed all things in measure, number, and weight* (Wis. 11:21).[42] William envisions all creation as bearing the characteristics of this triad, and, therefore, as good.

Why only *mensura, numerus, pondus?* These three alone, according to William, "are from God immediately," while all other created characteristics "are derived from them." Moreover, "in those three things rather than in other natural goods God is said to have disposed all things, since chiefly in these is the fullness and perfection of the universe of creatures considered *(attenditur)*."[43] With respect to this triad, he adopts the language of dispositive causality. He asserts, on the one hand, that, in as much as the sapiential triad, like the exemplary ideas, exists in God and is thus uncreated, the triad is an uncreated disposing cause: "all things are said to be created in [measure, number, and weight], as in a disposing cause." In this sense, the sapiential triad refers to a kind of divine attribute. And, according to William, for this reason Augustine called God "that Measure which gives measure or mode to each measured thing, that Number which supplies the form and limit of everything, and that Weight which bestows stability on all."[44] On the other hand, in as much

---

42. In Book II, Tractate 8, Chapter 2, William turns to the Genesis account of the six days, considering each individually in turn. Certain themes recur throughout: 1) Refutation of heretical positions; 2) Creation in the Word, who fully and openly speaks the goodness of God; who is the full and perfect Image of God; 3) God's goodness the motive for creation; 4) Creation as art. After addressing various issues related to the work of the six days, William concludes this tractate with a final question where he considers how the entire creation is disposed *in measure, number and weight* (Wis. 11:21).

43. SA II.8.2.9.2: 217,64.

44. Augustine, *De Gen. ad litt.*, IV, c.3, n.7 (PL 34.299): *"mensura omni mensurato modum seu mensuram tribuens, sive omnia terminans, numerus omni rei speciem prebens, pondus omnia ad stabilitatem trahens."*

as created things bear the imprint of their Creator, the triad can be seen as "dispositions or properties . . . which were left behind in created things from the disposition of God." In this sense, "all things are said to be created with [measure, number, and weight]" as their fundamental characteristic, "in the same way that a body is said to be made with color, since color occurs in a body as a property in a subject."[45]

In actual practice, William prefers the triad of "form, measure, and order," derived from and corresponding to the Salomonic triad of number, measure, and weight.[46] What precisely does he mean by form, measure, and order? Form *(species, numerus)* "is the orientation *(habitudo)* or natural habit *(habitus naturalis)* of operation or aptitude *(habilitas)* by which something is oriented to the use or work . . . for which it was created." More precisely, William sees *numerus* as a quasi-effect of *species:* "for species numbers things, that is, it discerns and distinguishes."[47] Form, then, gives to things their individuality, separating and distinguishing them as distinct from other things. It is, moreover, apparent from his definition that form is connected with the primary function or purpose *(utilitas)* of a given created thing, by which it is intended uniquely to manifest the divine glory. Measure *(mensura, modus)* pertains to a proper degree, intensity, or amount. Order *(ordo, pondus)* involves proper sequence, arrangement, and proportion. William sees or-

---

45. SA II.8.2.9.1: 213,12ff.

46. William in fact is acquainted with three different triads. The first is the Salomonic *numerum, pondus, et mensuram*, as already noted. The second, his preferred version—*modum, speciem,* and *ordinem*—is taken from Augustine's *De natura boni* (c.4 [PL 42.553]). A third, *armoniam, ordinem,* and *commensurationem*, is found in *The Divine Names* of Pseudo-Dionysius (c.4, n.23 [PG 3.724d; PL 122.1142b]). In general, he accepts the identification of these three triads, though with minor qualifications: SA II 8.2.9.2: "We say that measure, number and weight are the same things as *modus, species* and *ordo*. The association between measure and mode is clear. But species and number are the same thing, but yet they differ in this, that number is a quasi-effect of species; for species numbers things, that is, it discerns and distinguishes. Similarly, order is a quasi-effect of weight; for weight arranges and orders things in their proper places." Again, SA II 11.2.2.1: 327–28, 84ff.: "What Solomon called '*numerum, pondus, et mensuram*' is the same thing that Augustine called '*modum, speciem* and *ordinem*,' and Dionysius called '*armoniam, ordinem,* and *commensurationem*.' For in *species* is the *numerus* or discretion of a thing, in *pondere* [there is] order, since *pondus* is nothing other than that which inclines a substance toward its place; and it is clear that *mensura* is the same as that *modus*."

47. SA II 8.2.9.2: 217,69.

der as a quasi-effect of weight; "for weight arranges and orders things in their proper places,"[48] since *pondus* "is nothing other than that which inclines a substance toward its place."[49]

Yet, though William defines them individually, he prefers to describe the members of the triad in relation to each other:

> For in anything whatsoever, species *(species)* is called the condition *(habitudo)* or natural habit *(habitus)* by which something is perfected in the act toward which it naturally tends; through species, by its utility *(utilitas)*, in some fashion it imitates the divine activity or God [*in se*]; and in this there is said to be a harmony *(armonia)*, (in which through the species a consonance between the divine operation and other creatures arises), by which all things tend toward the utility of the universe. But since nothing has its species without measure *(mensura)*—since immense goodness pertains to God alone—for this reason everything naturally has its species *(speciem)* in measure *(in modo)*; and, since also it has its species for the utility of the universe, it therefore has it naturally in order *(in ordine)*.[50]

Thus, all created things ought to possess their form or species in measure and in order. When this occurs, a created thing has achieved its function or purpose *(utilitas)* in the universe and in some way it imitates the Creator. This is true, however, not only for individual things; for precisely as individual things achieve their form in measure and order they contribute to the *utilitas* of the whole creation, and a kind of universal harmony *(armonia)* emerges that also reflects the Creator.

In its most basic constitution, therefore, creation bears this objective threefold imprint of divine goodness and wisdom. We can speak then of the "symbolic sapience" of creation, the objective characteristics of divine wisdom which are manifest in the visible creation. Hence, symbolic theology, precisely defined, is the apprehension of divine wisdom within its created, visible effects.

A Definition of Beauty

From the foregoing, it may be surmised that William's interest in the sapiential triad extends beyond the mere fact of its presence in created

---

48. SA II 8.2.9.2: 218,93.
49. SA II 11.2.2.1: 327,84ff.
50. SA II 11.2.2.1: 326,50ff.

things. In fact, for him, the deeper significance lies in what its presence can reveal about the Creator. This revelatory aspect, moreover, pushes William beyond a simple ascription of goodness to creation, to an explicit association of the triad with beauty. On the basis of the presence of the sapiential triad in creation, he offers a definition of created beauty, employing his preferred triad of form, mode, and order *(species, modus, ordo)*: "these three constitute the beauty of a thing."[51] Again: "a thing is most beautiful *(res speciosa)* when it possesses its substantial form in proper measure and order."[52] Intriguingly, William envisions the relation between goodness and beauty in terms of a dynamic process. On account of the twofold ordination of created goodness—diffusing "downward" from, and striving "upward" toward, the *summum bonum*—a dynamic hierarchy emerges, in which each created form must find its particular ontological "location" and in some sense is always striving for or moving toward this proper "position" within the grand scheme of created goodness. It arrives there when its form possesses its proper measure and order. In particular, the notion of order *(ordo)* is crucial here. The goodness of a substance consists in the fact that it assumes its principal position *(principalis positio)* in its order and its measure. When this is the case, its goodness and beauty coalesce.[53] William summarizes: "There is therefore a goodness of every single substance in relation to its principal position in its order and measure, where its goodness and its beauty are the same substantially."[54] Every created thing, in moving toward its principal position, moves toward increasing degrees of order and measure, and thus increasing goodness, and, when it arrives at its proper place, it is simultaneously beautiful. When created goodness achieves its form in the right order and measure, then, precisely at that point, the good is the beautiful: "in the good of a thing its beauty shines forth."[55] William does not shy away from describing this as the perfection of created things:

51. SA II 11.2.2.1: 327,64–65.
52. SA II 11.2.2.1: 327,66.
53. Cf. Pseudo-Dionysius, *The Divine Names*, c.4, n.4 (PG 3.699; PL 122.1131a).
54. SA II 8.2.9.4: 222,19. *Est ergo uniuscuiusque substantie bonitas habitudo principalis positionis sue in ordine et mensura sua, ubi idem in ea eius bonitas et eius pulcritudo.*
55. SA II 11.2.2.1: 326,50.

Hence, it is clear that the perfection of anything whatsoever consists in these three things; and so something is perfect when it possesses these three things; and it is a beautiful thing *(res speciosa)* when it possesses its species in its measure and order.⁵⁶

Thus, with the complete presence of the sapiential triad, created things arrive at created perfection, and goodness and beauty, the good and the beautiful, coincide.

Precisely here, when through the presence of the triad goodness and beauty coalesce, created things reveal the Creator. Said otherwise, when divine goodness is perceived in creation, it is apprehended as beautiful. This is the epistemological correlate to the ontology of participatory goodness: because all created things participate in the uncreated divine goodness, they reflect that goodness as beauty when rightly perceived.⁵⁷ In sum, symbolic theology is the perception of the beauty of the visible creation, which chiefly reflects the divine wisdom in its measure *(mensura, modus)*, number *(numero, species)*, and weight *(pondere, ordo)*. "Chiefly in these is the fullness and perfection of the universe of creatures perceived *(attenditur)*."⁵⁸

The Dimensions of Symbolic Sapience

At various points throughout the *Summa Aurea*, William offers concrete examples of the beauty of sapience in the visible creation. The sapiential triad, for example, is manifest in physical bodies. William argues that the fullness and perfection of the created universe can be discerned *(censeatur)* and appreciated in the beauty of bodies, which not only have an attractive form *(species)*, but are also "characterized by a proper ordination of parts and of parts well-ordered with a proper proportion *(proportio)* and symmetry *(commensuratio)*."⁵⁹ For a body is beautiful *(speciosum)* when it possesses its species or natural color in the most beautiful measure and right mode and order *(in speciosa mensura et deb-*

---

56. SA II 11.2.2.1: 327,64. *Unde patet quod perfectio cuiuslibet rei consistit in hiis tribus; et tunc est res perfecta, quando habet hec tria; et tunc est res speciosa, quando habet speciem suam in suo modo et suo ordine.*
57. Arnold, *Perfecta communicatio*, pp. 111–14.
58. SA II 8.2.9.2: 217,66.
59. SA II 8.2.9.2: 217,89.

ito modo et ordine).⁶⁰ Again, a body is beautiful "when it has natural appearance *(species)* or color and its members are proportioned and arranged fittingly."⁶¹

While corporeal beauty attracts him, William's most favored examples pertain to the virtues and their acts.⁶² For William, the virtues are winsome or pleasing *(honestum)*, having a kind of aesthetic appeal. "A virtue is said to be good, that is, pleasing *(honesta)*. For the pleasing is that which attracts us by its beauty *(decore)* and draws us toward its goodness. For through itself *(per se)* it leads *(ductiva est)* us toward the first goodness."⁶³ Once again, William here links goodness and beauty in describing the attractiveness of the virtues. The perception of their presence in the soul fosters a certain pleasure or delight which leads the perceiver on to the source of its goodness.⁶⁴ Moreover, this *bonum honestas* "is the *decor* or *pulchritudo* of the soul" in the same way that the triad effects the beauty of bodies. For "just as the beauty *(pulchritudo)* of persons is from the becoming *(decenti)* ordination of their members and the loveliness *(venustate)* of their colors, so the beauty of the soul is from the becoming ordination of its acts and the loveliness of its habit *(habitu venusto)*."⁶⁵ Accordingly, the presence of virtue in the soul brings about a goodness that is also beauty.

More precisely, the presence of the theological virtues of faith and charity in the soul bring about its beauty. In the wake of patristic and early medieval tradition concerning the primacy of charity and the

---

60. SA II 11.2.2.1: 327,68.

61. SA II 8.2.9.2: 217,70ff.

62. It should be noted here that this type of sapience corresponds to the third form of the good, noted above, namely, the *bonum honestum*. Here, a caveat is required. Though strictly speaking moral beauty is spiritual, invisible, pertaining to the soul—and thus seemingly out of place in a discussion of visible beauty—yet for William moral beauty is not part of mystical theology. Moreover, moral beauty is revealed in its exterior, visible acts.

63. SA III 11.1: 173,74ff.

64. SA III 15.6: 285,35. "That is properly called *useful* which leads to beatitude, but which *a se* does not have a certain delight, such as sickness/sorrow *(egritudo)*, flagellations, and such like; the *honestum* is that which *in se* has delight, but not *ex se*, as the virtues; the delectable is that which has delight *in se* and *ex se*, and this is God alone. Taking *delectabilia* broadly, though, the *honestum* is delectable."

65. SA III 41.2: 787,143.

soul's predisposition for it, William gestures at the power of this virtue to decorate the soul through the presence of the sapiential triad. "For the love by which God is loved for his own sake with charity has its species *(speciem)* namely in this, that it loves God for his own sake *(propter se)*." That is, it has "order *(ordo)* by which it loves God above all things *(super omnia)*; [it has] measure *(modus)* since by it God is loved infinitely *(in infinitum)* above all things."[66] Charity "is the weight *(pondus)* of the soul" (according to Augustine), since it makes the soul "most lovely *(speciosam)*." Hence, Scripture compares it to gold: *Solomon built a throne and overlaid it with the finest gold* (1 Kgs 10:18).[67] Charity effects "*decor* or *pulchritudo* in the soul, since its acts are ordered and it is perfected with loveliness."[68] While William thus concedes that charity is indeed the form or species, the natural habitude of the soul, his predilection to give faith primacy among the virtues prompts him to see the soul's true form in that virtue instead. For, the principal act of a thing ought to determine its species, and for him the soul's principal act is apprehension of God through faith now, and through vision *in patria*.[69]

Moreover, from a virtuous, rightly ordered soul come virtuous, rightly ordered acts. To these also William grants the presence of moral sapience. These three things are required for acts to be meritorious: "first that they be done for God's sake, and so we have number or *species;* the

---

66. SA II 11.2.2.1: 329,123ff.

67. SA II 8.2.9.2: 222,3ff.

68. SA III 41.2: 787,143ff. By contrast, the absence of charity is defined by the absence of sapience. "[Libidinous love] truly *in se* lacks species, mode and order. For it loves created things too much, which it loves in order to have fruition; for God alone is to be loved in this way: thus a privation of mode. There is a privation of species, since such love lacks a proper end. For in as much as there is fruition of a creature, there is privation of a proper end; for this love delights in that only for its own sake, so not for God's sake. There is also a lack of order, since temporal things ought to be loved in their order, namely in a lower order" (SA II 11.2.1: 323,40ff). Cf. SA II 11.2.1: 324,68.

69. SA II 8.2.9.2: 223,19.ff. "Even though charity is the habitude or *habilitas* of the natural operation, since through it the soul is habituated to the act of loving God . . . yet it is not a species, since here not every disposition or *habilitas* toward an act is called a species, except toward that act toward which something is naturally and principally; but this [act] is to know *(cognoscere)*; for to know perfectly is perfect beatitude *in patria;* and to know imperfectly is imperfect beatitude *in via*. For Augustine said 'to believe is beatitude.' Hence faith rather than charity is the species; and even though charity makes the soul most beautiful; yet faith makes it even more beautiful."

second is that they be given as they ought to be given, and so we have measure or *modus;* the third is that they be given to whom they ought to be given, and when and where, and so we have *pondus* or *ordo;* for circumstances order actions."[70] In short, then, the moral sphere for William is a prime context in which the presence of these characteristics reveals the goodness and beauty of created things.

Finally, William defines evil not simply as the privation of the good, but precisely as the absence of form, measure, and order. "Since in those three things consists the perfection generally of anything either corporal or spiritual," and "evil is properly the privation or corruption of perfection in any particular corruptible thing," so "evil is better defined as the privation of these three things than the other goods."[71] Even here, though, William finds a sapiential vantage point from which to view this absence. For even such evil, though itself lacking order, is yet "well ordained." For "just as God at various points created darkness, and did so fittingly so that it might be fitting *(et ita decenter ut decet),* and just as we interpose silences in singing, so God the *Artifex* of all things rightly ordained evil within good."[72] Ultimately, a certain ordination exists in the providential order and fittingness of the coexistence of goodness and its absence.

The Trinitarian Manifestation of Sapience

For William, as noted at the outset of this chapter, the significance of the presence of wisdom within the visible creation is that it mediates a knowledge of God, namely, symbolic knowledge: knowledge of God

---

70. SA I 8.8.4: 173,26ff. William likens such an act to the three joints in a finger: "In every good work there are three quasi-joints, namely *numerus, mensura,* and *pondus,* or *species, modus,* and *ordo,* since God *has ordered all things in measure and number and weight* (Wis 11:21)." Conversely, if a moral act lacks the elements of sapience, it is corrupt: "But since this act lacks measure, form and/or order it therefore corrupts the natural human good" (SA II 11.1.2: 314,35).

71. SA II 11.2.2.1: 326–27,50ff.

72. SA II 11.1.1: 310,26ff. William uses a similar argument regarding the goodness or utility of prime matter: "[Prime matter's] utility or goodness is this alone, that it is the beginning of all corporal things and is the foundation of the harmony which God made in the *cythra* of the universe out of the alternation of the succeeding generations . . . just as in a material *cythra* a symphony is produced out of the succession of sounds with the interpolation of certain silences, as Augustine testified in *de musica*."

through the fittingness or appropriateness of created, visible things. This is the case because the sapiential triad is a created effect of the Trinity, bearing the imprint of its divine Exemplar, having a beauty that reveals the divine Beauty, corresponding in some fashion to its Source. On the basis of this relation, aspects and features of created reality can in some way be predicated of God. What knowledge of God does the sapiential triad mediate in William's view? A first answer is: knowledge of the whole Trinity. In a general sense, the sapiential triad is a *vestigium* of the Trinity: "Every substance in which these three things are found, like a created trinity, has in itself a *vestigium* of the uncreated Trinity."[73] In this sense, William allows for various associations between a given member of the triad and a member of the Trinity: "Each of these [number, weight, and measure] corresponds to each [of the three persons of the Trinity]." Yet, more precisely, by appropriation, William aligns the individual members of the triad with different persons of the Trinity. An artist needs "power, and art or an exemplar according to whose image he works, and a utility or good which moves him to do the work." Similarly, in the divine art, there is "power which is of the Father, art or wisdom which is of the Son, goodness which is of the Holy Spirit." Thus, even though number, weight, and measure are vestiges of the whole Trinity, by appropriation "each individual one is a vestige of the individual persons."[74] Corresponding to measure or mode is the Father's power; to species and number, the Son's wisdom and beauty; to order and weight, the Spirit's goodness. William elaborates: For "every creature according to its capacity possesses its great power *(virtus)*"; by its *species* "every creature represents the wisdom of God, which is the form making all things beautiful *(forma formicans)*"; by its *ordo,* "in which there is rest, in which it bears its fruit and its utility, every creature represents the goodness of God." And so "in these three things every creature imitates the uncreated Trinity."[75] In short, the sapiential triad is a *vestigium Trinitatis,* a created image in which the Trinity shines forth. The creation is or-

---

73. SA II 11.2.2.1: 327,83.
74. SA II 8.2.9.3: 221,23–25.
75. SA II 11.2.2.1: 328,84ff. "Every effect in which the creature imitates God is reduced to the Trinity, since in those things either the Father, the Son, or the Holy Spirit *is imitated.* Hence, God is in creatures, either through power which pertains to the Father, or through

dered, measured, disposed—in a word, beautiful—because God is and creaturely beauty is a self-revelation of the Creator. The very same sapiential and aesthetic qualities which for William characterize the Trinity *in se*—"the highest order and beauty"—are also found in the Trinity's created effects.[76] Beauty based on measure, number, and weight is suited for mediating the knowledge of the triune God: precisely these three dimensions allow a "trace of the Trinity" to appear.[77]

Conclusion: I have delighted myself in your works

Symbolic theology, therefore, perceives in the created sapience adhering in visible things the beauty of uncreated, invisible Wisdom. The self-diffusive *bonum* of the Trinity "overflows" out of its own dynamic fecundity as the bestowing good *(bonum conferens)* into its created tributaries and refractions, disposing all things in measure, number, and weight. These, in various intensities and according to diverse capacities, manifest the *vestigia Trinitatis*, the power, wisdom, and goodness of the Father, Son, and Spirit. But, for William, this perception is not complete—in some sense has not even occurred—unless it is an aesthetic perception, a perception of the good as the beautiful, and therefore as delectable *(bonum delectabile)*. Accordingly, the last theme in symbolic theology that must be emphasized is delight *(delectatio)*. *I have delighted myself in your works* (Ps 91:5), wrote the Psalmist, and William loves to quote him.[78] This is the scriptural warrant for a certain love of, and delight in, the *pulchritudo* of *visibilia* which is appropriate, that is to say, which perceives in *visibilia* the trinitarian *vestigia* and thus refers that goodness and

---

presence or wisdom which pertains to the Son, or through essence or goodness which pertains to the Holy Spirit" (SA I 14.2: 270,13–18).

76. Arnold, *Perfecta communicatio*, pp. 111–14.

77. SA I 3.1: 27,53ff.

78. From his treatment of beatitude: "In one way, we have fruition of God in himself, as through faith, hope, and charity, by which we are moved immediately toward God. In another way, we have fruition of God in creatures, namely, when we are delighted by the goodness of a creature, in as much as it is the gift of God and the way to God *(via ad Deum)*. For in this way the creature has fullness; but in itself it is empty. But in as much as it is the path to God it is delectable. Whence it is said, *I shall delight myself in your works, O Lord* (Ps 91:5). And the Apostle, *rejoice in the Lord* (Phil 1:20). For the soul is well disposed to find sweetness in all creatures" (SA IV 18.3.3.3: 518,58).

beauty back to its divine source and loves *visibilia* for God's sake. In this sense, symbolic theology itself is governed by a sapiential principle, for when it delights in created beauty for God's sake, then it too is an act characterized by *species, modus,* et *ordo.*[79]

In the last analysis, William's view of symbolic theology must be subsumed with the category of faith's apprehension. Ultimately, the object of faith's *aestimatio* or *visus* is the divine beauty, the *prima pulchritudo:* faith is an apprehension of the divine beauty, perceived as the delectable and beatifying end.[80] Moreover, the frequent examples William adduces from the perception of physical beauty[81] reflect his concern with this form of theology. Though, as will be seen, the symbolic perception of divine beauty is inferior to that of mystical theology—for faith only rests "when the believer sees the First Beauty unveiled before itself"[82]—yet William clearly considers it an important facet of the knowledge of God.

79. SA II 11.3.2: 343,30ff. "For if such an act has *speciem, modum, et ordinem,* it is good, since by its mediation man delights in creatures for God's sake, so it is possible to say: *I have delighted myself, Lord, in your works* (Ps 91:5)."

80. SA III 38.2: 718,36ff. "Corporal sight is delighted by corporal beauty; thus, how much more is spiritual sight, namely the intellect, delighted by the highest spiritual beauty, except by faith; hence, faith is essentially delighted by the first truth or the first beauty."

81. Cf. SA III 36.1.1. "There is delight in the vision of sensuous beauty; so there is delight in the vision of intelligible beauty."

82. SA II 8.2.9.5: 224,39.

CHAPTER 9

MYSTICAL THEOLOGY
Interior Perception of God's Effects

A FUNDAMENTAL PRINCIPLE in William's theology is that all knowledge of God is mediated through created things. As noted at the end of Part II, in a seminal discussion of this principle early in the *Summa Aurea*, William took up the Dionysian distinction between symbolic and mystical theology in order to distinguish two kinds of created effects and two corresponding forms of theology. As described in the previous chapter, symbolic theology knows God through external creatures. Mystical theology also pertains to creatures, but to those which William calls the "interior, hidden and more worthy effects" *(interiores et occultos et digniores effectus)* received from God. It "names God through that which it perceives *(sentit)* in secret concerning God, through intellectual vision or contemplation, as when it calls God sweet or beloved or things of this sort." And, William continues, "the soul imparts such names through the gift of wisdom *(donum sapientie)*, of which it is maximally and properly to know by experience what God is like *(maxime et proprie est cognoscere experimento qualis sit Deus)*."[1] Mystical theology, then, is a form of spiritual sensing *(sentire)*, wherein what William has elsewhere called the *delectabilia divina* are perceived; it is an experiential cognition *(cognoscere experimento)* of the divine nature; it entails both perception *(sentire)* and cognition *(cognoscere)*. In sum, it is a spiritual apprehension, a "savorous knowledge," which, as will be seen, is made possible by the soul's spiritual senses.

1. *SA* I 4.2: 40,117ff.

William's teaching on the spiritual senses, therefore, represents the climax of his unique account of mystical theology. The possibility of perceiving God through the spiritual senses emerges with the final gift of the Holy Spirit, the gift of wisdom, which is also the last in a three-stage process, along with knowledge *(scientia)* and understanding *(intellectus)*. The burden of this chapter is to explicate William's notion of mystical theology by charting the path that must be traversed in order to arrive at the gift of wisdom and its "spiritually sensuous" knowledge of God.

The Structure of Spiritual Apprehension:
scientia, intellectus, sapientia

The first words of the *Summa Aurea*'s Prologue are not William's own, but those of the Letter to the Hebrews: *faith is the substance of things hoped for, the argument of things not appearing* (Heb 11:1). The remainder of the Prologue reveals his fundamental intention for the work and sets its overall tone and trajectory, as William describes the basic structure and progression of faith's knowledge.

What is the relationship between faith and reason, theology and philosophy? Can Christian faith be rationally demonstrated or proven? Are philosophical arguments permissible within theological endeavor? These, of course, were not new questions at the turn of the thirteenth century; but they were agitating with new vigor, and reflective thinkers increasingly felt the need to reformulate answers in the wake of a rapidly changing, increasingly Aristotelian, intellectual milieu.[2] Precisely these

---

2. A substantial body of literature describes the various changes occurring in theological method before, during, and after William's time. Cf. Inos Biffi, *Figure medievali della teologia* (Milan: Jaca Book, 1992); M.-D. Chenu, *La théologie comme science au XIIIe siècle*, 3d ed. (Paris, 1957); Brian Gaybba, "Fifteenth Century Views on the Nature of Theology: An Outline of Its Characteristics and a Survey of the Printed Primary Sources," *Studia Historiae Ecclesiasticae* 20:1 (1994): pp. 106–19; P. Glorieux, *Les genres littéraires dans les source théologiques et philosophiques médiévales* (Louvain, 1982), and "L'enseignement au moyen âge," *Archives d'histoire doctrinale et littéraire du moyen âge* 43 (1969): pp. 65–186; John Jenkins, *Knowledge and Faith in Thomas Aquinas* (Cambridge: Cambridge University Press, 1997); U. Köpf, *Die Anfänge der theologischen Wissenschaftstheorie im 13. Jahrhundert* (Tübingen: Mohr, 1974); Albert Lang, *Die theologische Prinzipienlehre der mittelalterlichen Scholastik* (Freiburg: Herder, 1964); R. J. Long, "The Science of Theology according to Richard Fishacre: Edition of the Prologue to His 'Commentary on the Sentences,'"

issues inform William's opening remarks. Though not exhaustively elaborated, his response is clear, vigorous, and programmatic, not only for the *Summa Aurea*, but also for subsequent scholastic thinkers. "Just as God is loved with true love for his own sake, above all else," he argues, so

> faith rests in the first truth for its own sake, above all else *(acquiescitur prime veritati super omnia propter se)*: thus, nothing is more certain than faith.... For this reason the Apostle says in Hebrews 11 that "faith is an *argumentum* not a *conclusio,* proving not proven *(probans non probatum)*."[3]

With this "formula of beautiful density"[4]—"faith rests on the first truth for its own sake and above all else"—William asserts an absolute priority and autonomy for faith. Faith is an *argumentum,* not a *conclusio.* It is underived and prior to all else, having an unshakeable certainty that comes from direct adhesion to its divine object, the *prima veritas.*[5] The contrasting view—perverse, according to William—would attempt "to prove the faith or the articles of faith" by relying on "human reasons *(rationibus humanis)*" or "natural reasons *(naturales rationes)*."

This language is technical and significant. For William and his contemporaries, *argumentum* was not only part of the definition of faith in Hebrews, but also central to the methodology of Aristotelian science. There, it occupied the role of an underived, self-evident premise, from which further conclusions could be derived through logical analysis. As such, it was a useful "pivot" for articulating precisely the inversion of procedure in theology, as opposed to science or natural philosophy, which William advocates.[6] In theology, faith functions analogously as an

---

Medieval Studies 34 (1972); Walter Principe, *Introduction to Patristic and Medieval Theology,* 2d ed. (Toronto, 1982); J.-P. Torrell, "Le savoir théologique chez Saint Thomas," *Revue thomiste* 96 (1996): pp. 355–96; O. Weijers, ed., *Méthodes et instruments du travail intellectual au moyen âge* (Turnhout: Brepols, 1990); James Weisheipl, "The Meaning of *Sacra Doctrina* in *Summa Theologiae* I," *The Thomist* 38 (1974): pp. 49–80.

3. SA I Prol: 15,2.

4. Chenu, *La théologie,* p. 59: "Whence his definition of faith: *Fides est acquiescere primae veritati propter se super omnia.* A formula of beautiful density which will soon become law in the schools and which Aquinas will take over."

5. Several important scholastic "firsts" are present in this passage. First, the formulation "for its own sake and above all else" places faith on equal footing with charity, which was traditionally described with this formula. Second, William apparently coins the phrase "first truth *(prima veritas)*," a phrase that will become standard scholastic parlance.

6. See Chenu, *La théologie,* p. 36.

underived, self-evident, first principle. In no sense is it a conclusion; no reasoning is prior to it. In effect, then, William draws a line between theology and philosophy.

But then, what of reason, of William's *rationes naturales,* in theology? Are these ruled out of court? By no means. One of William's most significant contributions to subsequent scholastic theology is to have created a foundation and framework for a genuine theological science. Faith, he avers, can indeed be shown to be reasonable, not only as a defense against heretics and as an aid for the simple,[7] but also and primarily because natural reasons *(rationes naturales)* augment and confirm faith. For "God is not finally to be loved on account of temporal goods; yet such blessings augment and confirm charity in those who already possess it. They are the motivating and provocative cause of the love of God." Similarly, "natural reasons augment and confirm faith in the faithful."[8] Here, William creates an integral "space" for reason and argument within theological discourse. The believer's grasp of the truth of the faith does indeed involve the use of *rationes naturales.* These, however, are aids to faith already formed, augmenting and confirming it in the same way that temporal benefits augment and confirm the love of God in one already possessing charity. William stresses the point: "When someone has true faith and the reasons by which the faith may be demonstrated, he does not rest on the first truth on account of these reasons, but rather he rests in those reasons because they agree with the first truth and attest to it."[9] There are certain kinds of reasons—reasons which demonstrate the truth of the faith—which are neither the basis of faith's existence nor of its certainty; rather they confirm and augment faith's already existing adherence to the *prima veritas.*[10]

---

7. SA I Prol: 16,20ff. "The second reason is the defense of the faith against the heretics. The third is the promotion of the simple to our faith. For just as the simple are moved to the true love of God on account of temporal goods, so sometimes the simple are moved to true faith through natural reasons. On account of these three reasons, the highest prelate Saint Peter taught that they might *be prepared to offer to all those asking you a reason for the faith and hope which was in them* (1 Pt 3:15)."

8. SA I Prol: 15,16ff.

9. SA I Prol: 16,26ff.

10. William also offers a tropological exegesis of the Johannine narrative of Jesus' encounter with the Samaritan woman (John 4), which is a metaphor of faith's experience.

But how, then, should reason function in theology? Put simply, in the light of faith, reason provides insight into and understanding of the content of the faith. He describes faith as a quest for theological understanding *(intellectus)*:

> To whatever extent someone has faith, to that extent does he see *(videt)* with certainty and with clarity the reasons *(rationes)* of this kind, since faith is the illumination of the mind in order to see God and divine things *(ad Deum videndum et res divinas)*. The more the mind is illuminated, the more clearly does it see *(videt)*, not only *that (quod est)* what it believes is the case, but *how it is (quomodo)* and *why it is (quare)* that what it believes is the case; which is to understand *(intelligere)*. Whence, Isaiah says: *unless you believe you will not understand* (Is 7:9), for the mind *(mens)* is not able to see *(videre)* divine things clearly without the light of faith. And for this reason, it has been rightly said that "with Aristotle an *argumentum* is *ratio* making dubious things certain; with Christ, however, an *argumentum* is faith producing *ratio*."[11]

In this passage, William extends the definition of faith; faith is now a light *(lumen fidei)* and an illumination of the mind *(illuminatio mentis)* that enable spiritual sight and knowledge. Thus, a positive, expanded sense of faith as an *argumentum* appears. Faith is an *argumentum* not only negatively, as underived and thus precluding any prior process of ratiocination, but also as a starting point for a genuine, scientific body of theological knowledge. In the inversion of method, which William's view of theology entails, faith produces its own theological reasons, its own *ratio*, not, to be sure, a necessary demonstration, but a demonstration of

---

He is primarily interested in the response of the woman's friends and family, who, upon hearing about Jesus from the woman, go out to see him for themselves. After encountering him, they reply: *"We do not believe because of your testimony, but because we have seen and heard [Jesus] ourselves."* According to William, this is the proper attitude toward natural reasons on the part of those who believe properly. They believe not on account of natural reasons, but because through faith they have already "seen and heard Jesus themselves *(vidimus et audivimus)*" (SA I Prol: 16,29f.).

11. SA I Prol: 16,34ff. In the anonymous saying above, William is actually quoting Simon of Tournai (1190) from his *Expositio in Symbol Quicumque* (unedited: Ms. Paris, Nat. lat. 14886, fol. 73a): *Doctrina Aristotelis est de his de quibus ratio facit fidem, sed Christi doctrina de his quorum fides facit rationem. Hanc autem distinctionem doctrinarum christiane et aristotelice, naturalis philosophie et theologie, plerique non attendentes, in varios errores lapsi sunt, indifferenter in omni facultate ex ratione previa fidem querentes, et sic quod proprium est naturali facultati et doctrine aristotelice, theologie etiam christiane communicantes.* Moreover, the teaching is not of Aristotle, but Boethius.

the reasonableness, coherence, and intelligibility of faith claims—a theological demonstration of how and why.

Of greater significance, though, in the text quoted above, faith provides access to two different entities. As just noted, on the one hand, the mind is illumined to understand the reasons, the rationale undergirding those affirmations which it believes, namely, the articles of faith—e.g., Trinity, Incarnation, the human person's end in the triune God. In an important sense, it is the articles of faith that rest on and are illumined by the *prima veritas*. These function as an *argumentum* in the theological enterprise. In the Aristotelian parlance that William here adopts, this acquisition of understanding is the transition from knowledge *that* something is true *(scientia quia)* to knowledge of *why* and *how* it is true *(scientia propter quid)*. Gradually, faith comes to grasp the intelligibility and the coherence of the claims contained in the *articulos fidei*. At the same time, faith provides a form of spiritual perception *(videre)* of God and divine realities *(Deum et res divinas)*. Initially, William speaks of these two aspects in the same breath, with the same vocabulary. In the light of faith, the mind sees *(videre)* both *rationes* and *res divinas;* faith entails both theological understanding *(intellectus)* and spiritual perception *(visus)*. As he proceeds, however, a relationship emerges. Due to the effects of sin, he argues, "human beings have weak spiritual sight *(debilem visum spiritualem)*." In faith, accordingly, there are gradations *(gradus)* of spiritual vision, for as the soul is exercised and purged more and more it proceeds to greater and greater clarity, "so that finally it is able to direct its sight *(aspectum)* into eternal clarity itself *(eternam claritatem)*."[12] This spiritual vision of God, therefore, appears to be the climax of the entire process.

As a scriptural warrant for this theological method, William turns to the First Letter to the Corinthians, patterning faith's progress from *scientia* to *intellectus* to *visus* on Paul's remarks on the nature of Christian wisdom.

Faith begins with the articles nearest to the [physical] senses *(propinquis sensui)*, such as the Son of God was made man and that he was humiliated, gentle, and

12. SA I Prol: 17,47.

suffered, and things of this sort. Hence, the Apostle says in 1 Cor 2:2, *I consider myself to know nothing among you except Jesus Christ and him crucified,* so that through that clarity the intellect *(intellectus)* might be purged and exercised and solidified *(purgetur et exercitetur et solidetur)* so that it might see more clearly that *we are sons of God, heirs of God, and co-heirs of Christ* (Rom 8:17) and, finally, God himself. Whence, the Apostle in 1 Cor 2:6: *we speak wisdom among the mature.*[13]

Faith moves from a basic belief in the theological affirmations of the creedal articles *(scientia)*—which, significantly, pertain to Christological doctrines "closest to the senses"[14]—to an understanding *(intellectus)* of their salvific implications for human persons, and finally to a more direct and immediate vision of God himself, a knowledge to which William, following Paul, gives the name "wisdom *(sapientia)*" (1 Cor 2:6). In the process there is the crucible of purging, exercising, and solidification which William associates with the Cross.[15]

In the Prologue of his *Summa Aurea,* then, William outlines his view of the fundamental structure and process of Christian theology: from *scientia* to *intellectus* to *sapientia.* Starting with faith, the believer moves from simple affirmation and knowledge of the truth of the creedal articles *(scientia quia),* to an understanding *(intellectus)* of the theological reasons for these claims, their coherence and intelligibility *(scientia propter quid),* and from this, finally, to a direct and clarified *visus,* a perception of God and divine realities. The components of this triad are the fundamental elements in his concept of mystical theology: a science *(scientia),* leading to an understanding *(intellectus),* culminating in wisdom *(sapientia).*[16] The terms *intellectus* and *sapientia,* moreover, not only re-

---

13. SA I Prol: 17,51ff.

14. In the final analysis, William's interest in the doctrine of the spiritual senses of the soul seems to stem from a uniquely Christian, incarnational orientation, which values and upholds a "spiritually sensuous" knowledge of God precisely in light of the Incarnation and sensible appearing of God in human flesh. Perhaps William's doctrine of the spiritual senses is an appropriate response to the paradox of the divine becoming sensible and yet remaining divine and non-sensible.

15. William's concern with sin and resulting blindness suggests a link between virtue and theological endeavor.

16. Throughout the thirteenth century, scholastic theologians wrestled with the problem of how exactly theology should be conceived and defined. In the wake of an increasing Aristotelian influence, they considered whether theology is a "science"; in keeping

fer to stages in the knowledge of God, but also correspond to the two final gifts of the Holy Spirit. Accordingly, as will be seen below, William pioneers new territory in scholastic theology as he brings the gifts into the center of theological discourse.

But how precisely do these transitions occur? How does faith move from propositions to realities, from concepts to experience, that is, from science to wisdom? What is the relationship, if any, between speculative theology and spiritual experience? Where, finally, does the doctrine of the spiritual senses fit in? To these questions and to an analysis of these three components of faith's knowledge we now turn.

Scientia

When William turns to an extended analysis of the knowledge *(scientia)* of faith in Tractate 12 of Book III of the *Summa Aurea*, he builds upon the foundation laid in the Prologue. There, his remarks were largely methodological, pertaining to faith in its formal modality. Now, as he describes faith's material and concrete operation, he brings these formal aspects to bear in ways which reveal an even greater connection between

---

with earlier theological traditions, they also asked whether and in what sense theology could be termed a "wisdom." This discussion should be seen within the remote context of Augustine's distinction between active *scientia* and contemplative *sapientia,* where *scientia* pertains to the knowledge and use of created things or secular disciplines leading to the knowledge of divine things or *sapientia*. By the thirteenth century, the Augustinian wisdom/science division was crumbling, largely under the influence of Aristotle, whose "third wave" was now having its effect. In the *Nichomachean Ethics* (VI 6–7, 1141a), Aristotle calls *sophia* the highest knowledge in which one knows not only what can be deduced from first principles, but also intuitively possesses a firm knowledge of the principles *(archai)*. Thus wisdom includes both intuitive insight *(nous)* and knowledge derived from deduction *(episteme)*. From the thirteenth century forward, theological wisdom could be thought of as a science in the Aristotelian sense, and indeed as the highest science, and this combining of *scientia* and *sapientia* paved the way for a scientific approach to theology. As greater clarity emerged about the exact nature of Aristotelian science, scholastic method began to come into its own, as is evident in the move from an orientation around topics and rules to the full-blown use of Aristotle's concept of a science. Basic questions concerning the foundations of theological knowledge, its object, and its method emerged and were energetically debated. What is striking about this discussion is a certain lack of consensus. While most would allow the "scientific" character of theology, they disagreed about what made "theology" a "science." Similarly, while all insisted that theology is also a "wisdom," they frequently offered rather different explanations for the sapiential nature of theology. See the works cited in note 2 above for bibliography.

theological science and spiritual experience. As in the Prologue, in his *ex professo* consideration of faith in Tractate 12,[17] William invokes the Hebrews definition of faith and takes up its language of *argumentum* and *substantia* to elucidate its twofold emphasis.[18]

William begins briefly with *substantia*. Paraphrasing the biblical text, he argues that "faith is the foundation *(fundamentum)* of things to be hoped for." What is the sense of foundation? It is the anticipatory presence of realities not yet fully possessed: "through faith things hoped for are present *(substant)* in us." Intriguingly, but tersely, he construes the experience of these spiritual realities as a form of spiritual sensation: "by faith already we have a foretaste *(pregustamus)* of the sweetness of eternal felicity *(dulcedinem felicitas eterne)*."[19] Faith as *substantia*, then, entails an encounter with spiritual realities, which is analogous to physical sense perception.

With respect to *argumentum*, William is more expansive. He begins by asserting simply that faith is an *argumentum* in the sense of a demonstration or proof of the truth of things which are not apparent.[20] But in response to objections, he develops the thought. Faith, he claims, is an

---

17. After noting the many possible meanings of the word "faith"—referring variously to unformed or formed faith, to the full knowledge of the next life, to the act of belief, or finally to the articles of faith as a whole—he announces his intention to consider only formed faith. Cf. the discussion at SA III 12.11.1: 197,1ff.

18. Responding to an objection, William characterizes the Hebrews definition as theological rather than logical or philosophical: "We say that this definition is not logical or philosophical, but theological. For just as logic defines things through genus and differentia, as when it says: 'anger is an appetite contrary to sorrow'; and natural philosophy defines things through *materiam*, as 'anger is the rising of blood around the heart,' so theology defines things through their proper relation *(per habitudinem propriam)* which it has toward its final end, namely God" (SA III 12.1: 199,77).

19. SA III 12.1: 197,17ff.

20. SA III 12.1: 198,21ff. "The *evidence of things that appear not* is said in two ways, as is usually explained: first, since through it is demonstrated *(convincuntur)* that things not appearing actually are. So, the patriarchs, prophets, and apostles believed thus: the Father, Son, and Holy Spirit are one God; therefore, so it is. In the second way, faith is the *evidence of things that appear not*, since through faith it is shown *(probatur)* concerning things not appearing that they do not appear just as the church believes them; hence, so it is" (Argumentum non apparentium *dicitur duobus modis, ut solet exponi: primo, quia per eam convincuntur res non apparentes quod sint. Hoc modo patriarche et prophete et apostoli crediderunt ita: Pater et Filius et Spiritus Sanctus sunt unus Deus; ergo ita est. Secundo sic: fides est* argumentum non apparentium, *quoniam per fidem probatur de rebus non apparentibus quod non apparent sic<<ut>> Ecclesia credit hoc; ergo hoc non apparet*).

argumentum in a sense analogous to *(secundum similitudinem)* a major premise of a syllogism. He then identifies this *argumentum* with "the articles of faith,"[21] and refers to them as faith's "self-evident first principles" *(principia per se nota)*. These, like the first principles of any science, are axiomatic, requiring no prior demonstration. For, since it rests solely on the first truth, faith

> finds in the articles of faith themselves the reason why it believes them, namely God, just as in other faculties the intellect finds in this principle: "every whole is greater than its parts," the reason through which it knows that. For, if there were no principles in theology it would be neither art nor science *(ars vel scientia)*.

And thus, William continues, just as the above-noted principle has "a certain illumination through the mode of the natural illumination of the intellect, so this principle 'God is the rewarder of all goods,' as well as the other articles, have in themselves an illumination through the mode of grace *(illuminationem per modum gratie)*, by which God illumines the intellect."[22] William here posits the notion—radically new in his day, but

---

21. William offers the following definition of an article (SA III 12.7, qq. 1–5): (1) An article is so called from pressing together, contracting *(artando)*, since it draws or presses us toward those things which are to be believed *(artat nos ad se credendum)*. (2a) It concerns God and into God; (2b) it generates the fear *(timor)* of God through itself and directly; (2c) it generates the love *(amor)* of God through itself and directly. For through the fear of God we avoid evil and through the love of God we do the good; in which two things perfect righteousness consists which faith accomplishes in us. (3) The articles are *enuntiabilia* or propositions and not things, since properly speaking *credere* and *scire* are concerning complexes, and not concerning incomplexes. For it is improperly said: someone knows *(scire)* his house, that is, he cognizes. [Cf. M.-D. Chenu, "Contribution à l'histoire du traité de la foi. Commentaire historique de II^a–II^{ae}, q. I a. 2," in *Mélanges thomistes*, Bibliotheque thomiste, 3 (Paris, 1934), pp. 123–40: "For William of Auxerre, the articles of faith ... pertain to acts of judgment. This psychological argument will be taken up by Aquinas."] Across time the articles are the same formally, effectively, finally, but change essentially. (4) They pertain only to true things: nothing is subject to the virtue of faith except the true, since 'faith is an illumination of the mind by the first light for the seeing of spiritual and eternal goods.' But such an illumination is not, nor can it cause the sight of anything except that which exists *(ens)*; hence the virtue of faith concerns the articles, which are true. (5) They cannot be disbelieved without mortal sin. (6) They require deliberation and consideration before truly believed: *the invisible things of God are seen through that which has been made,* etc. Hence in order that someone might believe, it is necessary that he first consider visible things and by that infer their cause. Hence Aristotle said that 'to believe is to be persuaded' *(De anima* III 428a, 22–23). But the doing of all these things requires time.

22. SA III 12.1: 199,59ff.

soon to be standard scholastic doctrine[23]—that theology is a genuine science in a way that is parallel to the Aristotelian notion of *scientia*. Theological and Aristotelian science share a "magnificent analogy of structure."[24] Like Aristotelian science, theology too has first principles which are self-evident, requiring no extrinsic proof—namely, the articles of faith.[25] For the believer, the articles have in themselves a certain divine luminosity, through the mode of grace, which is analogous to the natural illumination of the intellect when it encounters a self-evident proposition, such as "every whole is greater than its parts." Later in the *Summa Aurea*, William will offer a similar description, this time emphasizing the role of the *prima veritas*. Faith is an apprehension of the articles through a graced illumination from the first truth. "For faith rests upon the first truth for its own sake and above all things; hence the cog-

---

23. Lang, *Die theologische Prinzipienlehre*, pp. 112–14. Lang observes that in the first half of the thirteenth century crucial methodological developments occurred when the articles of faith began to be seen as the first principles of the theological science, displacing past attempts to base theology on topical principles. Rapidly, this thesis became generally accepted, though it still had to overcome certain doubts and ambiguity. Only with the masters of the high scholastic period, above all Aquinas, did this thesis achieve final victory. These new currents and aspects, which animated thirteenth-century theology, emerged in particular at the University of Paris. Lang suggests that William of Auxerre is rightly credited with the merit of having first pointed out the principle-character of the articles of faith for theological science, though Lang cautions against exaggerating William's role. There are clearly traditional and common elements in his theology. William seems to assume, for example, a common Augustinian theory of illumination here. Also, he is not the only one pursuing these new methodologies. William of Auvergne, for example, was also clearly important in this regard.

24. Chenu, *La théologie*, p. 60.

25. Georg Wieland observes in this regard that William is influenced by Aristotle's *Posterior Analytics*, which stipulates the requirements for a true *scientia*. Increasingly in the newly established universities in the early thirteenth century, the various disciplines, including theology, attempted to justify themselves in accordance with this scientific ideal. Generally, the ideal stipulated that every genuine science has certain first principles, since an infinite regress is impossible, which are underived and serve as the basis for all other claims. In view of this challenge to designate the first principles of theological knowledge in order to protect the scientific character of theology, William of Auxerre is the first significant witness who submits theology to this standard of Aristotelian science, by specifying the articles of faith as theology's self-evident first principles. Despite the similarity, however, William stresses a basic difference, namely, that the articles of faith are only *per se nota* to believers through the graced illumination from the *prima veritas*, i.e., God. Georg Wieland, *Ethica-Scientia Practica: die Anfänge der philosophischen Ethik im 13. Jahrhundert*, Beiträge zur Geschichte der Philosophie und Theologie des Mittelalters, vol. 21 (Münster: Aschendorff, 1981), p. 76.

nition of God which faith is, is a kind of cognition of first principles." So, "the faithful soul finds in that first truth ... the cause of faith and no other cause is sought."[26]

In effect, William has imported into the theological sphere the Aristotelian assumption (passed on through Boethius, Gilbert of Poitiers, and Alan of Lille)[27] that every science has to proceed from underived and self-evident first principles.[28] For theological science, these are none other than the articles of faith. Faith's estimation of the *prima veritas* as beatifying good occurs in effect through its knowledge of, and assent to, these articles.[29] They are the individual truths to which faith assents, perceiving their verity in the light of the *prima veritas*.[30] They are guaran-

26. SA III 34.1: 650,30ff.

27. The eleventh- and twelfth-century schools began to develop a more scientific methodology in the spirit of *fides quarens intellectum* and based on the principles of authority and reason (e.g., the School of Bec: Lanfranc, Anselm of Canterbury, Ivo of Chartres, Berengar of Tours, Anselm and Ralph of Laon, Abelard—perhaps the first to use the word "theology" in the sense of a sacred discipline or body of knowledge concerning God, Gilbert of Poitiers, and Thierry of Chartres). At Chartres, scholars adopted a Boethian formulation of Aristotle's system of knowledge in which theology was classified as a theoretical science along with mathematics and physics. Also, thinkers like Gilbert of Poitiers, Alan of Lille, and Nicholas of Amiens suggested that each discipline has proper initial rules and attempted to guide theological processes from axioms and rules or "topics" to new propositions.

28. Much of the scholarly attention paid to William's theology in the past century is devoted to his pioneering accomplishments in this area. He is the first to attempt to put Christian theology on a methodological footing comparable to that of a true science in the Aristotelian sense of the word. Chenu notes repeatedly that the notion that the articles of faith are the *principia* of faith finds its first inspiration in William of Auxerre (cf. Chenu, *La théologie,* pp. 12–13 passim). On this point, Grillmeier calls William's *Summa Aurea* the "*Urtyp* of the new, classical *summas* of the thirteenth century." Alois Grillmeier, "Vom *Symbolum* zur *Summa*: Zum theologiegeschichtlichen Verhältnis von Patristik und Scholastik," in *Kirche und Überlieferung,* eds. J. Betz and H. Fries (Freiburg, 1960), p. 169.

29. William makes a distinction depending upon the subjective knowability of the articles of faith: "It should be known that certain principles are *dignitates*, others are *suppositiones*. The *dignitates* are seen *per se* without any discussion; the *suppositiones* are not seen without a certain light explanation. Similarly, the articles of faith are *per se noti* to some believers in the mode of a *dignitas*, namely to those whose intellects have been exercised in the things of God; to other believers they are *per se nota* in the mode of a *suppositio;* and for those a certain explanation is to be given so that they might believe in act" (SA IV 5.4.3: 115–16,76ff.). Those articles which are immediately self-evident he terms *dignitates;* those which require a certain explanation in order to be understood are called *suppositiones*. Lang suggests that the former might be identical to what the later Franciscan tradition called by the same name (*Die theologische Prinzipienlehre,* pp. 157–58).

30. "[For Aquinas] the formal object of faith is simply the first truth, which is God; the

teed by the *prima veritas* and this guarantee is the exclusive basis of their certainty.³¹ This allows them to function as self-evident first principles *(per se nota)*. In this way, William places his theological project within the framework of the absolute transcendence of the faith. Faith believes solely on account of its encounter with divine truth.³² In the Aristotelian parlance gaining currency in his time, he refers to this basic knowledge *(scientia)* of the revealed truths contained in the articles of faith as *scientia quia*, as simple knowledge that something is the case, that something is in fact true. Faith's *scientia* is that certain creedal affirmations are in fact true.³³

Fundamental to William's view of theological science (and almost completely neglected in secondary treatments of his theology) is the fact that, as described in Chapter 6, he construes faith's knowledge of its first principles as a theological perception *(sensus)*, or, more precisely, a perceptual judgment, a consideration in some sense analogous to the immediate recognition and judgment of physical sense perception. In this

---

material object is God and other things insofar as they are related to God. The human intellect, however, considers what is utterly simple, God, through considering what is complex. Thus faith consists in believing certain propositions, which are the articles of the Creed" (Jenkins, *Knowledge and Faith*, p. 162).

31. SA III 12.2: 201,47. "Faith is not only above opinion but also above science, and even above demonstrative science. For the intellect illumined by faith believes in the first truth more than in a syllogistic demonstration."

32. In this regard, Lang refers to a certain mystical aspect to William's theology (*Die theologische Prinzipienlehre*, pp. 157–58), as does Chenu (*La théologie*, pp. 12–13): "It is the scientific claim of theology which requires the mystical presence of faith. We limit ourselves to the question of whether theology is a science—that question posed by Thomas in the prologue of the *Summa Theologica* and the matter of articles 2 and 8—a double question which is only formally posed in the second quarter of the thirteenth century from a very fertile perception of William of Auxerre who assimilated the articles of faith in supernatural knowledge to the principles required in the construction of a science."

33. See Lang, *Die theologische Prinzipienlehre*, p. 120. The Parisian masters of the first half of the thirteenth century basically agreed on the argumentative procedure of theology, which proceeds from the articles of faith and is based upon their self-evident certainty. All these authors were conscious that the articles stand above natural principle-truths regarding intellectual insight. All refer to the fact that theology has a superior certainty over all other sciences by the illumination given in the *lumen fidei*. Therefore, according to Lang, theology does not arrive at the full stature of a *scientia*. The noetic evaluation of theology, i.e., whether it was a true science, was not yet the controlling problem. The character of a science in the full sense for theology was not yet taken up by any of these early thirteenth-century theologians, including William of Auxerre.

regard, he employs the technical term *aestimatio* to characterize faith's apprehension of its first principles. In the divine light which illuminates it[34] and with the immediacy and certitude of physical sense perception, the soul "sees" and knows the articles of faith: "just as through an argument one comes to the knowledge of a conclusion *(notitiam conclusionis)*, so through faith by a greater and greater illumination of the intellect one comes little by little to the perfect knowledge of eternal goods *(perfectam notitiam eternorum bonorum)* which are not appearing."[35]

This sense-like quality of faith's *scientia* becomes apparent as William wrestles with a technical dilemma regarding the nature of faith as a virtue. As noted in the chapter on faith, essentially and formally the object of faith's act is singular: the *prima veritas;* but concretely and materially, faith's immediate objects are the various creedal articles. Are there then multiple objects of faith, corresponding to the individual articles? If so, does not faith entail several distinct virtues, corresponding to and determined by these diverse objects, as a genus containing several species?[36] William rejects this view. But how to maintain the unity of faith in light of the plurality of creedal articles? William resolves the dilemma by positing a singular formal object of faith: all the articles have the same *ratio,* namely "because the first truth teaches it." Thus, the singular formal object of faith is God and all things related to God in the light of the *prima veritas.* On account of this singular object, William maintains that faith is a singular virtue or habit.[37] At the same time, however, he allows

---

34. William frequently refers to faith's illumination: "faith is the illumination of the mind in order to see God and divine things" (SA I Prol: 16,34); "faith alone first and *per se* illuminates the intellect" (SA III 12.1: 199,58); "faith is an illumination of the mind by the first light for the seeing of spiritual and eternal goods" (SA III 12.7.3: 224–25,62–63); quoting Augustine (Letter 120 nn.14–18), "faith is an illumination of the mind by which the mind is illumined by the first truth or by the true light so that it may see spiritual goods" (SA III 12.7.3: 223,5–6).

35. SA III 12.1: 198–99,55ff.

36. SA III 12.3: 202,5ff.

37. SA III 12.3: 202,27ff. "All things believed are concerning the same thing, namely God, since all the articles pertain to God . . . and they have the same *ratio,* since there is a single *ratio* of believing all the articles, for if one is asked why you believe this or that [article], there is only one response, namely, because the first truth teaches thus. For faith rests solely on the first truth, and it does not seek another mode of proving a certain article, since *faith is an argumentum, not a conclusion,* as the Apostle says. For faith has various modes of proving an article, yet it does not rest on them principally, but only on the

that from this singular habit come diverse acts of belief regarding the various articles of faith: "Cogitation is diversified according to the diverse things cogitated, and belief is diversified according to the diverse things believed; and thus the acts of faith are diverse in species *(diversi sunt motus fidei in species)*; yet faith is single in species *(unica est fides in specie)*."[38] Intriguingly, he appeals to physical sense perception for a parallel. "Just as diverse kinds of acts (e.g., seeing white or black) proceed from the natural habit of vision, so from the habit of faith proceed diverse kinds of acts *(diversi actus in specie)* (e.g., to believe the Son of God was born of a virgin, that God will punish the evil and reward the good in eternity)."[39] In effect, William posits both a primary, singular species of act, which issues substantially from the *habitus* of faith, as well as secondary, multiple subspecies of faith's acts. Corresponding to these diverse acts of belief are diverse spiritual delights *(delectabilia)*. Again, he appeals to physical sense perception, arguing that "just as there is one kind of delight annexed to vision when I see greenness, and another kind of delight annexed to vision when I see whiteness, so there is one delight annexed to the act of faith in which I believe God to be Creator and another in that by which I believe God to be Triune, and another in that by which I believe in the Incarnation."[40] As there is a unique aesthetic experience and pleasure in the vision of different colors, so William associates a unique spiritual delight with belief in individual articles of faith.[41]

In these passages, then, William describes faith as a singular habit or

---

first truth. For just as geometry is a single science, since it concerns a single subject, even though it proves various movements *(diversas passiones)* concerning that subject and in diverse ways *(diversis mediis)*, so much more is faith singular *(unica fides)*, since it concerns a single subject and has a single mode through which it arrives at this, that it believes whatever it believes."

38. SA III 12.3: 205,123f.   39. SA III 12.3: 204,71ff.
40. SA III 12.3: 205,125ff.

41. Informing this discussion is a generally Aristotelian view of virtue as a *habitus* with not only a substantial act, but also an associated passion or delight, which is unique to it, which arises from its encounter with its proper object, and which is neither the virtue itself nor its substantial act, but a kind of "second act." This model allows him to accommodate the demands of Christian faith by allowing diverse concrete acts of belief, diverse material objects, and diverse delights without compromising the unity and integrity of faith as a single virtue.

virtue, as singular in species, having a singular formal object *(ratio)*, the *prima veritas*. Yet an Aristotelian account of virtue allows him to speak of faith's *visus* in the singular, while also positing diverse acts of sight, each of which has an associated delight that in some way is "colored" by its corresponding object or article of faith. Hence, faith's primary act is vision; yet it contains diverse secondary acts of sight with diverse concomitant delights. William summarizes: in faith "there is essentially a manifold joy and a manifold refection, not only in the delectable multitude of things to be believed, but also in the very act of believing, since the *intellectus fidei* tends toward this."[42]

This initial knowledge of faith, though, has an inner dynamic toward increasing insight into, and penetration of, the truths of faith, toward an *intellectus fidei*, which culminates in a *visus* of non-appearing, revealed, spiritual goods or divine realities, *sapientia:* "faith is the illumination of the mind in order to see God and divine things."[43]

Excursus on the Gifts of the Holy Spirit and Theology

The second and third stages in William's understanding of spiritual apprehension—*intellectus* and *sapientia*—coincide with the final two gifts of the Holy Spirit and are best viewed within that context. Though our concern is these two gifts, his treatment of the topic generally merits a brief consideration. William charts new territory in scholastic theology when he explicitly includes the gifts of Spirit within the theological endeavor. He focuses in particular on the gifts of science *(donum scientiae)*, understanding *(donum intellectus)*, and wisdom *(donum sapientiae)*.[44]

For William, as for patristic and medieval tradition, the number and identity of the gifts of the Holy Spirit are derived from Isaiah 11:2–3. Properly speaking, wisdom *(sapientia)*, understanding *(intellectus)*,

---

42. SA III 11.3.1: 186,64.
43. SA I Prol: 16,30.
44. Beumer, *Theologie als Glaubensverständnis*, pp. 71–80. Curiously, the gift of knowledge has the function according to William of producing faith in others and defending it. It is considered as substantially identical to the virtue of prudence, differing only in that it has supernatural faith as a prerequisite. To that extent the other gifts, namely wisdom and understanding, must supply it with the reasons, so that it can produce and defend the faith. Hence, William does not include the *donum scientiae* within the constructive theological endeavor of seeking the understanding of the faith.

counsel *(counsilium)*, fortitude *(fortitudo)*, knowledge *(scientia)*, piety *(pietas)*, and fear *(timor)* are gifts[45] of the whole Trinity, yet through appropriation they are aligned with the Spirit, as they are conferred by divine goodness, which is appropriated to the Third Person.[46] Aside from this consensus, though, contemporary accounts of the gifts' nature and function vary widely. What precisely are they? How do they relate to the virtues? What role do they play in the spiritual life? While his answers to these questions are not always adopted by the later scholastics, his views shape later developments at crucial points.[47]

For William, the gifts govern the entire Christian life: "The seven gifts sufficiently govern human life, both the active and the contemplative."[48] With respect to the active life, William allocates five gifts: fear, piety, knowledge, fortitude, and counsel.[49] In contrast to other opinions, he sees the gifts essentially as virtues,[50] primarily because they operate like the virtues.[51] At the same time, he distinguishes them rationally *(ratione)* from both the cardinal or political virtues[52] and the theological

---

45. SA III 30.2: 593,63ff. William posits the following relational pairings between the gifts: understanding generates wisdom; counsel generates and regulates fortitude; knowledge generates and regulates piety. Fear, however, is not combined.

46. SA III 30.1.1: 585,5f.

47. Lottin, "Les dons du Saint-Esprit," pp. 41–43.

48. SA III 30.2: 591,17f. "As was demonstrated above, the seven gifts suffice for the regulation of the spiritual life, as much in the active life as in the contemplative."

49. SA III 30.2: 592,34ff. For William the active life consists especially in three things: in ceasing to do evil, in doing good, and in suffering adversity worthily.

50. SA III 30.1.2: 591,20ff. He thus rejects the view of Praepositinus—that only those gifts which pertain to the affection or appetitive faculties are virtues, namely, fear, piety, and fortitude, while the four which pertain to the intellect are not. He also rejects the view of Godfrey of Poitiers—that the gifts proceed from the virtues and facilitate their acts; and the position of Simon of Tournai—that the gifts are the seeds of the virtues which precede and prepare the soul for them. Rather, the gifts are the habits of the virtues and the Augustinian definition of a virtue can be applied to them.

51. Lottin "Les dons du Saint-Esprit," p. 43. "Will it be said, on the contrary, that the gifts are prior to the virtues, since they purify the heart of sin and thus prepare the way with infusion of the virtues? But, William notes, virtue itself has the same function to purify the heart, since it is directly opposed to sin. By saying that the gifts drive sin out of the heart, these authors thus acknowledge that the gifts are virtues. And it is with this position that William stops."

52. SA III 30.3: 595,38. "We say that in a righteous/just man the cardinal virtues and the gifts of the Holy Spirit are the same in essence, but they differ in *ratione*." William describes the following correspondence between the gifts and the virtues: the gift of fortitude and the virtue of fortitude; gift of knowledge and the virtue of prudence; gift of piety

virtues.⁵³ In particular, they differ in their mode of action and this in two ways. First, their motive for action is different: the political or cardinal virtues are inclined toward action according to motives taken from natural reason, while the gifts of the Spirit are inclined according to the reason of the supernatural order.⁵⁴ Second, the cardinal virtues, as they are "political," pertain to exterior acts which resist the vices. The gifts are those same cardinal virtues, but as providing an interior purification and disposition.⁵⁵ In this sense, the gifts are called purgatorial virtues.⁵⁶

Significantly, William describes this transition from the exterior political virtues to their interiorization through the gifts as facilitating an

---

and the virtue of justice; the gift of fear and the virtue of temperance. The gift of counsel, however, seems to have no corresponding virtue.

53. SA III 30.4: 600,39ff. Cf. SA III 34.2: 652,22. "The gift of understanding is a virtue, and wisdom and faith are similarly, since faith apprehends the first truth with assent, and understanding and wisdom similarly assent to the first truth for its own sake and to assent in this way is meritorious, since it is does not rest upon natural reasons but on the first truth alone."

54. SA III 30.3: 595,45. "The cardinal virtues move toward action from reasons taken from the natural law, while the gifts [move] from reasons of faith *(rationes fidei)*, which are spiritual." Cf. SA III 30.3: 596,56: "For the cardinal virtues are signified by the corners of the house, since they use *rationes* taken from natural law, and in this they are like the built foundation of the whole spiritual house; but the gifts are called sons, since they use the *rationes* of faith, through which we are sons of God." Cf. SA III 30.2: 592,34ff.: "They cause persons to act rightly through the supposition of spiritual reason *(per suppositionem spiritualium rationum)*. But the political virtues do not function in the same way; for the political virtues cause right action from the supposition of precepts of the natural law; and for this reason they are sometimes called natural virtues."

55. SA III 30.3: 596,46f. "The cardinal virtues are attended by exterior works, in as much as through exterior works they fight against the vices; but these same virtues are called gifts maximally in as much as they are in interior acts, by which they have already conquered in that very act."

56. SA III 30.3: 596,51. "These virtues are called gifts in as much they are purgatorial, hence they are called sanctifications of the soul." Cf. SA III 30.2: 591,20ff. "These seven are called gifts of the Holy Spirit through a certain appropriation, since on account of the prerogative they have of cleansing the soul first and principally from the capital vices, they are especially called gifts. Fear, through that which humiliates, expels pride; piety, through that which rejoices to honor a neighbor, expels envy; knowledge, by which we understand our neighbor to be a child of God or able to become one easily, expels wrath; fortitude, which excludes the impediments of the world, expels *accidie;* counsel, which teaches us to prefer eternal things to temporal things, removes avarice; understanding, through which we are delighted by spiritual goods, excludes gluttony; wisdom, by which we are delighted by God purely and in which there is the highest spiritual delight, excludes luxury, in which is the highest carnal delight, since, as St. Gregory said, 'by spiritual taste one renders empty all things fleshly.'"

interior detachment from exterior things so that the soul may begin to taste sweetness and perceive the delights of the interior life.[57] The completion, moreover, of this interiorization is construed as arriving at a perfected spiritual perception of the divine sweetness,[58] by which the purified soul rests definitively in God. The difference between the political virtues and the active gifts of the Spirit is the latter's interior perception *(sentire)* of divine sweetness: "When the purged soul begins to be recalled *(revocatus)* within, it begins to sense *(sentit)* [the sweetness of God]. But when he comes to the virtues of the soul already purged, at that time it perfectly senses the sweetness of God." This stage pertains to the contemplative life, and the final two gifts, understanding and wisdom: "in these two gifts perfect contemplation consists and therefore these last two gifts perfectly govern contemplation."[59]

In sum, the gifts of the Holy Spirit lead progressively from the exterior, active life (fear, piety, knowledge, fortitude, counsel) to the interior, contemplative life (understanding and wisdom). The active life purges the soul in preparation for the contemplative life, and this purgation entails preparation of the spiritual palate for the tasting of divine sweetness through wisdom.

Intellectus

As seen in the Prologue, the initial knowledge *(scientia)* of the creedal articles is not an end in itself, but leads to understanding *(intellectus)*.

---

57. SA III 30.3: 596,59. "Through the gift of fortitude we tolerate adversity sweetly *(dulciter)*, but the through the political virtue of fortitude, we [tolerate adversity] in a manly way only." Cf. SA III.30.3: 597,83ff. "The political virtues differ from the gifts of the Spirit on account of exterior works, since a person who has the political virtues does not taste the sweetness of God, and thus is not recalled from there to interior things, and therefore he is occupied as yet with exterior works; but when the person arrives at the purgatorial virtues he senses *(sentit)* [the sweetness of God] somewhat and is somewhat recalled to interior things. . . ." Again, in interior things, "there are greater pleasures *(delicias)*."

58. SA III 30.3: 597,88. "But when a person arrives at the virtues of the soul already purged, at that time he perfectly senses the sweetness of God." Cf. SA III 30.3: 596,62ff. "But they are called virtues of the purged soul, when those same virtues are already purged with respect to their state, which is after the consummated victory over the vices, when the purged soul perfectly rests in the embrace of the spouse, whence Origen said that Solomon taught the political virtues in Proverbs, the purgatorial virtues in Ecclesiastes, and the virtues of the already purged soul in the Song of Songs."

59. SA III 30.3: 597,88.

There, William spoke explicitly of an *intellectus fidei*. He cited the anonymous saying "with Aristotle an *argumentum* is *ratio* making dubious things certain; with Christ, however, an *argumentum* is faith providing *ratio*," and the well-known Septuagint text from Isaiah "if you do not believe, you will not understand." This stage of the knowledge of God, accordingly, involves *ratio* and pursues *intellectus*. In this context, the articles of faith function as first principles, but not merely because they are self-evident and objectively given. They also serve as the basis for a positive, constructive theological body of knowledge, entailing an intellectual penetration into the truths of the faith, a deeper appreciation of their meaning, coherence, and intelligibility—an understanding. William's theology is well described as an *intellectus fidei*,[60] an attempt within the sphere of faith to penetrate the deeper meaning of fundamental Christian doctrines, to make them intelligible, to grasp their individual credibility and to perceive their collective coherence.[61]

In order to appreciate William's thought here, his conception of the genesis of formed faith—or, more precisely, the transition from unformed to formed faith—must be briefly rehearsed. He distinguishes between natural *(naturalis)* and accidental *(accidentalis)* knowledge of God. Natural knowledge of God is twofold: before the Fall *(ante peccatum)*, Adam possessed a manifest *(aperte)* knowledge of God in the mirror of creatures; after the Fall *(post peccatum)*, however, Adam and all his

---

60. Beumer argues that William's view of theology is best characterized as *Glaubensverständnis (intellectus fidei)*, rather than *scientia* (which he associates with Aquinas) or even *sapientia* (which he associates with Alexander of Hales, Albert the Great, Bonaventure). He finds this approach to be typical among theologians in the first quarter of the thirteenth century, who, in a line stretching from Anselm of Canterbury and the Victorines to William and on to such authors as Peter Tarantasia, were bearers of an Augustinian tradition into the Middle Ages. He sees in this older approach not so much a contradiction as a difference in emphasis and perspective, which is in greater sympathy with the notion of *gnosis* among the Greek church fathers. Johannes Beumer, "Die Theologie als *intellectus fidei*: Dargestellt an Hand der Lehre des Wilhelm von Auxerre und Petrus von Tarantasia," *Scholastik* 17 (1942): pp. 32–49.

61. Beumer, *Theologie als Glaubensverständnis*, p. 59. According to Beumer, William expands and deepens this Augustinian approach to theology in novel and valuable ways, which in one form or another are taken up by subsequent theologians. The early Franciscan school (Alexander of Hales, Bonaventure) remained faithful to the Augustinian tradition on this point. The same is true for the Dominicans Albert the Great and Peter Tarantasia.

descendants possess a natural knowledge of God which is in a mirror *(per speculum)* and enigmatic *(in enigmate)*, since henceforth "*the darkness of sin was over the face of the abyss* (Gn 1:2), that is the human heart."[62] Accidental knowledge of God is threefold: that which is acquired through natural reasons *(per naturales rationes)*, the domain of philosophy; that which rests upon the testimony of Scripture or miracles, unformed faith *(fides informis)*; and that which is graced *(gratuita)*, formed faith.[63] For William, only the knowledge of formed faith, which occurs through illumination when the true light illumines the soul for seeing itself and other spiritual things *(ad videndum se et alia spiritualia)*,[64] can be considered the true knowledge of faith.

The advent of formed faith affects the soul's relationship to the prior forms of knowledge. As an immediate effect of divine illumination, formed faith *(fides gratuita)* entails a form of spiritual *visus:* "now the human heart believes, not on account of natural reasons, but on account of what it sees, namely the first truth." Faith assents, as noted above, to the first truth for its own sake and above all else.[65] Now, the other accidental forms of knowledge cease. Neither their acts nor their habits remain. For "there is a singular apprehension *(apprehensio)* of all accidental knowledge by which God is cognized."[66] The apprehension of formed

---

62. SA III 12.4: 208,55ff. These two kinds of knowledge differ from one another in the same way that a dignity *(dignitas)* and a supposition *(suppositio)* differ. A dignity needs no other demonstration or only a light persuasion *(levi persuasione)*; a supposition needs at least a light persuasion. Cf. SA III 12.4: 208,59ff.

63. SA III 12.4: 208,65f. Included in William's discussion of the knowledge of philosophers, heretics, and weak believers is also a brief question on the knowledge of the Jews (cf. SA III 12.8.2: 238,26ff.).

64. SA III 12.4: 208,65ff.

65. SA II 10.5: 293,75ff. "In order for someone to believe with formed faith, it is necessary that he deny himself, that is his own senses and carnal intellect in allegiance to Christ in obedience to God and the first truth, and that he rely on no *ratio*, but only on the authority of the first truth." Cf. SA II 10.5: 295,131ff. "As long as the human heart accedes through [extrinsic] modes in order that it may believe, that belief is only unformed faith, as long as it clings to testimonies and arguments of miracles; but in order that it believe fully and truly it is necessary to cling deeply to the first truth alone purely and nakedly, requiring no extrinsic certainty. This is possible only if it is illumined by the grace of faith, since, before true faith comes, man can still hesitate and be false; but when true faith comes, it exterminates and expels every hesitation. . . ."

66. SA III 12.4: 209,89. "All accidental cognitions of God have a single apprehension; and for this reason . . . it does not suffer any other apprehension to be present with it."

faith immediately supplants the acts of all other accidental cognitions.[67] The soul is no longer habituated to believe on account of reasons and testimonies as before; and so these other accidental cognitions disappear.[68] William compares the knowledge of unformed faith to the light of the moon which, once the sun of formed faith has risen, remains present but contributes nothing to the light that then shines.[69] This, therefore, is simultaneously a negative and positive, a destructive and constructive, moment in the genesis of faith[70]—cutting off all natural as-

67. SA III 12.4: 211,165ff. To explain the possibility of radically differing apprehensions of the same object, William offers a stock analogy: "it is customary to refer to the one who killed the father of Plato and fled, but after a long time returned, was so altered that Plato did not recognize him, and won the familiarity of Plato. In this sense, it is true that Plato both loved and hated him, but according to diverse apprehensions, since to the extent that he apprehended his father's killer in the state in which he is, he loved him; but to the extent that he apprehended his father's killer under the image in which he saw him when he killed his father, he hates him; and so he hates and loves the same thing according to diverse apprehensions."

68. SA III 12.4: 208,70ff. "With the arrival of such cognitions, all the prior accidental cognitions depart, both with respect to act and habit *(ad actum et ad habitum)*. . . . There is the same apprehension *(apprehensio)* of all the accidental cognitions by which God is cognized; and when that apprehension arrives in the soul, just as quickly faith takes over the act *(motus)* of all other accidental cognitions, if they were present; and so in the presence of faith, the human person is no longer habilitated *(habilis est)* for believing through reasons and testimonies *(per rationes et per testimonia)*."

69. M.-D. Chenu, "Pro fidei supernaturalitate illustranda," in *Xenia Thomistica*, ed. Sdoc Szabó, vol. 3 (Rome, 1925), pp. 300–301. Of unformed faith *(fides informis)* Chenu notes that William does not find it unformed because it is lacking in charity; rather, it is the boundary between the virtue of formed faith and unbelief. It is natural belief *(credere naturale)*, that is, *fides acquisita*. Formed and unformed faith do not differ in their object, but in their modes, since formed faith operates through an illumination directly infused by God, which forms conclusion through reason from them. Formed faith *(fides gratuita)* is free, meritorious, unshakeable, its own *argumentum*. By contrast unformed faith remains weak, like opinion, and although it possesses a supernatural object, in reality it is called human assent. Chenu notes that since William allows for the exterior confirmation of true faith by natural reasons, as well as an aid to belief for the simple, then there must be some connection between them. But this connection is only a connection of succession, not conjunction, since the acquired habit of belief disappears when true faith is infused, just as the light of the moon is obscured by, and does not add to, the light of the sun. Unformed and formed faith have the same object, but a different habit. And this, according to Chenu, is marvelous since William knows the Aristotelian definition of a *habitus*. But this has not deeply penetrated William's thought, and the Augustinian psychology compromises the Aristotelian notions.

70. Albert Lang, *Die Wege der Glaubensbegründung bei den Scholastiken des 14. Jahrhunderts* (Munster: Aschendorff, 1930), pp. 4–7. Lang argues that "at the beginning of the thirteenth century, the question of faith and reason is clarified on the negative side:

pects of the knowledge of God, yet also creating a new theological *visus*.[71]

William thus draws a sharp line between natural knowledge and supernatural knowledge—the realm of divine illumination and graced perception of faith, which alone yields true knowledge of God.[72] He consistently stresses the supernatural nature of faith. The deeper penetration into the truths of faith requires the presence of the Holy Spirit and the gift which It bestows, the *donum intellectus*.

What is the nature of this supernatural knowledge of faith and how is it related to prior forms? One might surmise prima facie that William sees no place for "natural reasons," the images and analogies drawn from the sphere of nature.[73]

Wishing, therefore, to show divine things with reason *(rationibus res divinas)*, let us proceed from appropriate reasons *(ex convenientibus rationibus)*, not from those reasons which are appropriate to natural things *(proprie rerum nat-*

---

every dependence of faith on reason for the internal understanding of faith's contents is rejected. Here, along with William of Auvergne, William of Auxerre plays an important role, strongly denying the possibility that reason can make the contents of the faith evident. The presence of evidence would remove all merit. The *fides virtus* creates a certainty like that of but separate from the first principles in the natural sciences. But faith's certainty is grounded in the supernatural illumination by the divine light. The separation is sharp, especially with William of Auxerre. He knows a rational ground of faith by outside proofs: by miracle, reading of Scripture, prophecies. It is based expressly on the syllogism: *Omne dictum a prima veritate est verum. Hoc sc. filium Dei esse hominem, est dictum a prima veritate. Igitur hoc est verum.* But this '*credere naturale*,' this *fides informis* has at most the meaning of a certain *confirmatio* of the '*credere gratuitum*,' of *fides infusa*; a substantial connection with the *fides infusa*, which rests solely on grace, does not exist. The organic interrelatedness of the *credibilitas externa* and the *fides infusa* is not yet found."

71. M.-D. Chenu, "La surnaturalisation des vertus," *Bulletin thomiste* 9 (1932), pp. 93–96. "William of Auxerre is the patron of the negative answer to the question—hotly debated throughout the scholastic period—whether *naturalia fiunt gratuita*. The patron of the positive answer is Hugh of St. Victor. William was par excellence the teacher of the supernaturality of faith, in formulas which will impregnate the vocabulary and the doctrines of Aquinas."

72. Heitz, *Essai historique*, pp. 92–98. Thus, William rejects much of the "Trinitarian rationalism" of the preceding century, notably that of Richard of St. Victor. Heitz claims that William is the first to oppose this excessive use of dialectic in theology and thus contributed in a particular but significant way to the delimitation of faith and science, of theology and philosophy.

73. Indeed, William does not put special value on natural correspondences; for example, he does not in his anthropology attempt to find correspondence between the human soul and the Trinity, a telling fact given his deep dependence on Augustine.

uralium). For in this way the heretics were deceived, since they desired to apply reasons proper to natural things to divine things, as if they wished to adequate nature with its Creator.... But the theologians argue from proper reasons in this way: The Father is God, the Son is God, the Holy Spirit is God; therefore, the Father, the Son and the Holy Spirit are one God. This difference of inference proceeds from the diverse properties of the things to which the words refer.[74]

The reasons proper to philosophy and those proper to theology appear to be incompatible. It would be hasty to conclude, however, that William rejects natural conceptions or philosophical arguments completely. Elsewhere, he expressly states: "with such considerations we precede according to those things which are as fitting to natural things as to divine things."[75] William, therefore, recognizes a valid use of natural conceptions for theological reasoning. In fact, his polemic is against the misappropriation of natural *rationes* to divine things. In the Prologue, he suggested that the entire *Summa Aurea* is an attempt to speak properly of God, that is, to use natural reasons fittingly and appropriately in the task of understanding divine things. The failure to do so has led to heretical views,[76] for example, those of Arius and Sabellius.[77] Behind this misap-

---

74. SA I Prol: 18,1.
75. Beumer, *Theologie als Glaubensverständnis,* pp. 74–75: "The words, 'that which is fitting to the natural and the divine,' probably allude to the Aristotelian concept of analogy, which will acquire greater importance in the theology of the Aquinas and the subsequent scholastics. William means basically the same thing." (The term *analogia,* however, does not appear in the *Summa Aurea*).
76. SA I Prol: 20,57ff. He argues that this misappropriation can occur in three ways: some attribute to God what they find in corporal creatures; some attribute what they find in spiritual creatures; and some attribute what they find neither in corporal nor spiritual creatures.
77. SA I Prol: 18,6ff. "Thus was Arius deceived. For since in natural things it is generally true that plural things are plural by nature, as of several men several humanities ... Arius wished to apply this rule to divine things thus: The Father, Son, and Holy Ghost are several, therefore, the several are of the same nature; but the Father has divinity and divinity is one single thing; therefore the Son does not have deity but another nature other than divinity.... In the same way Sabellius was deceived. For since it is true generally in things that one nature is of one single thing; but deity is one nature; therefore it is of one single thing; but the Father, and the Son, and the Holy Spirit are the same; therefore as the Father and the Son and the Holy Spirit are one thing *(unum),* so they are one person *(unus)*.... Therefore, Sabellius confused the persons by making one from three; but Arius separated the nature or the substance of the persons."

propriation is the heretics' failure to appreciate "that divine things infinitely exceed natural things."[78]

For his part, William conceives of a new perspective or orientation on the part of faith toward these *rationes naturales*, as well as a new use. In the divine illumination that produces formed faith, a new consideration of prior thought-forms emerges. Those reasons which had previously formed the basis of philosophical and unformed faith are not obviated with the advent of formed faith. They remain, not to generate faith, but rather to confirm and augment it. No longer are they the source of faith's experience:

> Human reason, that is, natural reason, does not supply the intellect with proof *(experimentum)*, since those reasons, which the intellect has, are not human but divine, since they are taken from faith, hence by consequence the understanding rests upon the first truth for its own sake and above all else.[79]

Rather, they provide a subsequent enhancement, an increase to faith by providing insight and understanding. They no longer ground faith; rather, faith now grounds them, giving them their theological intelligibility. In the light of faith, they are transformed into theological *rationes* and explanations. What William means by theological *rationes* is a speculative penetration into the truths of faith, thus an actual *ratio theologica*.[80] Theology has its own proper and appropriate reasons, reasons which are consonant with their divine object: "We, therefore, do not rely

---

78. SA I Prol: 19,23. "But if the heretics had considered that divine things infinitely exceed natural things, they would never have wished to apply reasons proper to natural things to divine things." See Chenu, *La théologie*, pp. 31–32: "The magisterial expression of this protest against the excessive introduction of reason into the sphere of faith in the very plan of theology is found in William of Auxerre, the guide and inspiration of this whole generation. It is the most marked trait of his thought that he is concerned to respect the transcendence of divine realities, and never to judge the divine according to the earthly measure of our concepts. The ideas acquired in the knowledge of nature, in science, cannot be transferred as such to God. As late as Lateran IV, whose intervention is situated in the center of the first flowering of reason, one can find this religious protest against a certain conceptualization of revealed gifts, in a sacred doctrine which would become scientific: '*Inter creatorem et creaturam non potest tanta similtudo notari, quin inter eos maior sit dissimilitudo notanda.*'"

79. SA III 34.2: 652,27.

80. See Beumer, "Die Theologie als *intellectus fidei*," and "Theologie als Glaubensverständnis."

upon the proper reasons of natural things, but with respect to divine things we will proceed from theological reasons *(ex theologicis rationibus)* and from reasons consonant *(consonis)* with that of which we speak."[81] Theological understanding, therefore, entails an appropriate use of reasons, of argument, of human concepts, created analogies and natural knowledge.[82] The gift of understanding pursues the internal reasons for faith's fundamental affirmations. Already in the Prologue, William suggested that "natural reasons" increase the faith, by providing an *intellectus fidei*. Thus, what he had ruled out of court in the genesis of faith—namely, the *rationes naturales*—he now ushers back onto center stage.

What precisely does understanding *(intellectus)* entail? In a word, a fuller understanding of the articles of faith. Using Aristotelian terminology, understanding emerges as faith passes from *scientia quia* to *scientia propter quid*, from the knowledge *that* something is the case to the knowledge of *why* and *on account of which* it is so. Understanding perceives the cause of those things which faith believes. He offers an analogy patently inspired by an Aristotelian antecedent, suggesting that faith differs from understanding "just as the naval science *(navalis scientia)* differs from that of astronomy *(astrologia)*":

For, those who have knowledge of navigation know concerning a certain star that *(quod)* it is immobile, and concerning other stars that they never set, but of the reason on account of which *(propter quia)* this is so, they are ignorant, while the astronomers know the reason on account of which this is so. Thus, faith knows that *(quod)* God rewards the good, but the understanding knows the reason why *(propter quid)*.[83]

Similarly, it is an article of faith that God rewards the good beyond merit; simple faith knows only the fact that this is so *(quia)*. The gift of understanding adds the theological insight that God rewards the good on

---

81. SA I Prol: 20,66ff.
82. Cf. SA I Prol. See Lang, *Die theologische Prinzipienlehre,* p. 145. Lang observes that "the *Summa Aurea* remains strongly linked to early scholastic thinking, so much so that Landgraf places it at the end of the early scholasticism." Lang, for his part, places it at the beginning of the *Hochscholastik* because of the new methodological approach.
83. SA III 34.1: 650,41ff. This will become a stock scholastic example of sub-alternation in theological science.

account of his own nature: "God is much greater than it is possible to understand; therefore he will reward the good more than it is possible to understand." Hence, understanding gives the reason *(ratio)* concerning this. Borrowing another Aristotelian distinction, William compares understanding to the knowledge of physics in relation to metaphysics: understanding *(intellectus)* "is a kind of physical cognition *(quasi cognitio phisica)*, since physics or natural philosophy treats *(phisica sive naturalis philosophia)* moveable things" and understanding "cognizes God in as much as God grants movement to all things, whence also at the end of Aristotle's *Physics* it is concluded that 'the first principle of motion is immobile and has no magnitude.'"[84] Understanding thus considers God "in an assembled way *(collative)*, namely, in relation to creatures."[85]

In sum, for William, speculative theological science has an inescapable supernatural character.[86] The *intellectus fidei* is actually and substantially effected by the *donum intellectus*. Theological science, accordingly, is parallel to, but radically separate from, its Aristotelian analogue.[87] William's is an intellectualist view of faith, though in no way a rationalistic one. The movement from *scientia* to *intellectus* requires supernatural insight into the basic structures of divine revelation within its created effects. The internal *rationes* are visible only in the light of supernatural illumination of faith. He posits an intimate link between deep theological understanding and the purging and exercising of the virtues and supernatural grace.[88]

---

84. SA III 34.1: 649,20ff.
85. SA III 34.1: 649,14. Cf. SA III 30.2: 593,64: The gift of understanding is properly "the cognition of spiritual gifts, which God confers to holy souls and to holy angels, by which both souls and angels are sanctified," and "by which God assimilates them to himself."
86. Beumer, "Die Theologie als *intellectus fidei*," pp. 40–41: "The history of theology knows of efforts, which, while striving to serve the interests of supernatural faith (like William of Auxerre), did not however sufficiently emphasize, at least in the manner of speaking, the difference between faith's understanding and rational evidence. One is reminded of the *rationes necesssariae* of Anselm or Richard of St. Victor from the period of early scholasticism. William of Auxerre brings the Augustinian trajectory to a certain termination and at the same time provides a fruitful initiative in a new direction. This pertains in particular to the supernatural quality of faith and in its connection with the gifts of the Holy Spirit."
87. SA III 34.5: 664,55f. "Wisdom and understanding properly speaking are not sciences, since a science, properly speaking, is a habit of cognition through a cause and through natural reasons having first *per se nota* principles *simpliciter* or naturally."
88. Beumer, *Theologie als Glaubensverständnis*, p. 78.

As is evident, William here introduces a rational dimension into the interior of sacred doctrine. He does this not for apologetic purposes, but for the benefit of the faith, which, far from being based on these "reasons," gives them consistency. Increasingly, gradually, faith acquires an understanding of the mysteries which it believes.[89] William is perhaps the first scholastic theologian to insist explicitly that the *rationes* taught by reason do not belong to the motive for faith but only to its energizing.[90] In this way, he furnishes the classical analysis and elaboration of the right of reason to argument in theology. With him, the notion of credibility is introduced into theological science. Faith remains intact in this reasoning, not resting on reasons in order to believe, but on the first truth, heard for itself.[91] By grounding a genuine theological science in the gift of understanding, William serves as a pioneer for subsequent scholastic reflection on theological method,[92] charting a path his successors will explore further.[93]

Sapientia

Finally, theological apprehension *(scientia* and *intellectus)* yields to the final stage in the knowledge of God, the gift of wisdom *(sapientia)*,[94]

89. Chenu, *La théologie*, pp. 35–36: "William cites of the aphorism of Simon of Tournai concerning the difference between Christian theology and Aristotelian philosophy. With Simon, William expressly enjoins the Poretian tradition on the diversity of methods according to diverse disciplines, based epistemologically on the protestation against the transfer of natural concepts to theology."

90. Lang, *Die theologische Prinzipienlehre*, pp. 144–46.

91. Chenu, *La théologie*, p. 34.

92. Lang, *Die theologische Prinzipienlehre*, p. 140: "The *Summa Alexandria* repeats nearly word for word the thoughts of William of Auxerre. Albert handles the problem in his doctrine of God and takes up William's and Praepositinus' justification for the use of rational arguments in theology. The early Dominican and Franciscan theologians also adopt William's solution."

93. Beumer, *Theologie als Glaubensverständnis*, p. 75. "In the linguistic expressions of the *Summa Aurea* one feels it as it were that the author penetrates into theologically new ground and struggles for the correct articulation of his thoughts."

94. See Chenu, *La théologie*, pp. 93–96. The notion that theology is a wisdom is venerable, at least in the sense that there has always been a close association between, if not identification of, the Logos and Wisdom. In the eleventh and twelfth centuries proponents of so-called "monastic theology" championed a sapiential approach to theology, in the sense of a gift of the Holy Spirit, involving a deeper, prayerful penetration of the mysteries of faith through contemplative/mystical experience. Chenu argues that the scholastic inclusion of the concept of wisdom in its methodological reflections on the theological

the last gift of the Spirit,⁹⁵ and the sphere of mystical theology. For William, the theological enterprise finds its fulfillment here, and here too his doctrine of the spiritual senses emerges. Whereas with faith and charity William privileged the senses of sight and touch, respectively, with wisdom the spiritual sense of taste comes to the fore, as he capitalizes on the etymology of *sapientia*.⁹⁶

What precisely William means by wisdom begins to emerge as he distinguishes it from understanding, comparing the two forms of knowing to the two different treatments of nouns by the classical grammarian Priscian. Understanding *(intellectus)* corresponds to "the science or cognition of nouns in relation to verbs *(in comparatione ad verbum)*," which is treated "in the minor volume of Priscian," a knowledge of God that William calls "assembled *(collative)*," derived "in relation to creatures *(in comparatione ad creaturas)*." But, "in the major volume of Priscian," the cognition of nouns absolutely *(nominis absolute)* is described, and William compares this with wisdom *(sapientia)*, an absolute knowledge of God *(cognitio Dei absolute)*. Moreover, whereas William had likened *intellectus* to physics, he here compares *sapientia* to metaphysics, suggesting that "since metaphysics treats of God absolutely by considering his proper dispositions *(proprias dispositiones)*," this absolute cognition of God "is a kind of metaphysics *(quasi methaphisica)*." He concludes that "the difference between wisdom and understanding is clear, for al-

---

enterprise represents the retention of an often overlooked Augustinian element, which should be seen as an intentional form of resistance to, or at least modification of, the inroads of Aristotelian science and its methods into the theological domain.

95. This gift corresponds to the seventh and final beatitude, peace *(pax)*. Cf. SA III 35.2.7: 681,62f. "Peace is aligned with the seventh petition, which is the last in time but the first in dignity, as well as the seventh gift, namely wisdom, in this way: *sanctify your name*, that is, give to us the 'spirit of wisdom' by which savor *(sapidus)* we are delighted by you, and thus *sanctify your name*, that is, let your name be confirmed in us, so that from Christ we may be called Christians and so may be sons of God, having his inheritance."

96. Grabmann, *Die Geschichte der scholastischen Methode*, vol. 2, p. 275. Grabmann observes that William's emphasis on the experiential dimension of the *intellectus fidei* and the connection posited between the *cognitio Dei* and the *gustare* of wisdom is similar to that found in earlier thinkers such as Hugh of St. Victor, William of St Thierry, and Anselm. These also spoke of an *experiri* and a *gustare* in the supernatural experience of the contents of faith. Moreover, Grabmann notes the underlying sympathy with such an approach in the great scholastics of the following generation, such as Aquinas, who assigned to the *donum sapientiae* a similar experiential function.

though they have the same subject matter *(materia)*, they do not, nevertheless, [have] the same *ratio*."⁹⁷ Most basically, then, the difference between *intellectus* and *sapientia* is formal, pertaining to the mode *(ratio)* in which each operates. Understanding is the knowledge of God in relation to creatures; wisdom pertains to God in himself.

Building upon this basic difference, William stresses the immediacy of wisdom's encounter with God, an immediacy which produces spiritual delight: "The gift of wisdom ... moves immediately toward God, whence it is more delectable, since it joins us more immediately to God."⁹⁸ It is, moreover, this delight born of immediacy that produces what is perhaps the hallmark of wisdom, namely its experiential nature. In wisdom there is "delight in the suavity of God, so that we might know God by experience *(experimento cognoscamus Deum)*."⁹⁹ Predictably, William prefers to describe this immediate, delectable experience in the language of the spiritual senses, in particular the sense of taste, given the etymology of *sapientia*. Wisdom is "the cognition of God through a foretaste of his sweetness *(per pregustationem dulcedinis)* and by this cognition we are delighted."¹⁰⁰ Expanding on this theme, he specifies that "properly speaking wisdom is not the cognition of God, but a certain kind of perception of spiritual taste through the mode of experience *(perceptio quedam gustus spiritualis per modum experiencie)*." For "God himself causes sweetness in the palate of the soul *(in palato anime)* which wisdom savors *(saporat)*, just as honey in physical taste; therefore wisdom is a certain kind of immediate perception *(perceptio)* or savoring *(saporatio)* of the sweetness of God *(dulcedinis Dei)*."¹⁰¹ In fact, it is precisely this element of spiritual sense perception that provides the essential and defining characteristic of wisdom:

Wisdom differs from faith in the way that the knowledge of something [received] through the hearing differs from the knowledge of something [received] through the sense of taste. For example: someone knows that a certain wine is good, and knows this from hearing; another knows that the wine is good and knows this from tasting. In this way these two kinds of knowledge differ. So,

---

97. SA III 34.1: 650,13ff.
98. SA III 41.3: 789,27.
99. SA III 30.2: 593,66.
100. SA III 30.1.1: 585,12.
101. SA III 42.2.3.2: 815,79f.

faith differs from wisdom, for faith is cognition [received] through hearing, . . . but wisdom is the cognition of God [received] through taste. Hence, wisdom is called knowledge by the savory taste of virtue, since the sweetness or suavity of God is tasted through wisdom, whence the Psalm, *taste and see that the Lord is good* (Ps 33:9). And this is the maximal cognition of God: cognition through wisdom, for if the Creator is known through [his] effects, he is maximally known through his maximal effects. . . . And this is in the gift of wisdom, hence through the gift of wisdom God is maximally known.[102]

In this passage, William contrasts the knowledge of faith—and what he means is that knowledge found in the first two stages of the knowledge of God, namely, *scientia* and *intellectus*—with that of wisdom. The former is knowledge through hearing: distant, remote, mediated by other things, with hearer and heard separated by distance. The latter is "tasted knowledge": immediate, intimate, direct, delectably experiential, with minimal distance and maximal apprehension between taster and tasted.

In wisdom, then, spiritual apprehension passes from *scientia quia* and *scientia propter quid* to *scientia per sensum*. Theological science and understanding pass over into spiritual experience; faith's *argumentum* arrives at its *substantia;* collative knowledge of God, in relation to creation, becomes absolute, in some sense more direct; *cognitio* passes over into *delectatio*.[103] Wisdom is a form of spiritual sense perception; it entails an experiential perception *(percipere)* and sensation *(sentire)* of God's maximal effects; it is mystical theology, which "senses *(sentit)* in secret concerning God"; it is contemplative, pertaining to the "interior and hidden

---

102. SA III 34.1: 650,46ff. *Fides autem differt a sapientia eo modo, quo scientia alicuis rei per auditum differt a scientia eiusdem rei per gustum; verbi gratia, aliquis scit quod hoc vinum est bonum, et hoc scit per auditum; alius scit quod hoc vinum est bonum, et hoc scit per gustum; et iste due scientie differunt; hoc modo differt fides a sapientia, fides enim est cognitio per auditum, quoniam fides ex auditu, ut dicit Apostolus, sapientia vero cognitio Dei per gustum; unde sapientia dicitur sapore virtutum condita, scientia, quia per sapientiam gustatur, dulcedo sive suavitas Dei, unde in Psalmo:* Gustate et videte, quoniam suavis est Dominus. *Et hoc est maxima cognitio Dei; cognitio per sapientiam, si enim creator cognoscitur per effectum, per maximum effectum maxime cognoscitur, et maximus effectus est dilectio, quam habemus in Deo per caritatem et intellectum per quam dilectionem habetur sapientia; et hoc est in sapientia dono, unde per donum sapientie maxime cognoscitur Deus.*

103. SA III 34.2: 652,32f. Understanding is properly speaking without delight or fruition, "since there is to be no fruition of creatures, the cognition of which is understanding; nevertheless we are able to delight in creatures, but in relation to God, as it says in the Psalm: *I have delighted myself, O Lord, in your works* (Ps 91:5)."

and more worthy effects which the soul receives above itself through the contemplation of God"; it is experiential, whose it is "especially and properly to know experientially *(cognoscere experimento)* what God is like."[104]

Conclusion: Wisdom's Banquet

At one point, William describes the relationship between the gifts of the Spirit and the theological virtues using the image of a banquet, to which both the gifts and the virtues are summoned. There is a hierarchy of guests, and the more excellent the gift or virtue, the greater its delight. For "everything whatsoever, if it is capable of delight *(capax delectationis)*, has rest and delight in its proper place." Near the top, he positions the theological virtues, while below them are the gifts and the other virtues. Together, the virtues and the gifts commingle in a feast of spiritual delight, where "the theological virtues give savor to *(condiunt)* the gifts with heavenly taste *(sapore celesti),*" and "are delighted with every gift and every virtue," and "feast with them." Atop the scale, though, is wisdom, "the most excellent gift," which alone has greater spiritual pleasures *(deliciis spiritualibus)* than the theological virtues.[105] This image nicely captures William's account of the knowledge of God. Spiritual apprehension involves the whole range of the soul's knowing capacities, the intellectual and the aesthetic, along with the gifts and virtues that enable them.

The triad of virtues and gifts, which are central to the structure and character of William's conception of human knowledge of God—*scientia, intellectus, sapientia*—are now in full view. These are the distinguishable moments in a unified apprehension of God: *sapientia* is the culmination of *scientia*, its personal and experiential appropriation.[106] This

---

104. SA I 4.2: 40,117ff. This linking of the spiritual *sentire* and *percipere* of mystical theology with the climax of speculative theology bears a striking similarity to the full text of 1 Corinthians 2:6–16, noted above, which William invoked in the Prologue as a justification for his theological method. There, after introducing the notion of wisdom "among the mature," Paul characterizes it as "secret and hidden" (v. 7), as revealed only through the Holy Spirit (vv. 10–12), as gifts bestowed by God (v. 13), and as entailing spiritual as opposed to worldly understanding (v. 13). In short, William's view of Christian theology entails an extended application of 1 Corinthians 2.

105. SA III 30.4: 600,39.

106. Accordingly, though in William's account faith's experience is personal and interi-

structure also unites faith's two objects—creedal articles and spiritual realities—within a common framework. From *argumentum* (speculative, creedal propositions), faith moves toward *substantia* (spiritual perception of divine realities). Wisdom, moreover, effects the highest and fullest knowledge of God *(maxima cognitio Dei)* by bringing faith and charity to fruition.[107]

What is perhaps most striking in all of this is that William envisions an arrangement wherein each successive moment subsumes the prior one. Wisdom does not abandon knowledge and understanding. Rather, *sapientia*'s experiential perception subsumes the conceptual aspects of *scientia* and *intellectus*.[108] The former is mediated by the latter. Faith entails the experiential perception of spiritual realities mediated by the articles of faith: beginning with *scientia*, it arrives at *sentire;* yet faith's *sentire* emerges out of and is structured by *scientia*. The intellect knows, for example, "that God greatly gives rest to holy souls, and from this it has wisdom in which God is greatly suave *(summe Deus suavis).*" And so, wisdom consists "not only in delight but also in cognizing God."[109] The result is a kind of experiential knowledge of God:

> For understanding . . . leads us to delight in the suavity of God, so that by experience *(experimento)* we might apprehend *(cognoscere)* God, which cognition is wisdom.[110]

---

orized, it is in no way privatized or individualistic, precisely because it is mediated by creedal affirmations, derived by the believing community, historically mediated through tradition, and corporately, even publically, affirmed. There is no supplanting of corporate piety by privatized, personal devotion. The scholastic enterprise is quite communal, not only as a shared discourse, but also as drawing on the corporate inheritance of the tradition found in the Creed.

107. SA III 34.1: 650–51,55ff. ". . . for if the Creator is known through his effects, he is maximally known through his maximal effects, and his maximal effect is *dilectio,* which we have in God through charity and understanding, through which *dilectio,* wisdom is obtained."

108. SA III 30.4: 600,42. Invoking Boethius as his authority, William observes that "whatever an inferior power can do a superior power can also do, but not vice versa."

109. SA III 34.5: 665,52f. Cf. SA III 34.5: 665,57f. "Wisdom, since it is a cognition, does not properly refer to the highest good, but to the highest truth. For wisdom is the cognition of the first truth, . . . [or] the cognition of the good as true."

110. SA III 30.2: 593,63. *Intellectus enim . . . ducit nos ad delectandum in suavitatem Dei, ut experimento cognoscamus Deum, que cognitio est sapientia.*

This, for William, is mystical theology: an apprehension of God, both scientific and sapiential, both speculative and mystical, both conceptual and experiential.[111]

111. Von Balthasar, *Glory of the Lord,* vol. 1, *Seeing the Form,* p. 76. "Few among today's 'exact' Biblical scholars, however, make any room at all in their Biblical science for the *fruitio* of the *sensus spiritualis,* to say nothing of assigning to it the place of honour. I say 'place of honour' because this act is the central act of theology as a science."

CHAPTER 10

TASTE AND SEE
The Spiritual Senses and the Eucharist

AS SEEN THROUGHOUT the preceding chapters, for William the goal of human life is an experiential apprehension of God that subsumes within itself the human capacities for spiritual cognition and perception, its intellectual and affective dimensions. In that apprehension, faith's delight and charity's desire collaborate to find fruition in the *delectabilia divina;* in that apprehension, creedal *scientia* is taken up through the gifts of the Holy Spirit into theological *intellectus* and finally into an experiential *sapientia*. To capture the fullness of this apprehension, William has employed the ancient doctrine of the spiritual senses of the soul. Thus, faith's *visus* moves from *argumentum* to *substantia*, from scientific concept to sapiential percept, and culminates in charity's *tactus;* wisdom, finally, tastes the worthiest effects of the Trinity itself in a direct manner. In William's theology, though, there exists a final locus for the activity of the spiritual senses, a locus that reflects these characteristics of spiritual apprehension and throws them into relief: the Eucharist.

Located in the fourth and final book of his *Summa Aurea*, Tractate 7, William's treatment of the Eucharist is, on the one hand, a systematic and technical discussion of various theological issues, both speculative and practical, including the reason for its institution, how Christ is present, how and when the Eucharist should be given, and who should receive.[1] At the same time, his treatment of these topics reveals that the Eu-

---

1. In certain respects, William's influence on sacramental theology, especially issues re-

charist is a focal point for the divine-human encounter. All the basic components of spiritual apprehension are present here. As the forms of bread and wine are encountered and incorporated physically, faith and charity collaborate in theological discernment of the Incarnate Christ, present in the Eucharist. Following the structure of spiritual apprehension, theological discernment leads to delightful immediacy as the believer experiences the presence of Christ and his salvific significance. Finally, delight in the Incarnate Christ leads ultimately to union with Christ—the goal of William's eucharistic theology. In this movement from discernment, through delight, to union, William describes the Eucharist as a mystical feast in which Christ's body and blood are encountered in a spiritually sensuous manner through the soul's spiritual senses. Not surprisingly, the dominant metaphor is eating and tasting *(gustus)*, yet he describes an experience of spiritual *visus, auditus, olfactus,* and *tactus* too. Eucharistic reception, which engages all the physical senses and involves a union between the forms of bread and wine and believer, provides both a ready symbol and an actual vehicle for spiritually sensuous apprehension.

---

garding the Eucharist, has long been noted. Scholars have investigated William's eucharistic theology for his views on such doctrines as transubstantiation and concomitance. James Megivern, for example, in his 1963 study of the doctrine of concomitance, notes William's important place in the development of that doctrine; James J. Megivern, *Concomitance and Communion: A Study in Eucharistic Doctrine and Practice* (Freiburg: University Press, 1963), pp. 174–78. Further, William's relation to preceding twelfth-century theologies of the Eucharist has been examined in Gary Macy's excellent treatment of the twelfth-century developments and schools of thought regarding the Eucharist, which concludes with a brief section on William's place in that evolution; see Gary Macy, *The Theologies of the Eucharist in the Early Scholastic Period: A Study of the Salvific Function of the Sacrament according to the Theologians, c. 1080–c. 1220* (Oxford: Oxford University Press, 1984), pp. 129–35. In other respects, however, William's writings have been relatively neglected in terms of their contribution to developments in eucharistic spirituality and devotion. Carolyn Bynum, for example, largely ignores William's influence while examining the thirteenth-century background for developments in eucharistic devotion among medieval women; Carolyn Bynum, *Holy Feast and Holy Fast: The Religious Significance of Food to Medieval Women* (Berkeley: University of California Press, 1987), pp. 31–112. Miri Rubin's recent book on the development of the feast of Corpus Christi pays scant attention to William's teaching; Miri Rubin, *Corpus Christi: The Eucharist in Late Medieval Culture* (Cambridge: Cambridge University Press, 1991). This present study seeks to ameliorate these omissions by approaching William's eucharistic theology with specific attention to its spiritual and experiential dimensions.

The Eucharist as Spiritual Food

Not surprisingly, the Eucharist for William is first and foremost spiritual food, and his theology is grounded in this metaphor. William's use of the analogy with ordinary food and its consumption allows him to integrate scholastic teaching concerning the nature of the Eucharist within an overall framework that is also richly experiential. At the outset, he sounds the theme of spiritual food: "the Eucharist is the food of the fully grown and confirmed *(cibus grandium et confirmatorum)*, as the Lord said to Augustine: 'I am the food of the fully grown; grow up and you will feed on me.'"[2] Shortly thereafter, he compares the Eucharist to the primal food of Eden: "just as it was said concerning that tree *on whatever day you eat from the tree of the knowledge of good and evil, you will truly die*, so of this bread John 6 says, *whoever eats this bread will live forever*." This theme remains prominent as he then considers the composition of the eucharistic elements. Bread and wine, he argues, have "a double likeness with the body of Christ." First, just as bread and wine are both composed of "the most pure *(ex purissimis)*" grains and grapes, so Christ's true body and blood are "most pure," and "the mystical body of Christ consists of the most pure faithful *(ex purissimis fidelibus)*, cleansed of mortal sin." Second, just as bread "greatly restores and strengthens *(maxime reficit et confirmat)* the body" and wine "gladdens *(letificat)*," so the body and blood of Christ "greatly restores and strengthens" and "gladdens and inebriates *(letificat et inebriat)*" the soul. Whence, *my overflowing cup which inebriates* (Ps 22:5).[3] Thus, the spiritual properties and benefits of eucharistic food correspond to their ordinary counterparts. Like ordinary bread for the body, eucharistic bread nourishes and restores the soul and brings it to maturity; like common wine, eucharistic wine gladdens and even inebriates the soul.

This construal of the Eucharist as spiritual food is fundamental. The

---

2. SA IV 7: 138,4–6. The full citation from Augustine's *Confessions* appears to be in William's mind as he proceeds: "And I heard as it were your voice from on high: 'I am the food of the fully grown; grow and you will feed on me *(Cibus sum grandium. Cresce et manducabis me)*. And you will not change me into you like the food your flesh eats, but you will be changed into me'" (*Conf.* VII, x, 16; trans. Chadwick).

3. SA IV 7.1: 141,56ff.

comparison with ordinary physical food is the source of the experiential dimension of William's eucharistic theology, providing the paradigm for the spiritual experience of eucharistic food. It is in this context, moreover, that William introduces the spiritual senses, which perceive the "bread of angels *(panis angelorum),*" possessing every delight. Just as ordinary food engages the physical senses, so the Eucharist will delight the spiritual senses. This conception of the Eucharist as spiritual food sets the stage for the next dimension of his eucharistic theology, where the ordinary act of eating becomes the primary interpretive framework for eucharistic eating.

The Framework of Eucharistic Eating

Standing at the center of William's theology of the Eucharist, as an extension of this food metaphor, is an analogy with the act of ordinary eating.[4] This analogy emerges in the context of a discussion concerning two forms of eucharistic eating: sacramental and spiritual.[5] "The body of Christ is eaten sacramentally *(sacramentaliter)* when it is eaten under the forms of bread and wine. It is eaten spiritually *(spiritualiter)* when we are incorporated into Christ by faith. Concerning this mode, Augustine said: 'believe, and you have eaten.'"[6] This basic distinction reveals the primary objective of William's eucharistic theology—union with Christ—as well as the necessary condition under which it occurs: faith. Here, all who physically receive the forms of bread and wine receive the body of Christ sacramentally. But not all who receive sacramentally also receive spiritually. Spiritual eating requires faith and results in union.

Two clarifications immediately follow, both regarding the appropriateness of Augustine's remark "believe and you have eaten *(crede, et manducasti).*"[7] First, William asks whether Augustine should rather have

---

4. SA IV 7.3: 150,23ff.

5. This distinction between *sumere sacramentalis* and *sumere spiritualis* was introduced and extensively developed by numerous theologians throughout the course of the twelfth century (see Macy, *Theologies of the Eucharist*, p. 133). Throughout his discussion, William uses several different words for eating or chewing—*sumere, comedere, manducare*—without any crucial or consistent difference in meaning.

6. SA IV 7.3: 149,2f.

7. Augustine, *In Johannes evangelium*, tr. 25, n.12 (PL 25.1602).

said, "love and you have eaten *(dilige, et manducasti)*." For "the sacrament of the body of Christ is the sacrament of the union of Christ and the church; and that union occurs through charity *(per caritatem)*. For, indeed, it is love, which, like cement, joins the stones which are the faithful into the spiritual house of God, that is, the church. Thus, we eat Christ through love; and so we ought to say: love and you have eaten, rather than: believe."[8] In response, William introduces the analogy between ordinary eating and spiritual eating. He notes: "in corporal eating *(manducatione corporali)* there are four acts: chewing *(masticatio)*, delight *(delectatio)*, assimilation *(assimilatio)*, and union *(incorporatio)*." Similarly, in spiritual eating *(manducatione spirituali)* the same four acts exist. He then argues that, properly speaking, all four acts in spiritual eating occur "through faith *(per fidem)*," not love. Spiritual chewing *(masticatio spiritualis)* consists in discernment *(diiudicatio)* of the body of Christ in the Eucharist (following Paul's admonition to the Corinthians), and this "happens through faith." Spiritual delight also occurs *"per fidem."* Citing Augustine's remark from *De Trinitate*—"all love is in cognition *(in cognitione est totalis dilectio)*"—William argues that, "if I love something, I do not yet delight in it, but if I perceive the good of that which I love, then I delight." Similarly, "[spiritual] assimilation occurs through faith, since *he gave them the power to become sons of God, to those who believe in his name* (Jn 1:12)." And finally, since "union occurs through assimilation," it too happens "through faith." William concludes that Augustine rightly said "believe and you have eaten," rather than "love." He hastily adds, however, that "charity moves toward *(movet ad)* that union more and more and conserves *(conservat)* it."[9]

The second clarification pertains to the subject of eucharistic eating. An objection argues that, since Augustine said "to believe in God is to go into God by believing and to be incorporated into his body," he therefore ought to have said: "believe and you *have been eaten (manducatus es)* [emphasis mine]." For, "to be incorporated is to be eaten" and so "to believe is to be eaten." Ought not it be said, then, that "Christ eats the faith-

---

8. SA IV 7.3: 149,6f.
9. SA IV 7.3: 150,23ff.

ful *(comedit fideles)*, that is, he incorporates [them] into himself *(sibi incorporat)*, since the faithful are changed into him *(in ipsum mutantur)*, and not he into them"? Is the believer the "eater" or the "eaten"? Which is Christ? In response, William argues for both. "We both feed on Christ *(comedimus Christum)* and Christ feeds *(Christus comedit)* on us."

> For regarding the spiritual chewing *(masticationem)* and delight *(delectationem)* which we have of Christ, we eat him, and this eating is understood when [Augustine] says: believe and you have eaten.

At the same time:

> in assimilation *(assimilatio)* and incorporation *(incorporatio)* Christ eats us, since he assimilates and unites us *(sibi unit)* to himself by his grace.

In effect, William divides the four acts of spiritual eating into two pairs, arguing that the subject of the eating switches between the first and the second. In spiritual chewing and delight, the believer feeds on Christ, and this is what William takes to be Augustine's meaning. Regarding assimilation and union, however, Christ can indeed be said to feed on the believer, since he assimilates and unites believers to himself. Hence, Christ is not only consumed by the faithful, but consumes them as well.[10]

With these two clarifications, the basic framework of William's eucharistic theology is now in view. The Eucharist is spiritual food, the spiritual eating of which facilitates union with Christ. Spiritual eating consists in these two pairs: discernment and delight, on the one hand, assimilation and union, on the other. The first pair consists in acts of the human recipient through faith and charity, and corresponds to the perceptual and experiential aspects of physical eating, namely, chewing and delighting. The second pair, where Christ is the subject, involves the less

---

10. SA IV 7.3: 150,13ff. William also argues for an assimilation of sinners to the devil in parallel fashion to the assimilation of believers to Christ: "However, it is the opposite among the wicked. For the wicked assimilate and unite themselves with the devil and thus eat him, whence, *you gave him as food to the peoples of Ethiopia* (Ps 73:14). For the devil does not unite nor assimilate them to himself except by prompting. Otherwise, the evil are said to delight in the devil, while the good delight in God, since the good delight in God himself and not in his works, but the wicked do not delight in the devil, but in his works" (SA IV 7.3: 151,49f.).

apparent but no less significant aspects of physical eating: assimilation and union.

Theological Discernment and Spiritual Delight: "We Feed on Christ"

Within this framework of spiritual eating, the first pair of acts—discernment and delight—provides the context in which William will employ the doctrine of the spiritual senses. As he introduced the fourfold framework of spiritual eating, William associated the first act, spiritual chewing *(masticatio spiritualis)*, with theological discernment *(diiudicatio)* of the body of Christ in the Eucharist. He advised believers "to discern what kind the body of Christ is, how noble, how life-giving, and the like." His remarks elsewhere in this treatise illuminate what he means by this discernment. At one point, he argues that the Eucharist was instituted so that faith might have the merit of discerning under the form of bread the true body of Christ, believing what it cannot see and trusting more in the first truth *(prima veritas)* than in the evidence of the physical senses or natural reason.[11] In the same discussion, he emphasizes the importance of the Eucharist as a commemoration *(commemoratio)* of Christ's passion, stressing the way in which eucharistic reflection on Christ's suffering stirs up love.[12] In another place, he interprets Paul's exhortation to the Corinthians in this way:

Concerning the mode of feasting the Apostle adds: *not with old yeast,* that is, in the corruption of vices. And he subdivides the yeast, saying: Neither *with the yeast of malice,* that is, by evilness of will, nor *with evil,* that is, with perverse belief. . . . He speaks of someone who lacks cognition or true faith. But *with the unleavened bread of sincerity, etc.,* that is, a sincere will, *and truth,* that is, true cognition or true faith. And even though cognition precedes the desired good, yet the Apostle places the desired good or the willed good before the cognition of the truth, since the fullness of cognition *(plenitudo cognitionis)* follows the good of desire.[13]

In this passage, several by-now-familiar themes emerge: the necessity of moral purging and virtuous disposition prior to success in the theological endeavor; the need for true faith or apprehension; the priority of

11. SA IV 7.1: 139,16ff.
12. SA IV 7.1: 139,2ff.
13. SA IV 7.3: 152,71ff.

faith and cognition of the true and yet the consummating necessity of a sincere will, love, and desire for the good. That which is to be discerned in the Eucharist, then, is the Incarnate Christ, especially his suffering and Passion. It occurs primarily through faith, a right apprehension and understanding of Christ's presence; yet charity is not omitted.

In the second act, theological discernment gives way to experiential immediacy in the act of spiritual delight, as the believer delights in the presence of Christ and his salvific significance. Here, too, William pays attention to the respective roles of knowledge and love, faith and charity. William interprets two biblical passages to evince this second act of eucharistic eating. He comments, for instance, on a passage from Isaiah 65: *my servants shall eat, but you shall be hungry; my servants shall drink, but you shall be thirsty.* He interprets this eating and drinking to be an allusion to the eucharistic delight of the servants of Christ: *they will eat* means "they will be delighted *(comedunt, id est delectabuntur).*" Shifting to the New Testament, William returns to Paul's exhortation in 1 Corinthians 5:

Christ our Paschal lamb has been sacrificed; therefore, let us keep the feast, and let us delight *(et delectemur).* And the Apostle infers the motive from the cause. For, since *Christ our Paschal lamb has been sacrificed,* since he has suffered for us, we ought to delight *(delectari)* in the goodness and great love which he showed us, when he suffered for us. For it is this which greatly inflames us *(maxime nos inflammat)* to love him.[14]

William's interpolation of an added exhortation into the biblical text— "and let us delight *(delectemur)*"—above and beyond Paul's exhortation *to keep the feast* reveals the importance of this theme. As he summarizes his exegesis of Paul's exhortation, moreover, he observes that to feast *with the unleavened bread of sincerity and truth* "is to delight in Christ *(delectari in Christo)* in love and understanding *(in dilectione et cognitione)* of him." And in this Christ himself is the example, since "he maximally delights in himself *(maxime delectatur in semetipso)* through knowledge and love of himself."[15] Significantly, then, *delectatio* assimi-

---

14. SA IV 7.3: 151,55ff.
15. SA IV 7.3: 152,83.

lates within itself the proper acts of faith and charity and issues from them. When faith's perception joins charity's desire, then *delectatio* emerges.

It should be noted that this eucharistic *delectatio* arises out of the basic theological affirmations concerning the salvific significance of the Incarnation. "To eat the body of Christ spiritually" is "through faith to delight in the fact that he was made man for us *(homo factus est pro nobis).* For his humanity is highly delectable to us *(delectabilis est nobis eius humanitas)."* Citing the First Letter of John—*this is the victory which overcomes the world, even our faith* (1 Jn 5:4)—William avers that the one who overcomes is "the one who believes that Jesus is the Son of God." Again, "to eat Christ spiritually is through the faith of his Incarnation . . . to delight in his humanity *(in eius humanitate delectari)."* For "through faith in the Incarnation we live spiritually."[16] Again, Christ himself is the example here, "since he is the highest knower *(maximus cognitor)* and highest lover *(maximus amator)* of himself, he greatly delights in his own humanity *(maxime delectatur in humanitate sua).*"[17]

The Eucharist and the Spiritual Senses

This eucharistic *delectatio*, arising from faith's discernment and charity's desire, finds its consummation in the activity of the spiritual senses. Just as physical food, upon being discerned and desired, delights the physical senses as it is received, so the spiritual food of the body of Christ engages and delights the soul's spiritual senses. At this point, William shifts out of his typical scholastic cadence. Reveling further in the metaphor of food, he cites various authorities in rapid succession: first, Psalm 22: *You prepare a table before me* (Ps 22:5); then Augustine: "so that man might eat the bread of angels, the Creator of the angels was made man" (*Enarratio in psalmum* 77, 17); finally, Wisdom 16: *you have provided them with bread from heaven without toil, possessing every delight within itself and every sweetness of taste* (Wis 20:16). He then observes:

Since this food is the highest sweetness, and since it has entirely every delight and every sweetness of taste, it would seem that it greatly delights him who has a

---

16. SA IV 7.4: 156,38f.
17. SA IV 7.4: 157,52f.

well-disposed palate of the heart, since extremely sweet corporal food delights extremely the well-disposed corporal palate. Therefore, since the body of Christ is an extremely delicious food, it delights to the full him whose palate of the heart is well disposed.[18]

Not surprisingly, the spiritual sense of taste is initially privileged here, as he speaks of "the palate of the heart," well disposed to encounter spiritual food possessing "every sweetness of taste." Discussing the reasons for the institution of the Eucharist, however, William moves beyond the language of spiritual taste. He portrays the Eucharist as a sumptuous spiritual feast or banquet in which the "bread of angels *(panis angelorum)*"[19] engages all the spiritual senses. The Eucharist, he argues, was instituted so that:

> we might celebrate the feast with the unleavened bread of sincerity and truth (1 Cor 5:8). . . . Of this bread it is most truly said that it has every delight in itself. For it delights the spiritual vision through beauty. Whence, *beautiful in form before the sons of men,* etc. (Ps 44:3). Moreover, it delights the spiritual hearing through melody, whence, *let me hear what my Lord God says to me* (Ps 84:9). It delights the affection through the spiritual aroma, whence the Canticle, *let us run in the fragrance of your ointments* (Cant 1:3). It delights the spiritual taste through sweetness, whence, *what great abundance [is your] sweetness* (Ps 30:20). It delights the spiritual touch through pleasantness, whence *taste and see that the Lord is good* (Ps. 33:9). It delights as riches, since *in him are hidden all the treasures of wisdom and knowledge of God* (Col 2:3).[20]

---

18. SA IV 7.3: 152,83ff. *Sed cum ist cibus sit summe delectabilis, et maxime cum habeat omne delectamentum et omnem saporis suavitatem, videtur quod maxime delectat illum qui habet palatum cordis bene dispositum, quia cibus corporalis summe dulcis summe delectat palatum corporale bene dispositum. Ergo cum corpus Christi sit cibus summe delectabilis, summe delectat illum qui habet palatum cordis bene dispositum.*

19. Some twelfth-century theologians associated with the school of Anselm of Laon utilized this phrase in discussions of the Eucharist (see Macy, *Theologies of the Eucharist,* pp. 73–78).

20. SA IV 7.1: 140,41ff. *Quinta causa est, ut epulemur in azimis sinceritatis et veritatis (1 Cor 5:8). Unde Psalmus: Parasti in conspectu meo mensam (Ps 22:5). Et Augustinus dicit:* "Ut panem angelorum manducaret homo, creator angelorum factus est homo" (*Enarr. In Ps.* 77, n. 17 [PL 36.995]). *De hoc pane in XVI Sapiente: Panem de celo prestitisti esi sine labore, omne delectamentum in se habentem et <<omnis>> saporis suavitatem (Sap. 16:20). De isto pane verissime diciture quod omne delectamentum in se habet. Delectat enim visum spiritualem per pulcritudinem. Unde: Speciosus forma pre filiis hominum etc (Ps 44:3). Delectat autem auditum spiritualem per melodiam, unde: Audiam quid loquatur in me dominus Deus meus (Ps 84:9). Delectat affectum per odorem spiritaulem; unde in Canticis, <<1>>:*

As is evident, this passage serves as a (nearly) lyrical summary of William's eucharistic theology. Here, William elevates the language of food and eating to that of feasting (again following Paul), describing a repast that engages all the spiritual senses.[21] The objects of spiritual delight, the *delectabilia divina,* expand beyond the domain of delicious food. The eucharistic bread is beautiful, melodious, aromatic, and pleasing to the touch. This passage, moreover, describes the primary goal of that form of spiritual eating in which the believer is the subject—delight in Christ.[22] Moreover, it is precisely the activity of the spiritual senses that facilitates the experiential nature of this delight.[23] William's use of

---

Curremus in odore<<m>> unguentorum tuorum (Cant 1:3). Delectat gustum spiritualem per dulcedinem; unde: Quam magna multitudo dulcedinis (Ps 30:20). Delectat tactum spiritualem per suavitatem; unde: Gustate et videte quam suavis est Dominus (Ps 33:9). Delectat ut divicie, quia in ipso sunt omnes thesauri sapientie et scientie Dei absconditi (Col 2:3).

21. Bynum's observations concerning the typical medieval meal are worth noting with respect to William's emphasis on the aesthetic aspects of the eucharistic feast. She observes that "the characteristic medieval meal was the feast, and it was more an aesthetic and social event than a gastronomic one" and that "the feast was a banquet for all the senses." Thus, "given such assumptions about and expectations of food," it is not surprising "that Christ's feast involved all the senses, since secular banquets did so" (*Holy Feast, Holy Fast,* pp. 60–61).

22. William also stresses this eucharistic delight in conjunction with the practice of viewing the sacrament instead of actually receiving it, and his discussion of the benefits of viewing the host is the first formal theological treatment of that topic. Since he was also the first commentator on the Mass to discuss the practice of the elevation of the host, it is quite likely that it is this practice which he has in mind here (see Macy, *Theologies of the Eucharist,* p. 135). In the seventh chapter, William addresses the question whether those who are already in a state of mortal sin, sin mortally by viewing the body of Christ. After offering several opinions which suggest that such viewing is, in fact, mortal sin, William argues against such a conclusion on the basis of the power of the sight of the sacrament to evoke in the viewer a love and delight in God: "We say that to observe the body of Christ is not sin, but always good, since, 'with love,' as Augustine says, 'there is the same desire to see and to enjoy God,' to observe the body of Christ is a provocation to the love of God. Hence, in things of this sort, to observe excites and prepares people for the love of God, and the request of many others are heard in that vision of the body of Christ; hence, grace is poured out to many in that event" (SA IV 7.7: 183,22f). Hence, for William, even viewing the consecrated host is an occasion for delight in this spiritual food.

23. Against an undue emphasis on delight, William raises the possible objection, in the *sed contra* of this section, that the bitterness of penance is the most fitting attitude toward the reception of the Eucharist: "On the other hand. It was specified in Exodus 12 *that the paschal lamb is to be eaten with bitter herbs;* which shows that the paschal lamb, who takes away the sins of the world, is to be fed upon with bitter penance. Therefore, he is not to be fed upon with extreme delight by the one who eats him as he ought." As a solution, William suggests that the bitterness of penance has its place, but only as a temporary

his authorities is also remarkable, as he takes up the language of Scripture, in particular, a Christological reading of the Old Testament (especially the Psalter), to describe and to justify this use of the spiritual senses with respect to the Eucharist. Yet, in spite of this, William has shifted the focus of the spiritual senses away from Scripture—their traditional focus throughout the patristic period—and toward the Eucharist, thus reflecting the emerging orientation of medieval spirituality and devotion toward the Eucharist as the locus of an experiential and, indeed, "sensuous" encounter with God. Finally, while in his eucharistic teaching William does not make any explicit references to the gift of wisdom, this passage concludes with an intriguing quotation from the Letter to the Colossians—*in [Christ] are hidden all the treasures of wisdom and knowledge.* Not linked with any particular spiritual sense, this final reference to the wisdom found in Christ recalls the sapiential climax of William's theological endeavor.

Assimilation and Incorporation

As noted above, William divided the four acts of spiritual eating into two pairs. With respect to the second pair, he shifted the subject of the eating, asserting that Christ eats the believer in the acts of assimilation and incorporation or union. This is the ultimate goal of his eucharistic theology. Before examining how this second kind of eating occurs, it is necessary to dwell briefly on William's specific formulation of the manner of Christ's presence in the Eucharist. William distinguishes between

---

check on excessive delight in this life: "That food in itself is the highest delight, and fully delights the angels in the fatherland. . . . But since we are on the way, it does not fully delight. For we are able to fall and we sin and we are able to fall away by pride, since with too much gladness pride is swollen with presumption; and for this reason, we have such a restraint, namely, the bitterness of penance. Just as in delicacies or medicines with too much sharpness a restraint is put in place, so also in the fellowship of our lamb bitter penance is put in place, in order to restrain that ineffable delight. Whence, in Psalm 85:11: *gladden my heart:* notice the gladness; *so that it may fear your name:* notice the restraint. Similarly in another Psalm: *Exalt the Lord with trembling.* And in Job 28: *who gave the wind its weight,* that is, to the spiritual ones he gives a restraint, lest they wither away in pride" (SA IV 7.4: 153,96ff.). Accordingly, while penance has its place in spiritual eating, William clearly wishes to see it in the service of the delight, which it temporarily restrains so as to prevent pride on the part of those whose extreme delight might prompt presumptuous self-exaltation.

two different bodies of Christ present in the Eucharist: the true body of Christ *(corpus Christi verum),* which Christ assumed from the virgin, and Christ's mystical body *(corpus Christi misticum),* which is the church.[24] In his view, the forms of bread and wine are only signs *(sacramentum tantum)* of the body of Christ taken from Mary. This first body of Christ is not only something *(res)* signified by the forms of bread and wine, but is itself a sign *(sacramentum)* of the second body, Christ's mystical body, which alone is signified *(res tantum)* and does not signify.[25] In his view, while the true body which Christ assumed at his Incarnation is the central object of the believer's spiritual feeding, the mystical body of Christ, though perceived neither physically (like the forms of bread and wine) nor spiritually (like the true body of Christ), is an equally significant reality present in the Eucharist. For it is into the mystical body of Christ that believers are assimilated as they feed on the Incarnate Christ.[26]

William refers to this assimilation into the mystical body of Christ, through a kind of mystical reversal, as Christ feeding on believers in the Eucharist. It occurs as believers delight in the eucharistic presence of the Incarnate Christ. This second kind of eating, therefore, is intimately connected to the first kind of spiritual eating. William puts it this way: "to feed on the body of Christ spiritually is, through faith in the Incarnation, to be united and assimilated to him *(ei uniri ei et assimilari).*"[27] For William, then, the acts of discernment and delight in the Incarnate

---

24. SA IV 7.1: 141,63ff. "Three things, moreover, are understood in this sacrament. The first is the form of bread and the form of wine. The second is the true body of Christ, which Christ assumed from the virgin. The third is the mystical body of Christ, which is the church. The first is a sign only; the second is a reality and sign; the third is a reality only. The first is a sign of the second; the second, namely the body of Christ, is a sign of the mystical body of Christ."

25. This threefold understanding of the structure of the Eucharist—*sacramentum, res et sacramentum,* and *res*—emerged in the twelfth century and was extensively developed by several important theologians associated with Laon and St. Victor (see Macy, *Theologies of the Eucharist,* p. 103).

26. This emphasis on the union of the faithful, the church, with Christ as the ultimate effect of the Eucharist had been stressed by earlier twelfth-century theologians such as Gerhoh of Reichersberg, Peter Abelard, and Peter Lombard (see Macy, *Theologies of the Eucharist,* p. 122).

27. SA IV 7.4: 156,37f.

Christ effect assimilation and incorporation into his mystical body. In short, union with Christ results from the delight made possible by, and experienced through, the spiritual senses.

Conclusion

William of Auxerre's eucharistic theology, therefore, is structured by this unified framework of spiritual eating with its two basic moments: eating spiritually and being spiritually eaten. In the first, the faithful feed on the body of Christ by discerning and delighting in It through faith and charity, which comes to a climax in a "spiritually sensuous" feast via the spiritual senses. In the second, wherein Christ himself feeds on the faithful, believers are united to the mystical body of Christ. In this kind of eating, as William observes, "Christ is not changed into the church, but the church is changed into Christ."[28]

As is evident, *delectatio* is the keynote of William's eucharistic theology. In this context, the primary function of *delectatio* is its capacity to nourish and sustain spiritually, that is, its food-like quality. This same theme is prominent generally in William's thought and it is tempting to see his eucharistic theology (and experience) informing other areas of his theology. In Book III, for example, he observes that "in faith itself there is essentially a manifold joy and a manifold nourishment or restoration."[29] He suggests something similar when commenting on a verse from Ecclesiaticus (Sirach): "Those who eat me shall still hunger." William remarks: "They eat through vision, yet they are hungry through charity. For they will have hunger, that is, the desire of charity, so that they might eat more delightfully."[30] Elsewhere, he remarks that those who love Christ truly, without ulterior motives, receive a kind of "spiritual bread" from this love, "namely, faith, hope, and charity and all the other virtues by which they are spiritually nourished."[31] But perhaps the most striking instance of this language, outside of his treatment of the Eucharist, occurs in Book I, where, at the conclusion of his treatment of the Trinity, he poses a question that is rather peculiar unless viewed from the vantage point of the Eucharist: "Are the Father and the Son, in

---

28. SA IV 7.2: 147,119.
29. SA III 11.3.1: 186,64.
30. SA IV 18.3.3.1: 502,168.
31. SA III 14.4: 262,146f.

as much as they are given, one bread or many?" Intriguingly, he argues that although the triune being of God is manifold with respect to human beings, "the goodness and attractiveness and sweetness which nourishes us is a single thing" in its origin and, therefore, the Trinity "is one bread, in as much as it is given."[32] The predominance, then, of metaphors relating to feeding on Christ and being nourished or healed by this encounter suggests a significant connection to William's eucharistic theology.[33]

In many respects, lastly, William's theology of the Eucharist is illustrative of his basic conception of spiritual apprehension. Within the framework of spiritual eating, the same pattern appears that characterized the acquisition of wisdom. In the Eucharist, the believer encounters the external created effects of bread and wine, and through these comes to perceive spiritually and interiorly the Incarnate and Crucified Christ. Here, moral purgation and preparation through the virtues is required. Here,

---

32. SA I 8.8.3.4: 171,4–5. William makes a similar point with respect to Christ's presence in the Eucharist: "For the flesh of Christ is the temple of the whole Trinity, in which is every grace. Hence it is just like a pix or medicinal vase, in which are all manner of spices and spiritual electuaries [medicine covered in a sweet tasting substance such as honey or syrup], through which God cleanses our souls through his ministers" (SA IV 4.1).

33. As noted above in note 4, in *Holy Feast and Holy Fast,* Bynum does not discuss William of Auxerre's theology of the Eucharist, neither in her treatment of the historical background of high medieval eucharistic devotion (Chapter 2), nor in her attempt to contrast male and female eucharistic devotion in terms of the centrality of food and food-related metaphors (Chapter 3). Perhaps that would have been a difficult task. William's consistent understanding of the Eucharist as food and the centrality of the fourfold framework of spiritual eating, modeled on the analogy with ordinary physical eating, seem to place him astride at least part of the line which Bynum draws between male and female eucharistic devotion. According to Bynum, even the few medieval male writers, mostly lay and eremitic, who utilized food metaphors in their eucharistic treatises and sermons "did not carry those images over into their spiritual writings as central metaphors for encounter with God" (p. 94). Not for even the most "affective, exuberant, lyrical" of male spiritual writers, such as Francis, Henry Suso, Richard Rolle, John Tauler, and Jan van Ruysbroeck, "was food a fundamental metaphor for encounter with God" (p. 105). To be sure, William says very little about the experience of hunger; nor is fasting an important aspect of his eucharistic spirituality. These are clearly crucial aspects of the kind of spirituality which Bynum is attempting to characterize, and, as far as they are concerned, William is no counterexample. But, unlike the medieval men whom Bynum surveys, William posits a eucharistic theology that has an essential affective and experiential dimension which is clearly grounded in what for him is its most fundamental metaphor—the multi-sensuous nature of food and eating. In this respect, William is something of a counterexample to Bynum's thesis.

too, the theological virtues of faith and charity are pivotal, collaborating to facilitate this spiritual perception of Christ. Here, there is the same movement from theological concept to spiritual percept, the same doctrinally mediated mystical encounter. One perceives the beauty, melody, fragrance, sweetness, and pleasantness of Christ only when, by faith, one has apprehended the fact of his Incarnation and understood its significance, and then through charity has come to love and desire him. Here, the spiritual senses provide the consummation of this spiritual apprehension, perceiving with maximal delight the divine self-manifestation. Here, finally, spiritual apprehension culminates with wisdom, which entails an assimilating union with the Trinity. In a sense, though William never states it this way, the Eucharist facilitates the movement from symbolic to mystical theology and its synaesthetic *sapientia*.

CONCLUSION

SPIRITUAL APPREHENSION
The Spiritual Senses and the Knowledge of God

THE FOREGOING has attempted to describe William of Auxerre's conception of human knowledge of God from the perspective of his teaching on the spiritual senses of the soul. This teaching is, in fact, central to his theology. The beatific vision enjoyed by the blessed in the next life is realized and consummated through the spiritual senses, such that that *videre* is simultaneously an *audire, odorari, gustare,* and *tangere*. A crucial aspect of William's teaching on the spiritual senses *in patria* is the intimate integration of spiritual sensation and conceptual cognition. This wedding of percept and concept can be summed up in the phrase "spiritual apprehension," a term which William himself does not explicitly use, but which attempts to capture both of these dimensions.

With his teaching on the beatific activity of the spiritual senses in the foreground, it is possible to appreciate more fully various other aspects of William's theology. Seen retrospectively, in the light of its conclusion, the rest of his theology can be seen as oriented toward this goal. His metaphysics of the good, Trinitarian theology, and doctrine of creation all lay a foundation and provide a warrant for conceiving of God as the manifold object of the spiritual senses. In relationship to spiritual apprehension, the central implication of William's teaching on these topics is that knowledge of God is mediated by the Trinity's activity *ad extra,* that is, in the encounter with Its created effects. Thus, while essentially the Trinity is a single Object of human knowing, effectively there are diverse objects for this encounter, namely, the *delectabilia divina*. More precisely, these *delectabilia* are the manifold activities of divine Wisdom who, as exemplar, art, and beauty of creation, makes all created things to be words and images and mirrors of uncreated goodness. This sapiential vision is possible, however, only as Wisdom is revealed and made manifest to the spiritual senses through the presence and activity of the Spirit. Accordingly, knowledge of God through the spiritual senses is the Spirit-facilitated perception of the *delectabilia divina* in the Son, or the delectable apprehension of sapiential goodness in the Son through the Spirit.

Regarding these created effects, William distinguishes between two kinds, visible and invisible, external and internal, and, borrowing (while transforming) a Dionysian distinction, he further delineates two corresponding types of theology, symbolic and mystical. In both symbolic and mystical theology (as well as in beatific knowledge of God), the theological virtues of faith and charity are crucial. Here, William appropriates a particular sense modality to each of these in order to describe their essential natures and acts. Faith is essentially a speculative, intellectual act, whose object is the true. To this act, he appropriates the spiritual sense of sight. Faith is spiritual *visus*. For William, moreover, faith has a definite priority in relation to charity. For following on faith's initial speculation of the true is its *aestimatio* of the true as its highest good, and this estimation, in turn, generates in the soul a desire for, and movement toward, the good. Precisely this desire and movement become the virtue of charity. Charity's derived status, however, does not render it insignificant in spiritual apprehension. Rather, its desire to experience and enjoy faith's *visus* leads William to describe it ultimately as a form of spiritual *tactus*. Charity's act culminates in contact and union between the soul and God. So, faith and charity collaborate in the delight provided by all the spiritual senses. Charity pursues "not only the delight which is in spiritual touch, but also the delight of every spiritual sense" and so propels faith to an act of synaesthetic spiritual *visus*. Charity's desire culminates in faith's delight through spiritual *visus, auditus, gustus, odoratus,* and *tactus.*

William brings all of the foregoing together in his description of the forms of spiritual apprehension possible in this life *(in via).* Symbolic theology, though not properly the sphere of the spiritual senses, is nonetheless an important component of spiritual apprehension. It sets the stage for its counterpart, mystical theology. With its three components, *scientia, intellectus,* and *sapientia,* mystical theology contains the basic framework wherein human persons come to know God. As seen, mystical theology culminates in wisdom, in some sense a direct, unmediated, spiritually sensuous encounter with *delectabilia divina.* Lastly, the sacrament of the Eucharist provides a crowning locus for William's conception of the spiritual apprehension made possible by the spiritual senses. Here, all the components of spiritual apprehension emerge in William's description of the believer's sacramental encounter with Christ.

Thus it is possible to appreciate what is perhaps the most distinctive feature of William's conception of human knowledge of God through the spiritual senses. As seen, spiritual apprehension comprises distinguishable moments or aspects. In William's discussion of the beatific vision, the triad of *cognoscere, percipere* and *sentire* was prominent; our treatment of mystical theology featured the triad of *scientia, intellectus,* and *sapientia.* These triads contain the same basic components and chart the same progression of steps in William's conception of the knowledge of God. Indeed, he often interchanges the terms and uses terms from both sets in the same discussion. In the main, he depicts a movement from concept to percept, from knowledge to wisdom, which is consistently reflected in his descriptions of knowing God. This movement is readily apparent in a crucial text cited earlier concerning the spiritual senses in beatitude:

By faith we see spiritually. By faith we hear what Jesus says. For *faith comes by hearing.* By faith we perceive scents spiritually. For by faith we cognize that the Son of God became incarnate for us, that he wept and was tormented for us, that he sorrowed and suffered. When we recall these benefits, we perceive the good odor of Christ as an aromatic perfume flowing from him. . . . When by faith we meditate upon these things which we know, as if by chewing *(masticando)* we taste the sweetness of God, and this is by faith. By faith we touch the suavity of God.[1]

---

1. SA IV 18.3.3.2.3: 510,60ff.

This text describes well the soul's apprehension of God through faith. Throughout, the acts of spiritual sensation are intimately linked with doctrinal affirmations. Faith's diverse objects of knowledge become its diverse experiences of spiritual sensation. The knowledge of Jesus' teaching, for example, is spiritual hearing; arising from the cognition of doctrines about God (e.g., that the Son of God became incarnate and suffered) is Christ's aromatic perfume perceived by faith; faith's meditation leads to a chewing and tasting *(gustus)* of divine sweetness; and the culmination is to touch *(tangere)* the divine suavity *(suavitatem)*. Elsewhere in his discussion of beatitude, William suggests similarly that when we cognize *(cognoscere)* that divine goodness has been bestowed upon created things:

> we perceive the odor *(odoramur)* of God spiritually; and when we meditate on this, we chew *(masticamus)* spiritually; and when we are inflamed toward the love of God by this then we touch *(tangimus)* God spiritually. For we touch the heat *(calorem)* of God.[2]

Here is the familiar path from theological affirmation, through intellectual meditation, to finally touching of God in some direct way. Again, when William describes the synaesthetic nature of the final *visio Dei*, the same pattern is present:

> By seeing God we will hear spiritually, since by seeing we will have cognition *(cognitio)*; and this is to hear by seeing *(audire videndo)*. We will assemble the goods given to us by God and this will be to perceive the odor *(odorari)* of God by seeing *(odorari videndo)*. We will know the internal *rationes* of God; and this will be to taste *(gustare)* spiritually. Likewise, by seeing God we will be inflamed by his love, of which it is said: *our God is a consuming fire* (Heb 12:29); and this will be to touch *(tangere)* him.[3]

Cognition becomes spiritual hearing; the collation of blessings received from God, spiritual smell; the knowledge of the internal *rationes* of God merges with spiritual taste, all of which, finally, culminates, once again, in spiritual touch *(tangere)*.

William, therefore, unites doctrinal theology and spiritual experience

---

2. SA IV 18.3.3.2.4: 515,86.
3. SA IV 18.3.3.2.4: 513,57ff.

in a scholastic mode.⁴ Rather than pitting doctrine against devotion, or privileging "experience" and then permitting doctrinal formulation to play merely the role of a second-order, conceptualizing "overlay," his thought works in the opposite direction. Sapiential experience is informed, structured, and mediated by a revealed *scientia*. Spiritual percept emerges out of theological concept, and doctrine is a necessary condition for mystical, even "spiritually sensuous," experience. *Scientia* provides the initial content, object, and material from which *sapientia* emerges; *sapientia*, for its part, effects an experiential, affective posture in the knower toward the trinitarian God so described by *scientia*. Ultimately, for William of Auxerre, knowledge of God is a spiritual apprehension of God—both a *scientia* and a *sapientia*—and thus a "tasted knowledge," a knowledge of God by experience.

4. See Joseph Wawrykow, "New Directions in Research on Thomas Aquinas," *Religious Studies Review* 27:1 (January 2001): pp. 32–38. One could refer to William's theology, like that of Aquinas, as "second-level," in the sense of "reflecting on religious experience and the conditions, including the necessary core beliefs, for its occurrence" (p. 34). Wawrykow's observation in regard to Thomas scholarship—"that the modern tendency to use an easy and clear-cut division between scholastic and spiritual writers and to set the two at (hostile) odds is more modern than medieval"—is equally apt in relation to William of Auxerre. For both William and Thomas, the "spiritual is not at the expense of the scholastic" (p. 35).

BIBLIOGRAPHY

Primary Sources

Ambrose. *De officiis.* PL 16.26A–194B.
Anselm. *Monologion.* PL 158.141–224A.
Aristotle. *De anima.* Ed. I. Bekker. 1831.
———. *Ethica Nicomachea.* Ed. I. Bekker. 1831.
———. *Metaphysica.* Ed. I. Bekker. 1831.
———. *Opera.* 5 vols. Ed. I. Bekker. Berlin, 1831–70.
———. *Physica.* Ed. I. Bekker. 1831.
Augustine. *Confessions.* Translated with an introduction and notes by Henry Chadwick. Oxford: Oxford University Press, 1991.
———. *Confessiones.* PL 32.659–868.
———. *De diversis questionibus 83.* PL 40.11–100.
———. *De doctrina Christiana.* PL 34.15–122.
———. *De Genesi ad litteram.* PL 34.245–486.
———. *De libero arbitrio.* PL 32.1221–1310.
———. *De moribus Ecclesiae et Manichaeorum.* PL 32.1309–78.
———. *De natura boni.* PL 42.551–72.
———. *De Trinitate.* PL 42.819–1098.
———. *Enarrationes in psalmos.* PL 36–37.
———. *Epistolae.* PL 33.
———. *In Johannes evangelium.* PL 35.1379–1971.
———. *Soliloquia.* PL 32.869–904.
Augustine (Pseudo-). *De spiritu et anima.* PL 40.779–832.
Bernard of Clairvaux. *Sermones super Cantica Canticorum.* Ed. J. Leclercq, C. H. Talbot, and H. M. Rochais. *S. Bernardi Opera,* 1–2. Rome, 1957–58.
Biblia sacra cum Glossa interlineari, ordinaria et Nicolai Lyrani Postilla. Lyranus, 1588.
Boethius. *De consolatione philosophiae.* PL 63.547–862.
———. *De Hebdomadibus.* PL 64.1311–14.
Cassiodorus. *De anima.* PL 70.1279–1308.
Dionysius Areopagita (Pseudo-). *De divinis nominibus.* PG 3.585A–996B; PL 122.1113A–72B.
———. *De mystica theologica.* PG 3.997A–1064A; PL 122.1172C–76C.
———. *Epistola IX.* PG 3.1104A–13C; PL 122.1188B–93A.
Gregory the Great. *Moralia in Iob.* PL 75.509D–76.782A.

Hugh of St. Victor. *De sacramentis Christianae fidei.* PL 176.173–618.
———. *Hugonis de Sancto Victore Didascalicon de Studio Legendi: A Critical Text.* Ed. Charles Henry Buttimer. The Catholic University of America Studies in Medieval and Renaissance Latin, 10. Washington, D.C., 1939.
———. *In hierarchiam caelestem S. Dionysii.* PL 175.923–1154.
Hugh of St. Victor (Pseudo-). *Summa Sententiarum.* PL 176.41C–174A.
John Scotus Eriugena. *De divisione naturae.* PL 122.441A–1022D.
Peter Abelard. *Introductio ad theologiam.* PL 178.979A–1114B.
———. *Theologia christiana.* PL 178.1123A–1330C.
———. *Theologia "scholarium."* Ed. Constant J. Mews. CCCM 13.
Peter Lombard. *Collectanea in omnes d. Pauli apostoli epistolas* [*Glossa Lombardiana*]. PL 191.1297A–1696C; 192.9A–520A.
———. *Sententiarum libri IV.* Quaracchi-Grottaferrata, 1971, 1980.
Richard of St. Victor. *De Trinitate.* PL 196.887C–992B.
Simon of Tournai. *Expositio in Symbol Quicumque* (unedited: Ms. Paris, Nat. lat. 14886, fol. 73a).
Seneca. *L. Annaei Senecae: Ad Lucilium Epistulae Morales.* 2 vols. Ed. L. D. Reynolds. Oxford: Oxford University Press, 1965.
Tertullian. *De resurrectione carnis.* PL 2.837C–934C.
William of Auxerre. *Summa Aurea.* Ed. Ph. Pigouchet, Paris, 1500 and 1518 (reprint, Frankfurt [Minerva], 1964); ed. Fr. Regnault, Paris, 1500, and Venice, 1591; ed. J. Ribaillier (Spicilegium Bonaventurianum, vols. 16–20, Magistri Guillelmi Altissiodorensis, *Summa Aurea, Liber Quartus*), Paris-Grottaferrata, 1980–87.

Secondary Sources

Aertsen, Jan A. *Medieval Philosophy and the Transcendentals: The Case of Thomas Aquinas.* Studien und Texte zur Geistesgeschichte des Mittelalters, vol. 52. Leiden: Brill, 1996.
Arnold, Johannes. *Perfecta communicatio: die Trinitätstheologie Wilhelms von Auxerre.* Beiträge zur Geschichte der Philosophie und Theologie des Mittelalters, vol. 42. Münster: Aschendorff, 1995.
Baladier, C. *L'essence de la charité d'après Guillaume d'Auxerre: étude comparative avec quelques théologiens contemporains.* Ph.D. dissertation. Rome (Angelicum), 1953.
Beumer, Johannes. "Die Theologie als *intellectus fidei*: Dargestellt an Hand der Lehre des Wilhelm von Auxerre und Petrus von Tarantasia." *Scholastik* 17 (1942): 32–49.
———. *Theologie als Glaubensverständnis.* Würzburg: Echter, 1953.
Biffi, Inos. *Figure medievali della teologia.* Milan: Jaca Book, 1992.
Breuning, Wilhelm. *Die hypostatische Union in der Theologie Wilhelms von Auxerre, Hugos von St. Cher und Rolands von Cremona.* Trierer theologische Studien, vol. 11. Trier: Paulinus, 1962.
Brown, Stephen. "Declarative and Deductive Theology in the Early Fourteenth Century." In *Was ist Philosophie im Mittelalter*, ed. Jan A. Aertsen and Andreas Speer, 648–55. Berlin: Walter de Gruyter, 1998.

———. "The Intellectual Context of Later Medieval Philosophy: Universities, Aristotle, Arts, Theology." In *Routledge History of Philosophy*, 3, *Medieval Philosophy*, ed. John Marenbon. London: Routledge, 1986.
Bynum, Caroline. *Holy Feast and Holy Fast: The Religious Significance of Food to Medieval Women*. Berkeley: University of California Press, 1987.
Canévet, Mariette. "Sens Spirituel." In *Dictionnaire de spiritualité ascétique et mystique doctrine et histoire*, ed. Marcel Viller, assisted by F. Cavallera, J. de Guibert, et al., 599–617. Paris: Beauchesne, 1937.
Châtillon, Jean. "De Guillaume d'Auxerre à saint Thomas d'Aquin: L'argument de saint Anselme chez les premiers scolastiques du XIIIe siècle." In *D'Isidore de Séville à saint Thomas d'Aquin: Études d'histoire et de théologie*, 209–31. London: Variorum Reprints, 1985.
Chenu, M.-D. "L'amour dans la foi." *Bulletin thomiste* 9 (1932): pp. 97–99.
———. "Contribution à l'histoire du traité de la foi. Commentaire historique de II^a–II^{ae}, q. I a. 2." In *Melanges thomistes*. Bibliothèque thomiste, 3, 123–40. Paris, 1934.
———. "Pro fidei supernaturalitate illustranda." In *Xenia Thomistica*, ed. Sdoc Szabó, vol. 3, 297–307. Rome, 1925.
———. "La surnaturalisation des vertus." *Bulletin thomiste* 9 (1932): 93–96.
———. *La théologie comme science au XIIIe siècle*. 3d ed., rev. and enl. Bibliothèque thomiste, 33. Paris, 1957.
Colish, Marcia. "Early Scholastic Angelology." *Recherches de théologie ancienne et médiévale* 62 (1995): 80–109.
———. "*Habitus* Revisited: A Reply to Cary Nederman." *Traditio* 48 (1993): 77–92.
———. "Parisian Scholastic Theology, 1130–1215." *Manuels, programmes de cours et techniques d'enseignement dans les universités médiévales: actes du Colloque internationale de Louvain-la-Neuve (9–11 September 1993)*, ed. Jacqueline Hamesse. Louvain-la-Neuve: Institut d'Études Médiévales de l'Université Catholique de Louvain, 1994.
———. *Peter Lombard*. Brill's Studies in Intellectual History, vol. 41. Leiden: Brill, 1994.
Conlan, William J. "The Definition of Faith According to a Question of Ms. Assisi 138: Study and Edition of Text." In *Essays in Honour of Anton Charles Pegis*, ed. J. R. O'Donnell, 17–69. Toronto: Pontifical Institute of Mediaeval Studies, 1974.
De Bruyne, Edgar. *Études d'esthétique médiévale*, 3 vols. Bruges, 1946.
Decker, Bruno. *Die Entwicklung der Lehre von der prophetischen Offenbarung von Wilhelm von Auxerre bis zu Thomas von Aquin*. Breslauer Studien zur historischen Theologie, vol. 7. Breslau: Müller & Seiffert, 1940.
De Clerck, E. "Le dogme de la rédemption: De Robert de Melun à Guillaume d'Auxerre." *Recherches de théologie ancienne et médiévale* 14 (1947): 252–86.
Duhem, Pierre. *La crue de l'Aristotélisme*, part 3. In *Le systèm du monde: Histoire de doctrines cosmologique de Platon à Copernic*, vol. 5. Paris: Hermann et Fils, 1917.
Eco, Umberto. *Art and Beauty in the Middle Ages*. Trans. Hugh Bredin. New Haven, Conn.: Yale University Press, 1986.

Englhardt, G. *Die Entwicklung der dogmatischen Glabuenspsychologie in der mittelalterlichen Scholastik vom Abelardstreit (um 1140) bis zu Philipp dem Kanzler (gest. 1236)*. Beiträge zur Geschichte der Philosophie und Theologie des Mittelalters, vol. 30. Münster: Aschendorff, 1933.

Fields, Stephen, S.J. "Balthasar and Rahner on the Spiritual Senses." *Theological Studies* 57 (1996): 224–41.

Gaybba, Brian. "Fifteenth Century Views on the Nature of Theology: An Outline of Its Characteristics and a Survey of the Printed Primary Sources." *Studia Historiae Ecclesiasticae* 20:1 (1994): 106–19.

Gillmann, F. *Zur Sakramentenlehre des Wilhelm von Auxerre: Zugleich ein Beitrag zur Sakramentenlehre der Fruhscholastik*. Wurzburg: Bauch, 1918.

Gilson, Etienne. *The Philosophy of St. Bonaventure*. Paterson, N.J.: St. Anthony Guild Press, 1965.

Glorieux, P. "L'enseignement au moyen âge." *Archives d'histoire doctrinale et littéraire du moyen âge* 43 (1969): 65–186.

———. *Les genres littéraires dans les source théologiques et philosophiques médiévales*. Louvain, 1982.

Grabmann, Martin. *Die Geschichte der katholischen Theologie seit dem Ausgang der Väterzeit*. Freiburg, 1933.

———. *Die Geschichte der scholastischen Methode*. 2 vols. Reprint, Graz, 1957.

Grillmeier, Alois. "Vom *Symbolum* zur *Summa*: Zum theologiegeschictlichen Verhältnis von Patristik und Scholastik."In *Kirche und Überlieferung*, ed. J. Betz and H. Fries. Freiburg, 1960.

Hayes, Zachary. *The Hidden Center: Spirituality and Speculative Christology in St. Bonaventure*. New York: The Franciscan Institute, 1992.

Heinzmann, R. *Die Unsterblichkeit der Seele und die Auferstehung des Leibes: eine problemgeschichtliche Untersuchung der frühscholastischen Sentenzen und Summenliteratur von Anselm von Laon bis Wilhelm von Auxerre*. Beiträge zur Geschichte der Philosophie und Theologie des Mittelalters, vol. 40. Münster: Aschendorff, 1965.

Heitz, T. *Essai historique sur les rapports entre la philosophie et la foi: de Bérenger de Tours à S. Thomas d' Aquin*. Paris: Librairie Victor Lecoffre, 1909.

Jenkins, John I. *Knowledge and Faith in Thomas Aquinas*. Cambridge: Cambridge University Press, 1997.

Knoch, W. *Die Einsetzung der Sakramente durch Christus: eine Untersuchung zur Sakramententheologie der Frühscholastik von Anslem von Laon bis zu Wilhelm von Auxerre*. Beiträge zur Geschichte der Philosophie und Theologie des Mittelalters, vol. 24. Münster: Aschendorff, 1983.

Köpf, U. *Die Anfänge der theologischen Wissenschaftstheorie im 13. Jahrhndert*. Tübingen: Mohr, 1974.

Krebs, E. *Theologie und Wissenschaft nach der Lehre der Hochscholastik*. Beiträge zur Geschichte der Philosophie und Theologie des Mittelalters, vol. 11. Münster: Aschendorff, 1912.

Landgraf, A. M. "Beobachten zur Einflusssphare Wilhelm von Auxerre." *Zeitschrift für katholische Theologie* 52 (1928): 53–64.

Lang, Albert. *Die theologische Prinzipienlehre der mittelalterlichen Scholastik.* Freiburg: Herder, 1964.

———. *Die Wege der Glaubensbegründung bei den Scholastiken des 14. Jahrhunderts.* Beiträge zur Geschichte der Philosophie und Theologie des Mittelalters, vol. 30. Münster: Aschendorff, 1930.

Long, R. J. "The Science of Theology according to Richard Fishacre: Edition of the Prologue to His 'Commentary on the Sentences.'" *Mediaeval Studies* 34 (1972): 71–98.

Lottin, O. "Les dons du Saint-Esprit chez les théologiens depuis Pierre Lombard jusqu'à S. Thomas d'Aquin." *Recherches de théologie ancienne et médiévale* 1 (1929): 41–61.

———. *Psychologie et morale au XII et XIII siècles.* 6 vols. Louvain and Gembloux, 1942–60.

———. "La théorie du libre arbitre au treizième siècle." *Revue thomiste* 32 (1927): 359ff.

MacDonald, Scott. "Goodness as a Transcendental: The Early Thirteenth-Century Recovery of an Aristotelian Idea." *Topoi* 11 (1992): 173–86.

Macy, Gary. *The Theologies of the Eucharist in the Early Scholastic Period: A Study of the Salvific Function of the Sacrament according to the Theologians, c. 1080–c. 1220.* Oxford: Clarendon Press; New York: Oxford University Press, 1984.

Mandonnet, Pierre. "Date de la mort de Guillaume d'Auxerre (3 Nov. 1231)." *Archives d'histoire doctrinale et littéraire du moyen-âge* 7 (1932): 279–300.

Marrone, Steven P. *William of Auvergne and Robert Grosseteste: New Ideas of Truth in the Early Thirteenth Century.* Princeton, N.J.: Princeton University Press, 1983.

Martineau, R.-M. "Le plan de la 'Summa Aurea' de Guillaume d'Auxerre." In *Études et recherches publiees pare le college dominican d'Ottawa*, 2, 79–114. Ottawa: Editiones du Levrier, 1937.

———. "La 'Summa de officiis ecclesiasticis' de Guillaume d'Auxerre." In *Études d'histoire litteraire et doctrinale du XIII siecle*, 2d series, 25–58. Publications de l'institut d'études medievales d'Ottawa, 2. Paris, Ottawa: Institut d'Études Medievales, 1932.

McGinn, Bernard. *The Growth of Mysticism*, vol. 2 of *The Presence of God: A History of Western Christian Mysticism*. New York: Crossroad, 1994.

Megivern, James J. *Concomitance and Communion: A Study in Eucharistic Doctrine and Practice.* Freiburg: University Press, 1963.

Michaud-Quantin, Pierre. *Études sur le vocabulaire philosophique du Moyen Age.* Rome: Ateneo, 1970.

Minges, Parthenius. "Die theologischen Summen Wilhelms von Auxerre und Alexanders von Hales." *Theologische Quartalschrift* 97 (1915): 508–29.

Minnis, A. J., and A. B. Scott, eds. *Medieval Literary Theory and Criticism c. 1100–c. 1375: The Commentary-Tradition.* Rev. ed. Oxford: Oxford University Press, 1991.

Nederman, Cary. "Nature, Ethics, and the Doctrine of *Habitus*: Aristotelian Moral Psychology in the Twelfth Century." *Traditio* 45 (1989): 87–110.

Ottaviano, Carmelo. *Guglielmo d'Auxerre (d. 1231): la vita, le opere, il pensiero.* Biblioteca di filosofia e scienze, 12. Rome: L'Universale Tipografia Poliglotta, 1931.

Potts, Timothy. *Conscience in Medieval Philosophy.* Cambridge: Cambridge University Press, 1980.

Pouillon, Henri. "La beauté, propriété transcendentale chez les scolastiques (1220–1270)." *Archives d'histoire doctrinale et littéraire du moyen-âge* 15 (1946): 263–329.

———. "Le Premier traité des propriétés transcendentals, La 'Summa de bono' du Chancellier Phillipe." *Revue néoscolastique de philosophie* 42 (1939): 40–77.

Principe, Walter. *Introduction to Patristic and Medieval Theology,* 2d ed. Toronto, 1982.

———. *William of Auxerre's Theology of the Hypostatic Union.* Vol. 1 of *The Theology of the Hypostatic Union in the Early Thirteenth Century,* Studies and Texts no. 7. Toronto: Pontifical Institute of Medieval Studies, 1963.

Rahner, Karl. "The Doctrine of the 'Spiritual Senses' in the Middle Ages." In *Theological Investigations* 16, 104–34. New York: Seabury, 1979.

———. "The 'Spiritual Senses' According to Origen." In *Theological Investigations* 16, 81–103. New York: Seabury, 1979.

Ribaillier, J. "Guillaume d'Auxerre." In *Dictionnaire de spiritualité ascétique et mystique doctrine et histoire,* 6, 1192–99, ed. Marcel Viller, assisted by F. Cavallera, J. de Guibert, et al. Paris: Beauchesne, 1937.

Rorem, Paul. *Pseudo-Dionysius: A Commentary on the Texts and an Introduction to Their Influence.* Oxford: Oxford University Press, 1993.

Rubin, Miri. *Corpus Christi: The Eucharist in Late Medieval Culture.* Cambridge: Cambridge University Press, 1991.

Solignac, Aimé. "Oculus." In *Dictionnaire de spiritualité ascétique et mystique doctrine et histoire.* Ed. Marcel Viller, assisted by F. Cavallera, J. de Guibert, et al. Paris: Beauchesne, 1937.

St. Pierre, Jules. "The Theological Thought of William of Auxerre: An Introductory Bibliography." *Recherches de théologie ancienne et médiévale* 33 (1966): 146–56.

Stock, Brian. "Experience, Praxis, Work, and Planning in Bernard of Clairvaux: Observations on the *Sermones in Cantica.*" In *The Cultural Context of Medieval Learning,* ed. John E. Murdoch and Edith D. Sylla, 219–68. Dordrecht, Holland: D. Reidel, 1975.

Strake, Joseph. *Die Sakramentenlehre des Wilhelm von Auxerre.* Forschungen zur Christlichen Literatur und Dogmengeschichte, 13, 5. Paderborn, 1917.

———. "Die scholastiche Methode in der 'Summa aurea' des Wilhelm von Auxerre." *Theologie und Glaube* 5 (1913): 549–57.

Swanson, R. N. *Religion and Devotion in Europe, c. 1215–1515.* Cambridge: Cambridge University Press, 1995.

Tatarkiewicz, Władysław. *Geschichte der Äesthetik.* Vol. 2: *Die Äesthetik des Mittelalters.* Basel/Stuttgart: Schwabe & Company, 1980.

Tedoldi, Fabio M. *La dottrina dei cinque sensi spirituali in San Bonaventura.* Rome: Pontificum Athenaeum Antonianum, 1999.

Torrell, J.-P. "Le savoir théologique chez saint Thomas." *Revue thomiste* 96 (1996): 355–96.

———. *Théorie de la prophétie et philosophie de la connaissance aux environs de 1230.*

La contribution d'Hugues de Saint-Cher (Spicilegium Sacrum Lovaniense, fasc. 40). Louvain, 1977.
Tugwell, Simon, O.P. *Albert and Thomas: Selected Writings.* New York: Paulist Press, 1988.
Tummers, Paul. "Geometry and Theology in the XIIIth Century: An Example of Their Interrelation as Found in the Ms. Admont 442: The Influence of William of Auxerre?" *Vivarium* 18 (1980): 112–42.
Turner, Denis. *Eros and Allegory: Medieval Exegesis of the Song of Songs.* Kalamazoo, Mich.: Cistercian Publications, 1995.
Van Hove, A. "Doctrina Gulielmi Altissiodorensis de Causalitate Sacramentorum." *Divus Thomas* (Piacenza) 33 (1930): 305–24.
Vanneste, A. "Nature et grâce dans la théologie de Guillaume d'Auxerre et de Guillaume d'Auvergne." *Ephemerides Theologicae Lovanienses* 53 (1977): 83–106.
Von Balthasar, Hans Urs. *The Glory of the Lord: A Theological Aesthetics.* Vol. 1, *Seeing the Form.* San Francisco: Ignatius Press, 1982.
———. *The Glory of the Lord: A Theological Aesthetics.* Vol. 2, *Studies in Theological Style: Clerical Styles.* San Francisco: Ignatius Press, 1984.
Von Israel, Peri. "*Omnia Mensura et Numero et Pondere Disposuisti*: Die Auslegung von Weish 11,20 in der Lateinischen Patristik." In *Miscellanea Mediaevalia: Veröffentlichungen des Thomas-Instituts der Univerität zu Köln.* Vol. 16: *Mensura, Mass, Zahl, Zahlensymbolik im Mittelalter,* 1–22. Berlin: de Gruyter, 1983.
Wawrykow, Joseph. "New Directions in Research on Thomas Aquinas." *Religious Studies Review* 27:1 (January 2001): 32–38.
Weijers, O., ed. *Méthodes et instruments du travail intellectual au moyen âge: études sur le vocabulaire.* Turnhout: Brepols, 1990.
Weisheipl, James. "The Meaning of *Sacra Doctrina* in *Summa Theologiae* I." *The Thomist* 38 (1974): 49–80.
Wicki, Nicholas. *Die Lehre von der himmlischen Seligkeit in der mittelalterlichen Scholastik von Petrus Lombardus bis Thomas von Aquin.* Freiburg: University Press, 1954.
Wieland, Georg. *Ethica-Scientia Practica: die Anfänge der philosophischen Ethik im 13. Jahrhundert.* Beiträge zur Geschichte der Philosophie und Theologie des Mittelalters, vol. 21. Münster: Aschendorff, 1981.
Wolfson, Harry A. "The Internal Senses in Latin, Arabic, and Hebrew Philosophical Texts." *Harvard Theological Review* 28 (1935): 250–314.

INDEX

accident, 28, 59, 101, 105–6, 115, 118, 124, 148, 203–5
Aertsen, Jan A., 14, 55, 242
affection *(affectio)*, 11, 23–24, 61–62, 64–65, 68, 116, 131, 139, 141, 144–45, 155, 200, 227
Alan of Lille, 1, 50, 74, 162, 189
Albert the Great, 1, 10, 12, 23–24, 28, 165, 203, 210, 247
Alcher of Clairvaux (pseudo), 16, 24, 28, 125
Alexander III, 123
Alexander of Hales, 1, 12, 24, 28, 165, 203, 207
Ambrose, 62, 78, 241
analogy, 9–10, 29, 33, 36, 42–43, 74, 85–86, 91, 99–104, 113, 121, 124, 127, 132–33, 142, 156, 186, 192–94, 196, 205–7, 209–10, 220, 222, 232
Anselm of Canterbury, 73, 95, 195, 203, 210, 212, 227, 241, 243–44
arbitrium, 126
archetype, 92–94, 97, 102–3
argumentum, 123, 186, 188–89, 192–93, 197, 203, 205, 214, 216, 218
Aristotle, 4–5, 8–9, 13, 33, 36, 41–44, 46, 55, 58, 62–64, 69, 80, 95, 105, 115, 117–29, 131–32, 134, 145, 146, 169, 171, 185–86, 188–91, 193–196, 198–99, 203, 205, 207, 209–12, 241, 243, 245
Arius, 102, 207
Arnold, Johannes, 74–75, 77–78, 80–81, 100–101, 166, 177, 182, 242

art *(ars)*, 82–83, 88–90, 98, 124, 167–68, 170, 173, 181, 193, 236
articles of faith *(articulos fidei)*, 4–5, 14, 186, 189–90, 192–98, 202–3, 209, 216. *See also* creed
artist *(artifex)*, 83, 97–98, 168–69, 180–81
assimilation, 222–24, 229–31
Augustine, 4, 9–10, 13–17, 24–25, 28, 30–31, 33–34, 38, 40–41, 60–62, 73, 78, 81, 84, 91, 95, 97, 113, 120, 125, 127, 130, 133, 142, 144, 153, 157, 165–66, 173–74, 179–80, 191, 194, 197, 200, 203, 205, 206, 210, 212, 220–23, 226, 228, 241
Averroes, 125
Avicenna, 58, 123, 125–26

Baladier, C., 242
beatitude *(beatitudo)*, 3–4, 18, 21–27, 45, 47, 49, 53, 57, 65–67, 70–72, 76–78, 82, 84, 86, 90–91, 107–8, 111–16, 133–35, 137, 139, 148, 154, 156–57, 178–79, 182, 212, 237–38
beauty *(pulchritudo)*, 3–4, 22, 24, 26, 29, 39, 45, 47–48, 60, 62, 72, 76, 82–83, 88, 90–91, 98, 104, 111, 133, 136, 138, 141, 143, 155, 157, 162–68, 170–71, 175–83, 186, 227–28, 233, 236. *See also honestum*
Bede, 166
being *(esse)*, 33, 54, 57–61, 73, 78, 81–82, 85, 89, 95, 97, 100–101, 103–5, 163, 169–70, 172–73, 206, 232; *(ens)*, 102–3, 105, 193
benevolence *(benignitas)*, 76–77, 84

249

Bernard of Clairvaux, 7, 10, 18, 28, 78, 122, 127, 241, 246
Beumer, Johannes, 8, 10, 12, 199, 203, 208, 210–11, 242
Biffi, Inos, 185, 242
Boethius, 27, 56, 58, 60–61, 74, 125, 166, 195, 216, 241
Bonaventure, 2, 15, 23–24, 73, 91, 95–97, 99, 161, 203, 244
bread, 7, 40, 86, 88, 90, 219–21, 224–28, 230–32
breath (*spiramen*), 84, 87–88, 189
Breuning, Wilhelm, 242
bride, 16, 22–23, 45
bridegroom, 24, 45
brightness (*candor*), 28, 60, 82, 167
Brown, Stephen, 9, 14, 242
Bynum, Caroline, 219, 228, 232, 243

Canévet, Mariette, 2, 16, 243
Cassiodorus, 36, 41, 166, 241
cause, 82, 93–94, 101, 106, 115, 141–44, 146, 155, 173, 187, 193, 195, 209–10; efficient, 33, 97, 103, 116, 142, 146, 150, 154, 172; exemplary, 83, 97; final, 96, 102, 146, 172; formal, 32–33, 83, 89, 116, 167; material, 96, 102
charity (*caritas*), 4, 23–24, 26, 30–33, 40, 46, 62–71, 77–79, 111–13, 115–20, 118–19, 131, 133, 139–58, 178–79, 182, 186–87, 205, 212, 214, 216, 222–23, 225–26, 231, 233
Châtillon, Jean, 73, 243
Chenu, M.-D., 13, 156, 185–86, 193–96, 205–6, 208, 211, 243
chewing (*masticare*), 38, 43, 47–48, 53, 111, 221–24, 237–38. *See also* eating
church, 22–23, 26, 45, 78, 113–14, 146, 192, 203, 222, 230–31
Cistercian, 10, 14–15, 123, 165
cognition (*cognitio*), 4–7, 27–28, 30, 32–33, 35–36, 38, 40, 46–48, 64, 79–80, 89, 111, 117, 120–21, 128–32, 136–37, 140–42, 145, 149–50, 155, 157, 184, 194, 210, 212–14, 216, 218, 222, 224–25, 235, 238. *See also* intellect; knowledge; understanding

Colish, Marcia, 97, 115, 122–23, 243
commemoration, 224
communication (*communicatio*), 77–81, 84–85, 166
concept, theological, 5–6, 10–11, 23, 47–49, 55–56, 58, 80–81, 83, 93, 99, 103, 124, 164, 171, 191, 207–9, 211, 216–17, 233–35, 237, 239
concupiscence, 146
concupiscible, power of the soul, 23–24, 26, 30, 32, 62–65, 67, 111–12, 116, 120, 139–40, 145–48, 150, 156–57
Conlan, William J., 131, 243
creation, 91–108
creed, 197, 202, 216, 218. *See also* articles of faith
cross, 15, 190

De anima, 34, 36, 41, 64, 95, 105, 125, 129, 193
De Bruyne, Edgar, 132, 161–64, 243
Decker, Bruno, 243
De Clerck, E., 243
delectabilia, 5, 7, 29, 32, 35–39, 45–47, 53, 64–65, 72, 90, 111, 115, 119, 135, 164, 178, 184, 198, 218, 228, 235–37
delectable, 26, 29–31, 41, 62–67, 69–70, 72, 88–90, 103, 108, 111–12, 117, 119–21, 127–29, 132–33, 137, 139, 141–42, 146–47, 151, 153–54, 171–73, 178, 182–83, 199, 213–14, 226, 236
delight, 1, 4, 23–26, 28–35, 37, 39–44, 46–47, 49, 63–68, 70, 77–80, 86–89, 105, 111–12, 114–19, 121, 127–42, 145–57, 164, 171, 178–79, 182–83, 198–99, 201–2, 212–16, 218–19, 221–31, 233, 236
desire, 28, 30–33, 39, 46, 59–70, 78, 117, 120, 127–32, 140–43, 145–46, 171–72, 207, 218, 224–26, 228, 231, 233, 236
De spiritu et anima, 10, 34, 126
dialectic, 13, 206
Dionysius Areopagita (Pseudo-), 10–11, 60, 74–75, 80, 95, 104, 106, 119, 127, 130, 133, 162–63, 171, 174, 176, 182, 236, 241–42, 246

discernment, 15, 58, 131–32, 140, 162–63, 174, 177, 219, 222–26, 230, 231
Duhem, Pierre, 58, 243

eating, 26, 30, 34, 60, 148, 153–54, 219–26, 228–32. *See also* chewing
Eco, Umberto, 162–63, 243
effects, (divine, created), 10, 46, 53–54, 70, 89–91, 95–107, 118–19, 135, 162, 168–70, 172, 175, 181–82, 184, 204, 210, 214–16, 218, 232, 235–36
end *(finis)*, 18, 40, 59–61, 63–69, 81, 89–90, 105, 115–21, 128–32, 134, 136, 140–42, 144–48, 150–51, 154–56, 158, 161, 179, 183–84, 189, 192, 202, 209–10
endowments *(dos, dotes)*, 21–26, 30, 35, 46–47, 111, 113
Englhardt, G., 119–21, 127–28, 131–32, 143–44, 156, 244
equality *(equalitas)*, 25, 77–78, 82–84
essence, 34–37, 39–41, 55–58, 94–97, 99, 101–2, 105, 118, 143, 156, 170, 182, 200
estimation *(aestimatio)*, 42, 68–70, 117, 121–33, 136–37, 141–42, 147, 151–52, 154, 183, 195, 197, 236
eternity *(eternitas)*, 74, 77, 81, 84, 93, 95, 97–98, 153, 161, 198
Eucharist, 4, 7, 12, 15, 153, 218–33, 237, 244–45
Exemplar, 36, 83, 88–99, 102–4, 167–68, 170, 173, 181, 236
experience, 1, 3–7, 15, 21, 26–27, 29–33, 38, 41–42, 44, 46, 65–67, 69–70, 72, 77, 79, 99, 103, 107, 112, 114, 116, 124, 130, 132, 135–37, 140, 145–47, 152–46, 158, 163–64, 184, 187, 191–92, 198, 208, 211–21, 223, 225, 228–29, 231–32, 236, 238–39
eye *(oculus)*, 27, 114

faculty, 1, 29, 46, 123–25, 135, 188, 193, 200
faith, 111–38
Father, 27, 72–76, 79–84, 86–88, 92–93, 96, 98, 102, 143, 166–68, 170, 181, 192, 207, 231

fecundity *(fecunditas)*, 74–78, 92, 103, 182
Fields, Stephen, S.J., 2, 244
fittingness *(convenientia)*, 30, 32–33, 92, 99–101, 106, 162, 165–66, 178, 180–81, 206–7, 228
food, 30, 33, 60, 86, 148, 153, 219–21, 223, 226–29, 231–32
fruition *(fruitio)*, 4, 15, 22–33, 46–47, 53, 63–64, 70, 84–86, 88, 105, 111–12, 116, 133–35, 139–40, 146–49, 152–55, 157–58, 179, 182, 214, 218–20
fullness *(plenitudo)*, 28–29, 45, 74, 77, 113, 161, 173, 177, 182, 218, 224

Gaybba, Brian, 185, 244
generosity *(liberalitas)*, 74–76, 97, 99, 119
gift *(donum)*, 182; name of Spirit, 76, 79, 84–85, 170; of Spirit, 40, 57, 87, 106–7, 154, 184–85, 191, 199–202, 206, 208–15, 218, 229; wedding, 23–23, 45
Gilbert of Poitiers, 10, 58, 80, 195
Gillmann, F., 244
Gilson, Etienne, 94–96, 98, 161, 244
Glorieux, P., 185, 244
Glossa Ordinaria, 16, 28, 38, 113
good *(bonum)*, 53–71
Grabmann, Martin, 11–12, 212, 244
grace, 27, 54, 56–57, 70, 85–86, 88–90, 112, 137, 143, 193–94, 204, 206, 210, 223, 228, 232
Gregory of Nyssa, 15
Gregory, Pope IX, 8–9,
Gregory the Great, 15–17, 28, 125, 201, 241
Grillmeier, Alois, 195, 244

habit *(habitus)*, 13, 39–40, 43–44, 102–3, 113, 115, 133, 135, 137, 144, 174–76, 178–79, 192, 197–98, 204–5, 210
Hayes, Zachary, 91, 244
hearing, spiritual *(auditus)*, 1, 3, 6, 28–29, 34, 37–38, 40–41, 43, 45, 47–49, 53, 65, 70, 75, 111, 113, 134, 137, 188, 211, 213–14, 219, 227–28, 236–38
heart, 85–88, 99, 114, 130, 137, 145, 153, 192, 200, 204, 227, 229

heat *(calor)*, 41, 43, 45, 48, 91, 238
Heinzmann, R., 244
Heitz, T., 9, 13, 206, 244
Henry Suso, 232
Holy Spirit, 16, 57, 72, 74, 76–77, 79–80, 82, 84–90, 95, 98, 102–4, 107, 114, 118, 143, 146, 166, 169–70, 181–82, 185, 191–92, 199–202, 206–7, 210–12, 215, 218, 236
honestum, 62, 164, 171, 178. *See also* beauty
hope, 8–9, 17–18, 32, 40, 45, 68, 115–16, 119–20, 142–43, 148, 151, 153, 156, 165, 182, 185, 187, 192, 231
Hugh of St. Cher, 12, 23–24, 28
Hugh of St. Victor, 11, 78, 92, 121, 123, 127, 131, 206, 212, 242
hunger, 26, 31, 149, 153–55, 231–32

image *(imago)*, 36, 42, 74–76, 82, 90, 92–97, 100, 102, 105–6, 167, 170, 173, 181, 205–6, 232
incorporation, 222–23, 229, 231
intellect, 1, 11, 15, 32–38, 40, 42, 44, 46, 62–64, 82, 97, 105, 111–12, 115–19, 121, 124–36, 141–42, 144, 151, 154–55, 157, 161–62, 183, 190, 193–97, 200, 204, 208, 216
interrelatedness *(germanitas)*, 79, 166, 206
irascible, power of the soul, 26, 116, 120, 140

Jenkins, John I., 185, 196, 244
Jesus Christ, 3–4, 6–7, 15–16, 23–28, 37–38, 43, 45, 47–48, 86–87, 90, 111–14, 137, 142, 146, 187–88, 190, 203–4, 212, 218–33, 237–38
John of Treviso, 26, 28
John Scotus Eriugena, 58, 125, 242

Knoch, W., 244
knowledge *(scientia)*, 1–11, 13–15, 18, 21–23, 26–28, 32, 37–38, 44–48, 49, 53, 60–61, 70–73, 77, 79–82, 87–91, 97–99, 103–8, 111, 117–18, 122–24, 127, 131–32, 138, 154–58, 161–64, 180–85, 188–92, 193–97, 99–206, 208–16, 218, 220, 225, 227, 229, 235–39, 243. *See also* cognition; understanding
Köpf, U., 185, 244
Krebs, E., 14, 244

Landgraf, A. M., 209, 244
Lang, Albert, 185, 194–96, 205, 209, 211, 245
Lateran IV, 15, 208
light, 33–34, 60–61, 64, 70, 82, 115, 119, 132, 144, 162, 167, 169, 188–89, 193, 195, 197, 204–6, 208, 210
Long, R. J., 185, 245
Lottin, O., 12, 56, 115, 117, 121, 126, 143, 200, 245
love, 11, 16, 22–23, 25–26, 30–33, 40, 43, 46, 48, 53, 60–64, 66, 76–80, 84, 86–87, 106, 114, 117, 120, 126, 129–33, 137, 139–50, 149–57, 179, 182–84, 186–87, 193, 205, 222, 224–26, 228, 231, 233, 238; *amor*, 16, 23, 31, 63–64, 66, 76–78, 120, 133, 144, 152, 155, 157, 193; *dilectio*, 22–27, 30, 46, 78–80, 105, 107, 111, 139–40, 145–46, 150, 179, 214, 216, 222, 225
loveliness, 178–79. *See also* beauty; honestum

MacDonald, Scott, 55, 245
Macy, Gary, 219, 221, 227–28, 230, 245
Mandonnet, Pierre, 245
manifestation, 4, 45, 80, 83, 98, 119, 157, 161–62, 165, 167, 170, 233
Marrone, Steven P., 10, 245
Martineau, R.-M., 245
McGinn, Bernard, 16, 245
measure *(mensura)*, 78, 113, 164–66, 173–77, 179–82, 208
Megivern, James J., 12, 219, 245
metaphysics, 10, 54, 57, 59–60, 69–70, 72, 88ff., 93, 98, 103, 121, 163, 171, 210, 212, 235; Aristotle's *Metaphysics*, 120, 161
Michaud-Quantin, Pierre, 122–24, 126–27, 245
Minges, Parthenius, 245
Minnis, A. J., 1, 245

mirror *(speculum)*, 75–76, 79, 82–83, 88, 90–91, 103, 107, 161–62, 167, 170, 203–4, 236
monastic, 7, 15, 46, 211
mouth. *See* palate
movement *(motus)*, 39–41, 62, 66–67, 113, 115, 129–30, 136–37, 140–41, 148, 150, 154, 198; women's *(Frauenwebegung)*, 14; dualist, 165
multiplex, 86, 95, 98, 118–19, 168
mysticism, 15–16

names, divine, 73–75, 80–81, 84, 87, 101, 106, 162–63, 174, 184
nature, 27, 57, 66, 112, 142, 206–8; divine, 4–7, 29, 45, 47–48, 54, 70, 72–73, 75–76, 79, 87, 94, 96, 99, 102–5, 113, 166, 184, 210; of the good, 55–56, 69, 90; human, 26, 77, 114, 120; of the soul, 36, 46, 105; of the spiritual senses, 45
Nederman, Cary, 115, 243
number *(numerus)*, 164–66, 169, 173–74, 177, 179–82

odor *(odoratus)*, 4, 13, 29, 37–38, 40, 43, 45–48, 53, 55–56, 59, 72, 78, 111, 116, 137, 142, 151, 156, 231–32, 236, 237–41
order *(ordo)*, 164–65, 174, 176–77, 179–81, 183
Ottaviano, Carmelo, 245

palate, 114, 137, 202, 213, 227
Paris, university of, 2, 8, 23, 165, 194
patria, 3, 18, 21, 23, 27–28, 40–41, 45–46, 49, 53, 90, 157, 179, 235
Paul, the apostle, 95, 156, 190, 215, 228
perception *(percipere)*, 1, 4–7, 15–16, 28, 30–32, 35–38, 40, 42, 46–48, 70–72, 79–80, 89–90, 98, 106–8, 111, 113–14, 117, 124–26, 128, 130, 132–33, 135–38, 147–48, 151, 155, 162, 164, 178, 182–84, 189–90, 192, 196–98, 202, 206, 213–14, 216, 218, 226, 233, 236
Peter Abelard, 10, 78, 92, 119, 122–23, 126, 131, 195, 229, 242, 244

Peter Lombard, 78, 112–13, 121–23, 142–43, 153, 167, 230, 242–43, 245, 247
Philip the Chancellor, 11, 54–56, 119, 165, 244
pleasantness, 29, 227, 233. *See also* suavity
pleasure *(iocunditas, delicia)*, 5, 64, 76–80, 114, 119, 145–47, 152–53, 164, 178, 198, 202, 215. *See also* delight
Posterior Analytics, 13, 194
Potts, Timothy, 4–5, 244
Pouillon, Henri, 54–56, 162–63, 244
power *(potentia)*, 41, 73–75, 81, 84–85, 95, 100, 102–3, 119, 169, 180–81, 216, 222; of the soul, 5, 23–27, 29–30, 32, 35, 42–43, 46, 62–67, 70, 111–12, 115–16, 120, 132, 132, 134, 137, 139–40, 144–48, 150, 155–57, 164, 169, 179, 181, 228
Praepositinus of Cremona, 12, 81, 121, 127, 200, 211
Principe, Walter, 8, 12–13, 56–58, 101, 186
principles, first *(principia)*, 13–14, 191, 193–97, 203, 206, 210
properties *(notiones)*, 80–81, 83, 91, 99, 106, 164, 174, 207, 220
proportion *(proportio)*, 26, 42, 99–101, 153, 155, 163, 165, 173, 177–78

radiance. *See* splendor
Rahner, Karl, 2–3, 16–17, 28, 113, 244, 246
reason *(ratio)*, 27, 44, 73, 93, 115, 124, 127, 131–32, 140–41, 187–88, 193, 195, 201, 205–6, 208–11, 218, 224
reasons *(rationes)*, 186–90, 199, 201, 204–11
rest *(quies)*, 62, 105, 116–18, 121, 128–31, 136, 141, 150–51, 157, 172, 181, 187, 189, 201, 206, 215–16, 235
Ribaillier, J., 242, 246
Richard Fishacre, 73, 145, 185, 245
Richard Rolle, 232
Richard of St. Victor, 74–75, 77–78, 206, 210, 242
Roland of Cremona, 23–24
Rorem, Paul, 10–11, 246
Rubin, Miri, 219, 246

sacrament, 12–13, 21, 57, 218–19, 221–22, 228, 230, 237
savor, 6, 8, 48, 131, 153–55, 184, 212–15
scent, 37–38, 47–48, 111, 237
Scott, A. B., 1, 245
Seneca, 77, 242
senses *(sensus)*, 4, 7, 15–16, 29, 31–32, 35–36, 40–44, 46, 70, 113, 125, 134–35, 137, 152, 196–97
sensorium, 3, 29, 48, 112, 134
sensuous, 4–5, 64, 69, 70, 115, 133, 135, 151–53, 158, 183, 185, 190, 219, 229, 231–32, 237, 239
sensus communis, 43, 48, 134
sheep, 121, 124, 126, 128, 133, 141–42
sight *(visus)*, 1, 27–29, 43, 49, 53, 64–66, 70–71, 75, 112, 124, 132–35, 161–62, 183, 188–89, 191, 193, 196, 199, 208–10, 212, 236
Simon of Tournai, 58, 80, 188, 200, 211, 242
sin, 81, 92, 114, 126, 189–90, 193, 200, 204, 220, 228–29
smell, spiritual *(olfactus)*, 1, 4, 16, 29, 38, 40–41, 45, 48, 54, 65–66, 113, 135, 219, 238
smoothness *(levitas)*, 43, 45, 48
Solignac, Aimé, 16, 246
Solomon, 174, 179, 202
Son, 37–38, 47, 72–77, 79–84, 86–88, 102–3, 111, 143, 166–70, 181–82, 189, 192, 207, 226, 231, 236–38
Song of Songs, 1, 11, 16, 78, 202
soul, 1–3, 5, 15–16, 22–23, 26–30, 32–36, 39, 43–46, 49, 53, 60, 63–65, 67, 71, 84, 86, 95, 103, 106–7, 111, 114–16, 125–27, 129–30, 134–35, 137, 139–41, 144–45, 148–58, 164, 178–79, 182, 184, 189–90, 195, 197, 200–202, 204–6, 210, 213, 215–16, 218–20, 226, 232, 235–36, 238
species, 39–40, 32, 66, 83, 101, 117–18, 164–65, 167–68, 172–81, 183, 197–99
speculation, 6, 12, 16, 23, 66–67, 117–18, 121, 127–29, 131–32, 136–38, 191, 208, 210, 215–18, 236

splendor, 82, 163, 167, 170
St. Pierre, Jules, 11, 246
Stephen Langton, 24, 28, 56, 80, 119, 121, 127, 145
Stock, Brian, 7, 246
Strake, Joseph, 246
suavity *(suavitas)*, 4, 29, 34, 38–39, 45, 47–49, 68, 72, 86–87, 91, 103–4, 111, 119–21, 134, 141, 145, 151–52, 155, 213–14, 216, 227–28, 237–38. *See also* pleasantness
substance, 12, 26, 58–59, 64
Swanson, R. N., 14, 246
sweetness *(dulcedo)*, 4, 29–30, 33–34, 38–41, 45, 47–49, 60, 64, 68, 70, 72, 85–86, 91, 103–4, 107, 111, 114–15, 119, 124, 134, 137, 145–46, 149, 155–56, 182, 184, 192, 202, 213–14, 226–27, 232–33, 237–38
symbol, 106–8, 162–67, 169–70, 175, 177, 180, 182–84, 219, 233, 236
symmetry *(commensuratio)*, 166, 174, 177
symphony *(simphonia)*, 28–29, 45, 47, 91, 104, 111, 180
synaesthesia, 41, 49, 137, 157, 233, 236, 238

taste, spiritual *(gustus)*, 1, 4, 6–7, 16, 29, 34, 38–40, 43, 45, 47–49, 54, 60, 65–66, 111, 113–14, 134–35, 137, 148, 151, 157–58, 192, 201–2, 212–15, 218–19, 226–28, 232, 235–39
Tatarkiewicz, W., 163, 165, 246
Tedoldi, Fabio M., 2, 246
Tertullian, 22, 242
theology: method, 6, 10–13, 72, 185–86, 186–83, 191, 194–95, 209, 211–12, 215, 243, 245; mystical, 184–217; negative, 10, 205; practical, 118, 121, 218; speculative, 6, 12, 117–18, 121, 127–29, 131–32, 136, 138, 191, 208, 210, 215–18, 236, 243; symbolic, 161–83
Torrell, J.-P., 17, 186, 246
touch, spiritual *(tactus)*, 1, 4, 6–7, 16, 28–29, 34–35, 38, 41, 43, 45, 47–49, 53–54, 64–71, 111–13, 125, 134–35, 137,

139, 146, 148–49, 151–53, 154–56, 158, 211–12, 218–19, 227–28, 236–38
transcendentals, 54–55, 69, 162
Trinity, 5, 72–75, 77–90, 92–93, 96–98, 102–4, 111–12, 114, 121, 135, 157, 161–62, 166–68, 170–71, 181–82, 189, 200, 206, 218, 231–33
truth *(veritas)*, 14, 34, 39, 49, 61–64, 66, 116–20, 122, 127–30, 132–33, 136, 138, 140–41, 144–45, 148–50, 167, 183, 186–87, 190, 192–99, 201, 203–4, 206, 208, 211, 216, 224–25, 227, 244
Tugwell, Simon, 10, 247
Tummers, Paul, 247
Turner, Denis, 1, 247

understanding *(intellectus)*, 1, 4–7, 10, 13, 16, 21–22, 26–27, 30, 32–33, 35–36, 38, 40, 44, 46–49, 61–63, 65–67, 81–82, 87, 105–7, 117, 121, 127, 129, 131–33, 135, 141–42, 147, 151, 156, 184–85, 188–90, 195–96, 199–203, 206–16, 218, 225, 230, 232, 237–38. *See also* cognition; knowledge
union, 26, 30, 60, 70, 87, 117, 132, 139, 150, 152, 154–56, 158, 219, 221–24, 229–31, 233, 236

Van Hove, A., 247
Vanneste, A, 247
Verbum, 75–76, 79, 82–83, 92, 97–98, 166–68, 212
via, in, 18, 21, 40, 42, 44, 46, 49, 53, 107, 112, 179, 236

virtues, cardinal, 57, 114, 200–201; theological, 24, 35, 55, 65, 67–68, 70, 114–15, 119–20, 131, 134, 137, 142, 178, 215, 233, 236; *See also*, faith; hope; love
visio Dei, 3, 18, 21, 27, 49, 157, 238
vision *(visio)*, 3–4, 18, 21, 23–29, 31–34, 36, 40–41, 43, 45, 49, 53, 78, 82, 90, 106–7, 115, 127, 129, 132–33, 136–37, 140–41, 143, 146, 148–50, 152, 154, 157, 161, 163, 179, 183–84, 189–90, 198–99, 209–28, 231, 235–38
Von Balthasar, Hans Urs, 217, 247
Von Israel, Peri, 247

Wawrykow, Joseph, ix, 239, 247
weight *(pondus)*, 122, 164–65, 169, 173–75, 177, 179–82, 229
Weijers, O., 186, 247
Weisheipl, James, 186, 247
Wicki, Nicholas, 22–25, 27–28, 247
Wieland, Georg, 194, 247
William of Auvergne, 2, 10–11, 13, 23–24, 127, 165, 194, 206, 245
William of St. Thierry, 10, 16, 28, 123, 127
wine, 7, 16, 85–87, 146, 213, 219–21, 230, 232
wisdom *(sapientia)*, 4–6, 10, 44, 82–84, 87–90, 92, 97–98, 102, 107, 119, 124, 153, 164–71, 173, 175–85, 189–91, 199–203, 210–18, 226–29, 232–36, 239
wolf, 122, 124, 126, 128, 133, 141–42
Wolfson, Harry A., 123–125, 247

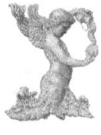 *Knowing God by Experience: The Spiritual Senses in the Theology of William of Auxerre* was designed and composed in Minion with Requiem display type by Kachergis Book Design, Pittsboro, North Carolina; and printed on 60-pound Glatfelter Natural and bound by Edwards Brothers, Inc., Lillington, North Carolina.

www.ingramcontent.com/pod-product-compliance
Lightning Source LLC
Chambersburg PA
CBHW051939290426
44110CB00015B/2036